THE UNIVERSITY OF MICHIGAN
CENTER FOR CHINESE STUDIES

SCIENCE, MEDICINE, AND TECHNOLOGY IN EAST ASIA

VOLUME 2

Nathan Sivin, General Editor

Traditional Medicine in Contemporary China

A Partial Translation of
Revised Outline of Chinese Medicine (1972)
With an Introductory Study on
Change in Present-Day and Early Medicine

By Nathan Sivin

CENTER FOR CHINESE STUDIES
THE UNIVERSITY OF MICHIGAN
ANN ARBOR

SCIENCE, MEDICINE, AND TECHNOLOGY IN EAST ASIA
VOLUME 2

Printed and made in the United States of America

⊗ The paper used in this publication meets the requirements
of the American National Standard for Information Sciences—
Permanence of Paper for Publications and Documents
in Libraries and Archives ANSI/NISO/Z39.48—1992.

Library of Congress Cataloging-in-Publication Data

Sivin, Nathan

Hsin pien Chung I hsüeh kai yao. English. Selections.
Traditional medicine in contemporary China.
(Science, medicine, and technology in East Asia; v. 2)
Partial translation of: Hsin pien Chung I hsüeh kai yao.
Bibliography: p.
Includes index.
ISBN 0-89264-073-1 (alk. paper)
ISBN 0-89264-074-X (alk. paper) (pbk.)
1. Medicine, Chinese.
I. Sivin, Nathan.
II. University of Michigan. Center for Chinese Studies.
III. Title: Revised outline of Chinese medicine.
IV. Title. V. Series.
[DNLM: 1. Medicine, Oriental Traditional—China.
W1 SC744 v. 2 / WB 50 JC6 HC56]
R601.H692513   1986   610'.951   86–31730

TO CAROLE
for endless inspiration

You know that medicines when well used restore health to the sick; and they will be well used when the doctor together with the understanding of their nature shall understand also what man is, what life is, what constitution is and what health is. Understanding these well he will also understand well their opposites and when this is the case he will know well how to heal.

Leonardo da Vinci, *Codex Atlanticus*

CONTENTS

CONTENTS OF INTRODUCTORY STUDY

CONTENTS OF TRANSLATION

Contents

SCIENCE, MEDICINE, AND TECHNOLOGY IN EAST ASIA

The Series publishes books on traditional and modern science, medicine, and technology in China, Japan, and Korea, based on research in primary sources in the languages of those societies or on the study of artifacts. It applies the highest standards of refereeing, technical editing, and production to books which combine scientific and East Asian content. Its aim is to produce books of the highest scholarly quality at prices nonspecialists can afford.

Inquiries regarding the submission of manuscripts for consideration and similar matters should be addressed to: Professor Nathan Sivin, 1 Smith Hall, University of Pennsylvania, Philadelphia, PA 19104–6310.

Orders and inquiries about the availability of titles in print should be addressed to: *Michigan Publications on East Asia*, Center for Chinese Studies, 104 Lane Hall, The University of Michigan, Ann Arbor, MI 48109.

ACKNOWLEDGMENTS

I acknowledge with gratitude support for this research from the National Library of Medicine of the National Institutes of Health, the Japan Society for the Promotion of Science (Nihon gakujutsu shinkōkai), and the School of Arts and Sciences, University of Pennsylvania. Over the years that it was in progress, my work was furthered by the kind hospitality of the Sinologisch Instituut, Rijksuniversiteit te Leyden; the Research Institute of Humanistic Studies (Jimbun kagaku kenkyūsho), Kyoto University; the Taniguchi Foundation; the Chinese Academy of Sciences, and especially the Institute for the History of Natural Science, Beijing; the China Institute for the History of Medicine and Medical Literature, Academy of Traditional Chinese Medicine, Beijing; the East Asian History of Science Library, Cambridge, England; and the Master and Fellows of St. John's College, Cambridge.

I have been greatly aided by frequent conversations with colleagues about the matters discussed here, particularly with Pan Jixing (Beijing), Nakayama Shigeru (Tokyo), Miyasita Saburō (Osaka), Lu Gwei-djen and Joseph Needham (Cambridge), Manfred Porkert (Munich), and Ma Boying, M.D. (Shanghai). I have received useful suggestions and ameliorations from Hans Ågren, Caryn Bern, M.D., David Cowhig, Kenneth J. DeWoskin, Judith Farquhar, Marta Hanson, Renée Fox, David Powlison, and Melinda Whitman Shenk. The editorial services of Janis Michael and (at an earlier stage) Barbara Congelosi at the Center for Chinese Studies, University of Michigan, have been invaluable. Carole Sivin and Virginia G. Dalton have as always helped in too many ways to enumerate.

PREFACE

The second half of this book, its focal part, is a partial translation of the *Revised Outline of Chinese Medicine* (Hsin pien Chung-i-hsueh kai yao 新 编 中 医 学 概 要), a handbook of traditional medicine published in Beijing in 1972. These chapters set out the fundamental conceptions of the body, its normal functioning, and its disorders: the conceptions that underlie diagnosis and decisions about therapy. The first part is an extended introductory study. It incorporates my commentary on the book's content, on the circumstances in which it emerged, and on the changing state of traditional medicine in contemporary China.

The chapters of the handbook translated here are clear and systematic. They summarize themselves. There is no need for me to restate what they say. I seek rather to convey what this book suggests about the past, present, and future of the millennial Chinese medical tradition.

I do so necessarily on the basis of very limited understanding. I have made only brief visits to the country I am writing about, and maintain contact with colleagues there primarily through correspondence. I am not a physician of the old or new type. I am a student of history and other humanistic dimensions of science, moderately familiar with the literature and history of Chinese medicine. I see my sources differently from the way they would appear to clinicians or policy analysts. My viewpoint, like theirs, is obviously not a balanced one; but perhaps it complements theirs.

Ancient and Modern Change

The *Revised Outline* presents itself as a statement of authoritative knowledge, timeless except when it occasionally mentions old maxims and old errors, and problems to be solved by future research. The theme of this introductory study is process, the transformation of knowledge. One of my major aims has been to demonstrate that documents presented as timeless, if they are understood in relation to process, are useful in thinking sensibly about the future. I am not interested (nor will most readers be) in the confident but often vacuous predictions that keep Kremlinology and its sinological equivalent in the news. My concern with the future in the introductory study is to identify problems and contradictions that already exist but have not yet been faced. If they are faced early enough it may be possible to minimize the trouble that they cause.

When I planned this book I thought it would be sufficient to relate the account of doctrine in the *Revised Outline* to alterations in theory over the past thirty-five years, the period in which occupational structures and educational qualifications for most medical practitioners were effectively regulated on the mainland of China for the first time in history. My studies gradually led me to understand that change has been the norm in traditional medicine over its entire history. The evolution of practices and concepts has been a neglected topic in Western writing on the history of Chinese medicine. In order to discuss whether current changes in fundamental ideas differ in kind from earlier evolutionary processes, I have examined several exemplary concepts over the past two thousand years.

Purpose

So much misinformation about Chinese medicine crowds the shelves of European and American bookshops that a Chinese account is badly needed. The Chinese books translated earlier have been primarily reference works on therapy. These provide a dangerously unbalanced picture, dangerous in that they are likely to mislead people beginning to learn acupuncture. Anyone familiar with Chinese medicine knows that it is not a grab-bag of techniques that can be picked up and used with a few days or weeks of training, but rather a system of practices for deducing a coordinated program of therapy from analysis of the patient as a whole person—a psychosomatic unity, connected with his environment. A list of acupuncture points and directions for inserting needles are about as useful, even to an M.D., as written instructions for thoracic surgery would be to someone ignorant of anatomy and physiology. It is quite possible for an acupuncturist who knows only techniques to mortally harm the patient.

The training of a traditional physician still begins with an introduction to theoretical concepts and their clinical use. Lacking a deeply informed account of these foundations, Western readers with normal critical capacities are bound to remain frustrated by the disjointed character of what most books about Chinese medicine tell them.

This book is meant for those who want to comprehend traditional medicine for their own non-medical purposes and for those who want to think in an informed way about its uses in clinical research or practice (I should say at the outset that this book does not contain directions for therapy). The attempt to meet both needs at the same time has led to some compromises that will no doubt make the book less than ideal for either readership. Some physicians, for instance, will be offended that I have avoided modern medical terminology in my explanations. Some specialists on China, I know, become acutely uncomfortable when discussions of medicine move away from government policy and social relations, and take up what doctors thought and did. I suspect, nonetheless, that there is something to be said for a book that physicians will not find entirely sinological and that those interested in Chinese thought will not find overwhelmingly technical. That is not to say that I avoid scientific and philological issues. It is impossible to look past the surface of the *Revised Outline* without encountering complexities that must be patiently unraveled. I have unraveled a few complexities in front of the reader's eyes in order to demonstrate how it is done. I have kept a diverse readership in mind when deciding what needs to be explained and how to explain it.

I need not apologize, I trust, for a way of looking at my subject that does not conform to any current fashion in anthropology, cross-cultural studies of medicine, history, and other disciplines on which I have drawn. I do regret that I have not devoted more adequate attention to social aspects of doctrinal change. What the book I am introducing demands above all is explication of ideas and what they signify. That is as much as I can hope to contribute in a volume of reasonable size. The social matrix of the Chinese medical art calls for analysis in depth, but that is another book.[1]

---

[1] A study of the social relations of curing in traditional China is in the works. I have discussed my method of approach to such questions in an essay published in 1977 (see bibliography B).

My lack of explicit concern with therapy is also not a trivial limitation. Several poorly informed Western authors have argued that theory is irrelevant to praxis in traditional medicine. These arguments have been largely shaped by the awesome taboo against using written primary sources, long observed by anthropologists who do field work in literate societies. This orthodoxy amounts to treating civilizations as internally diverse and sophisticated as that of China as though they do not differ in any essential respect from that of the Kalahari bushmen. It has begun to disappear as young anthropologists insist on learning the written languages of the peoples they study. But principled ignorance of the role of writings has encouraged putting the question in a singularly unprofitable way.

Theory is not a separate entity that may or may not appear in one region or another on the map of Chinese medicine. It *is* diagnostic and therapeutic reasoning. It has rarely been divorced from clinical work. Some doctors with little education may have had little theory at their disposal, but those who knew it used it, and those who wrote on it did so with therapy in mind. That point is unmistakable in the literature, old and new. It is still emphasized by experienced traditional physicians. It explains the preponderant concern with theory in clinically oriented Chinese journals of traditional medicine today. It is patent throughout this book. When I discuss concepts abstractly, using the tools of conceptual analysis, I do so because I must make them clear for a readership to whom they are novel.

This book does not purport to describe the day-to-day clinical reality of China. Like all expositions of doctrine it stresses ideals and principles. A systematic, concrete study of how theoretical constructs are used in clinical settings, compiled for readers outside China, is also desirable for those who want to avoid a romanticized view of a contemporary clinic. Fortunately Judith Farquhar has begun to fill this need with a splendid anthropological dissertation that was completed as this book was being typeset.[2]

---

[2] Farquhar 1986. Kleinman 1980 has done work in Taiwan with important implications for social research.

Approach

This book lets contemporary Chinese authorities speak for themselves, outlining in their own words, and according to their own organization of ideas, how the body works, what can go wrong, how symptoms are related to form a diagnosis, and how the pattern of a disorder, once recognized, suggests a program of therapy. I have not translated the chapters of the *Revised Outline* on therapy. A full translation would require a couple of additional volumes this size. It would be better done by someone learned in pharmacology and experienced in its clinical application.

The book chosen for translation is one of many handbooks and textbooks of traditional medicine that I have considered. It is the best, in my judgment, for Western readers who have not previously studied Chinese medicine and who want a single clear summary of the foundations.[3] It is far from ideal. There are many minor inconsistencies of terminology and other signs of compilation by committee. I have occasionally omitted repetitious or uninformative material. I have excised two short sections describing the course of the circulation system.[4]

---

[3] Its choice is explained below, pages 30–35. The works from which it was chosen are listed in appendix A.

[4] Examples of uninformative case material are Sections 6.2.2.4 and 8.6. The omitted sections on the circulation system are 4.2.1 and 4.2.2. Better expositions are mentioned at that point in the translation. One section included in the table of contents of the *Revised Outline* does not appear in the original book (5.3). Prescriptions are not given for some compound medicines mentioned in the text, and some medicinal plants mentioned are not discussed in the chapters on therapy.

Numbers in the form that appear in this footnote are references to sections in the *Revised Outline* and in its translation here. I have occasionally added a number that is not explicit in the original. A zero (as in 5.0) refers to the introductory section of a chapter.)

The circulation tracts are not a major topic of the *Revised Outline*, and these descriptions are markedly inferior to several readily available in European languages. Despite its imperfections, the *Revised Outline* provides an excellent overview of the founda-

In many details the *Revised Outline* is out of date. Traditional medicine has changed a great deal since 1972, as has the Chinese nation. The changes in medicine have mainly affected the organization of its practice and the penetration of influence by modern medicine. The larger outlines of doctrine remain more or less intact while the details change. My concern for accuracy did not lead me to choose a more recent book because, given the rapid pace of transition, even those just published are obsolescent in detail, and will be obsolete before long. The state of the art is best seen in research reports, not in textbooks. More important for the present purpose are the comprehensiveness of the *Revised Outline* and its ability to speak clearly to a non-Chinese readership.

Problems of Translation

Translating a book of this kind is not a simple matter even for someone competent in Chinese and conversant with the literature. The terminology of traditional medicine is in some ways more complicated than that of modern medicine, especially since often a single term may have two or three meanings, depending on when it was used, and in reference to what. There is much overlap between the terminologies of traditional and modern medicine, but a great deal less overlap in their meanings. *Je* 熱 , the ordinary word for "hot" in Chinese, means "fever" in modern medicine, and that is how every common dictionary defines it. In traditional medicine, however, it does not ordinarily refer to elevated body temperature determined by the doctor, but to internal sensations of heat, a symptom reported by the patient.[5]

This traditional terminology, which evolved gradually over more than two millennia, is not accommodated in English without a good deal of thought. For example, *shang han* 傷 寒 in modern medicine is the exact equivalent of "typhoid." In traditional medicine, however, the word refers to a large class of what modern doctors would call exogenous, infectious febrile diseases—but not to all such diseases. At the same time it is the name of one particular

---

tions of medicine as seen by experienced and learned contemporary practitioners.

[5] See below, pages 107–8.

member of that class.[6] Neither the broad nor the narrow meaning is close enough to any single concept of modern medicine to have a readymade English equivalent.

In order to translate or even explain one must therefore create a technical vocabulary in English. Several colleagues have made a good start in this work for the special aspects of traditional medicine on which they have written. The major contributions so far have been by Manfred Porkert (on the traditional equivalent of physiology) and Lu Gwei-djen and Joseph Needham (on acupuncture and certain other topics). These authors have attempted to make rigorous terminologies for use in the study of ancient writings. Porkert's standard ("normative") terms are in Latin; Lu and Needham freely use Greek and Latin roots to invent new English words that cannot be confused with familiar modern medical terms.[7] If translations using these approaches read here and there like English treatises of the seventeenth century, that is not inappropriate in a translation from an early source.

The present concern is with modern writings on traditional medicine, in which seventeenth-century locutions would be out of place. I have used translations originated by Porkert and Lu and Needham (and by others engaged in this common effort such as Hans Ågren and Ulrike and Paul Unschuld) when suitable for my purpose. I have also consulted several recent dictionaries of traditional medicine. The best Chinese-Chinese dictionaries are helpful in understanding modern writings, but are not compiled on historical principles, and are unreliable for reading premodern medical books. The Chinese-English dictionaries I have examined are in general considerably inferior to those with Chinese definitions.[8]

My own approach has been to find terms that straightforwardly translate the senses of the Chinese words into plain English and that at the same time are unlikely to be confused with modern

---

[6] See below, page 84.

[7] On differences of viewpoint that underlie these two approaches, see Needham and Lu 1975 and Porkert's appended rejoinder.

[8] The only dictionary of traditional medicine that can be recommended for reading current sources is Chung-i yen-chiu-yuan 中 医 研 究 院 et al. ed. 1982, the third in a series of preliminary editions (*idem* 1973, 1979). The best Chinese-English dictionary, to be used with considerable caution, is Xie Zhufan and Huang Xiaokai ed. 1984.

medical language. For instance, I translate *shang han* literally as "Cold Damage Disorders" in the first traditional sense and as "Cold Damage Disorder" in the second. The word "Disorder" is a flag for traditional syndromes or diseases, and initial capitals are an additional reminder that a traditional term should not be confused with modern ones.

The old terms *nei shang* 內 傷 (due to internal disturbance) and *nei yin* 內 因 (inner causes) sometimes refer to etiologic agents in a way similar to the modern term "endogenous" (in modern Chinese, *nei sheng* 內 生 or *nei yuan* 內 原). At other times they differ from it in ways too important to let the senses be jumbled together in translation. "Inner causes" (5.0) informs the reader at a glance that he is not encountering a modern term.

Some technical words are simply untranslatable. No English counterpart shorter, perhaps, than a paragraph can express their meaning while avoiding confusion with conceptions already established in the English language. Rather than translating such words into Latin or inventing a new English word, I leave a few such words in Chinese, and explain them.[9]

Other Chinese words untranslatable in classical medicine have become translatable as the influence of modern medical thought has changed their meaning. *Hsueh* 血 , for instance, has always meant "blood," but that was only part of its meaning. In classical medical discourse, with its emphasis on functions over materials and structures, this word referred more consistently to yin vitalities, the physical form of which was irrelevant, than to the familiar fluid that flows red from wounds.[10] When *hsueh* is translated in such writings as "blood," they may sound properly "modern," but a great deal of what they say no longer makes sense. In early writings *hsueh* is least confusing when left untranslated.

This is no longer the case in recent writings on traditional medicine. In China today, as in modern medicine, materialism is a Good Thing. The identification of *hsueh* with blood in medical doctrine is now unqualified, even though the stress on function reasserts itself once the identification has been made and the discussion proceeds (as in section 3.2 below). One cannot do justice to the historic shift from functionalism to materialism by maintaining rigid

---

[9] For instance, see the extensive discussion of *ch'i* 氣 below, pages 46–53.

[10] This point is made clear below, pages 152–61 and section 3.2.

consistency. I translate *hsueh* as "blood" in the body of this book, but leave it untranslated in the introductory study when discussing early conceptions.

The authors of the *Revised Outline* use a good deal of modern medical terminology in their explanations. I translate these words into their accepted English equivalents.

Sometimes a term that might be understood in either a traditional or modern sense is ambiguous in context. Some translators may prefer to give doubtful examples a modern interpretation, in order to emphasize the overlap between traditional and modern concepts and make the strongest possible case that Chinese medicine is not exotic. Since it seems to me that that point has long since been acknowledged by those who are informed about the tradition, I prefer in ambiguous cases to meet a more immediate need—to remind the reader that traditional and modern meanings differ. This often implies choosing the older, less familiar sense. I follow no inflexible rule.

Conventions

Two conventions for transcribing Chinese script compete for acceptance. Neither has much to recommend it except currency. The Wade-Giles system is a century-old compromise designed for use with English, French, and German at the cost of easy pronounceability in any of the three. The pinyin system was worked out a quarter-century ago, in the golden age of Sino-Soviet friendship, for use with the Cyrillic alphabet. It has been converted mechanically for use with Latin letters, making it phonetically less consistent than the Wade-Giles system for Western European or Anglophone users—and even less pronounceable.[11]

The best argument for Wade-Giles is that most important humanistic scholarship on medicine in Western languages uses it. That may not matter to sinologists, who must master both systems. But it is not lightly ignored by authors who want to avoid forcing a

---

[11] For instance, in pinyin the vowels in *ju* and *chu* are entirely distinct in pronunciation; in *ji* and *zhu* the consonants are pronounced identically. Wade-Giles, for all its faults, does register these differences and similarities. It writes the first pair as *chü* and *chu*, and the second pair as *chi* and *chu*.

general readership to do mental conversions between two systems. Pinyin has in its favor official adoption by the government of the People's Republic of China, which implies that—unless that government replaces it with a system that is not as linguistically anomalous—it is likely eventually to become the worldwide standard.

The two choices seem to me equally justified, at least for the time being. I insist for the moment on sitting on the fence and contemplating the poses of the most pugnacious combatants. Because virtually all official and popular publications in English now use the pinyin place names promulgated by the Chinese government, I use them here. Since authors are entitled to decide how their own names are to be spelled when they publish in alphabetic languages, I reproduce authors' names from the title pages when I cite their works in Western languages.[12] When I transcribe names, titles, phrases, etc., from Chinese, I use the Wade-Giles system so that they will be recognizable to non-specialists who have encountered them before. The result of these choices is an inconsistency that sinologists will notice. For those who find it difficult to cope with, I have provided a conversion table for the two transcriptions in appendix F.

No such painful choice is necessary for Japanese. I use the prevalent Hepburn system.

Orthography poses another painful choice, between classical Chinese characters and the simplified forms that have been officially adopted in the last generation.[13] I deal with this problem by taking my orthography from my sources.

That decision also holds some potential for confusion. A technical term may occur in classical script in the introductory study

---

[12] Thus an author who signs her English writings Qin Xiaozhu (a pinyin form)—or, for that matter, Sally Qin—would be so cited in bibliography B, but her name in Chinese at the head of an essay in that language would be transcribed as Ch'in Hsiao-chu, according to the Wade-Giles convention. Like many colleagues, I omit certain features of Wade-Giles, mainly alternate spellings and diacritics, that perform no discriminatory function.

[13] Since the end of the Cultural Revolution, during which anything old was suspect, a number of scholarly reprints, commentaries, and editions are again being published in unsimplified script. This is true in medicine as in other fields.

where I quote an early text, and in simplified characters in the body of the book when I cite the *Revised Outline*. That cannot confuse people who do not read Chinese. Those who do, if they are unable to read both orthographies, will find the index helpful in locating a form they can read.

I avoid citing recent editions in simplified characters of Chinese books written before 1900. They are translations. There is an inevitable loss of information in any translation (manifested in recent editions by one simplified character standing for two or more original characters).[14] There are some excellent critical editions of classics printed in simplified characters. I mention them in bibliography A, but in the body of this book, with a couple of unavoidable exceptions, I give page references to the best available version in the original orthography of each book.

The *Revised Outline* mentions a number of acupuncture loci (also called "points," although far from infinitesimal). As usual in Chinese publications, it refers to them by name. There are no generally accepted translations for these names, since evidence for many original meanings is lacking. A set of standard abbreviations is desirable for readers of this book who find names in romanization difficult to remember. Again one must choose between competing systems of abbreviations, principally the system used in China (mainly in books written for foreigners), and the one prevalent in Europe and adopted in Lu and Needham, *Celestial Lancets*, the best book on acupuncture published outside China.[15] I cite the European abbreviations, and list Chinese equivalents (for points cited only) in appendix E.

Botanical reference works are far from uniform in the Latin and English equivalents that they provide for Chinese plant names. The recent handbook of Chinese materia medica by Shiu-ying Hu is a competent attempt to solve the problem. I follow it whenever pos-

---

[14] For instance, the meanings of *li* 裡 and *li* 里 , both common words, have been collapsed into the latter.

[15] See Lu and Needham 1980: 53–59 for an index. I do not mention the United States because in this country the standards of acupuncture training, practice, and scholarship are considerably lower than in Europe—where they can hardly be called high.

sible.[16] When prescriptions are mentioned, I provide cross-references to the untranslated later chapters of the *Revised Outline* that discuss materia medica and prescriptions in detail. There is no satisfactory compendium of traditional Chinese prescriptions in any Western European language.[17]

In the translation, parenthetical phrases from the *Revised Outline* are left in parentheses; cross-references are also inserted in parentheses. Explanatory phrases inserted by the translator are enclosed in square brackets. Words such as *ch'i* 氣 or "heteropathy" clearly implied by the Chinese text are, when necessary for clarity, made explicit in the translation without further encumbering the page with brackets.

---

[16] For plants not covered in Hu 1981 I cite Chiang-su hsin i-hsueh-yuan 江苏新医学院 ed. 1977–78, which provides Latin but not English names.

[17] A reference book by Manfred Porkert is forthcoming to meet this need. For prescriptions not given in the *Revised Outline*, those who can read Chinese are referred to Chung-i yen-chiu-yuan 中 医 研 究 院 et al. ed. 1983.

PART I

INTRODUCTORY STUDY

Chapter I

TRADITIONAL MEDICINE IN
CONTEMPORARY CHINA

In health and illness, anywhere in the world, one human body is much the same as another. Its shape and parts vary within only narrow limits. What we witness of pain and illness in other cultures does not suggest different vital functions, nor does medical research make national distinctions of lesion or infection. Certain diseases, for instance tuberculosis, are, to be sure, found much more often in one part of the world than in others. Schistosomiasis remains an important public health problem in China, while most German doctors never encounter a case. But the same range of signs and symptoms announces schistosomiasis in China or Germany. These manifestations vary from case to case; but they may differ more in two neighbors than between two people a continent apart.

Differences of that kind become negligible when we consider with what lack of unanimity physicians and other curers at various times and in various societies have perceived the body and explained health and illness. To say that all are concerned with the same body is to lose sight of how differently they identify the internal processes that maintain vitality or threaten it. On this understanding depends, of course, how drugs and other means can be used to restore health.

Chinese medicine, like the classical medical doctrine of Europe, is concerned above all with the dynamic balance of the whole organism.[1] This emphasis differs from that of modern medicine, in

---

[1] By "Chinese medicine" or "traditional medicine" I mean the doctrines and practices called *Chung i* 中 医 in China today; the official translation is "traditional Chinese medicine." This term refers to the doctrines and practices that evolved over more

3

which the examining physician attempts to determine the organ or body system affected by the illness, the identity of the case, and the extent of impairment. In the traditional Chinese view the body is not a biochemical factory (or a living machine, to use the metaphor of the European Enlightenment) but a congeries of vital processes that makes possible the activities of a social person. Health is a physiological, emotional, and moral balance, maintained in all three spheres or not at all, for the three are inseparable. It is disturbances in this balance that challenge the judgment of the physician. As a most exalted amateur of medicine, Emperor Hui-tsung 徽 宗 (r. 1101–26) of the Sung, put it, "One yin and one yang [i.e., their constant alternation] are called the Way; bias toward yin or bias toward yang is called disease. None save those who clearly understand the Way have ever been able to cure man's diseases. . . . With the median comes felicity; with excess comes calamity; with license comes disease."[2]

---

than two millennia and were passed down by China's educated elite—as scientific, however that may be defined, as premodern European medicine, but continuously influenced by popular therapeutic practice. This tradition was simply called i, "medicine," until Occidental influence made it inevitable that what previously was thought universal be identified as native. I use "classical medicine" for ideas and methods that have not survived modern reinterpretation. Although a few physicians knew a little about the European art as early as the seventeenth century, little of its content affected the Chinese mainstream until very recently. For practical purposes the dividing line between classical and "modern traditional" medicine must be drawn somewhat after 1900. For twentieth-century medicine the traditional/modern distinction is no doubt more to the point than the Chinese/Western distinction, as Joseph Needham has emphasized (1970: 404). Modern medicine, despite European assumptions built into its discourse, is used and advanced by every people. Nevertheless Chinese remain keenly aware of which system is native and which is not, and almost always speak of modern medicine as Western.

[2] *Sheng chi ching* 聖 濟 経, preface by Hui-tsung, page 1. The role of yin-yang theory in medicine is explained below.

The clinical physician, faced with the endless profusion of signs and symptoms, looked through and beyond the particulars to find the imbalance:

> In diagnosis and therapy it is finding the essential unity that we value most. All the diseases in the world, in all their variation, have a single basis. All the remedies in the world, despite their multiplicity, are one in their effect on the manifestations. No matter what the doctrine of therapy, one must be certain that the disorder is of the cold type (7.2.1) before dispersing the cold heteropathy (5.1.2), or that it is of the hot type (7.2.2) before clearing the hot heteropathy (5.2.2). Once the root [of the disorder] has been dug out, all the manifestations will be relieved. Thus the *Inner Canon* says "to cure illness it is essential to find the root." This being so, in examining patients it is always necessary to investigate the root of the disorder before prescribing. If you are not able to perceive it exactly, it is better to wait a while, and then to make another detailed examination.[3]

---

[3] *Ching-yueh chüan shu* 景 岳 全 書 (1624), *1*: 35a (*Ch'uan chung lu* 傳 忠 錄 , *chüan* 1). "Heteropathy," Manfred Porkert's term for *hsieh* 邪 , the pathogens of traditional medicine, is discussed below, page 49. The *Inner Canon of the Yellow Lord* [*Huang ti nei ching* 黃 帝 內 経], the most authoritative source of traditional medical doctrine, is actually several collections, each containing originally heterogenous writings. Recent studies indicate that the *Huang ti nei ching* was probably written over a century or more and brought together in the first century B.C. or the early first century A.D. Research in progress by David Keegan has already clearly shown that none of the several extant books that transmit parts of the original *Inner Canon* represent its form and structure, although on the whole they quote its words in a consistent way. They must be considered distinct texts. The two books traditionally accepted by Chinese physicians as extant parts of the *Inner Canon* did not exist in their present form before the eighth century. These are the *Basic Questions* (*Su wen* 素 問 , cited as SW) and the Divine

If we were to survey the cure of ailments the world over we would see an even greater variety of conceptions underlying therapy. Some of the world's traditions are popular, based on oral teachings and often on religious world-views. Others are rational in the sense that illness is caused by objective, abstract forces rather than by the wills of divinities. Some of these rational conceptions are classical, passed down cumulatively in writing so that every author is consciously adding to the ideas of predecessors. In large and diverse cultures there may be several therapeutic traditions, representing different localities or different types of education, and, of course, different clinical priorities. These have commonly interacted, challenging and enriching each other.

Modern medicine, on the other hand, has certain basic characteristics that can be seen anywhere it is practiced, despite great variation in its social organization and in the way it is understood by laymen. Its innovations largely apply knowledge gained by research in other disciplines, especially biology, chemistry, and physics. It uses elaborate surgery, asepsis, anesthesia, and powerful drugs to overcome life-threatening traumas, infections, and biochemical dysfunctions that no traditional system can control. It is associated with a complex of technological, economic, social, and political forces that, as they spread around the world, leave no scope for long survival of the educational institutions that create traditional curers and give them the confidence of their patients. Modern medicine has been adopted in one country after another not simply because patients who have experienced its therapeutic superiority champion it, but because political decisions have given special status to its curricula, licensing, and professional prerogatives. Such decisions themselves are usually based not on the

---

Pivot (*Ling shu* 靈 樞 , cited as LS). The *Grand Basis* (*T'ai su* 太 素 , cited as TS) was probably compiled 666/683. Despite its chronological priority it has had little influence on medicine. Since it often provides superior readings, however, I generally cite it first, and note only significant discrepancies. The reference in the quotation is to SW, *2* (5): 27 (i.e., *chüan* 2, chapter 5, page 27) = TS, *3* (1): 3, in TIZ ed. only. For editions see the bibliography. Section numbers in parentheses in the text of this introductory study (i.e., 7.2.1) are cross-references to explanations in the translation that follows.

statistical outcomes of clinical tests in local circumstances, but on a commitment to modernization across the board.

Why should traditional notions of the body and its ills be so diverse? Is there not a single truth that any sensible person should have found? The variation cannot be explained by indigenous healers' lack of intelligence or proneness to error. Medical anthropologists and historians of medicine have given us no reason to believe that such practitioners on the whole are less intelligent or more careless than the average European or American physician. But it is the need to cure, not the abstract search for truth, that shapes medical conceptions and makes them manifold.

If we compare traditional medical systems with each other rather than with the modern medicine that is challenging and replacing them—certainly a more informative kind of comparison— we can acknowledge that there are many ways to slice the spectrum of suffering into symptoms and diseases. Each repertory of medical disorders will depend on how those who create it experience not only the body but society and nature. These tend to mirror each other in traditional societies that expect experience to fit together into a coherent whole. For a society that does not practice dissection, ideas about what goes on inside the body may reflect the structure of the village; whether the body is an inseparable, interacting unity or a collection of practically autonomous parts may depend on whether individuals in the social group, and phenomena in nature, are seen as tightly or loosely linked. Whether the body's parts or subsystems are seen as subordinated in a tight hierarchic order, or as cooperative but independent agents, is apt to reflect political ideals.[4]

A rich understanding of the body and its ills, adequate to relate symptoms, syndromes, and therapy, can evolve within very wide limits of this kind. A great many such understandings may make equally efficient use of limited resources for aiding the ill to recover. Which views become traditional will depend on other criteria, less narrowly medical but no less important, such as how well a given set of conceptions prepares people to comprehend what they are ex-

---

[4] The relation between cosmology and social structure is a major theme in sociology and anthropology, explored in such classic writing as Berger and Luckmann 1966. The most seminal work so far on its extension to the body is Douglas 1970.

periencing and to act in ways conducive to recovery; all of the symbols of a culture can be brought to bear on this preparation.

The process that brings modern medicine into traditional societies places their futures in the hands of people no longer traditionally educated. This process validates the views of nature and society that accompany it when it enters, not the prevalent views. The result is powerful influences that traditional medical systems can hardly ignore, and that often leave them discarded and forgotten in a generation or so.

Whether this fate awaits the classical tradition of Chinese medicine—which this book is about—it is too early to say (although there is no scarcity of strong opinions, positive and negative). Four centuries have passed since European medicine was first introduced into China in a form that had little influence. It has been a century since the foreign art became widely known, and a generation since, in its modern form, it began to play an important role in primary health care throughout Chinese society.

What is remarkable is that traditional medicine still plays a large role in the official health care system, and even enjoys a vogue in the rest of the world. Its position is more secure than that of most traditional therapeutic systems elsewhere, at least in the short term. While it has survived, the other sciences that grew up alongside it over the past two thousand years in China (astronomy, mathematics, geomancy, alchemy, and the rest) have perished or are dying out.

Why Study Traditional Medicine?

What is the point of studying any traditional medical system, and that of China in particular? A humanist might well argue that any system of thought and practice on a large scale, incorporating centuries of talent, is worth understanding for its inherent interest and for the light it casts on human potentialities, apart from its therapeutic usefulness. Someone concerned with the advancement of medicine might claim that we are bound to learn from such a rich fund of experience if we approach it comprehendingly and critically; to ignore it without scrutiny and test is no more scientific than to accept it without scrutiny and test. Thus Manfred Porkert has argued for "the thorough and consistent appraisal of each system as a whole and in its own right" and "the comparative empirical verification of accepted data" before reaching conclusions about how Chinese and modern medicine ought to be combined.[5]

Both of these positions call for general comprehension of traditional Chinese medicine—its social and theoretical as well as practical sides. Other interests in Chinese medicine are narrower, especially among physicians who are busy with other matters. Some who have learned a little about some aspect of traditional medicine see it simply as a source of techniques, the value of which does not depend on the structures of knowledge that held them together; such theoretical entities as yin-yang "can be left to historians."[6] This view assumes that the ideas and social arrangements of modern medicine need no improvement, or at least none that could conceivably come from investigation of old ideas or "folk" traditions.

The humanist view does not need elaborate justification; this book will enable the reader to decide whether it applies. The notion of Chinese medicine as an exotic garden of unrelated techniques is not the result of an overall understanding. It presupposes that such an understanding would be useless to modern medicine. Even those who believe that competence and learning excuse arrogance will have little patience for arrogance so righteous and badly informed. Porkert and his predecessors have long since shown in easily accessible writings that the traditional physician's every technical act

---

[5] Porkert 1977: 11.

[6] Frederick F. Kao in Jenerick ed. 1974: 110. Dr. Kao also opined that "the classical points [i.e., acupuncture loci] were worked out about the second or third century A.D., that those people never mentioned five elements [i.e., Five Phases] or Yin-Yang. That goes further back, about 3,000 years ago." In the same discussion, Mitsuo Numoto, not to be outdone in public display of ignorance, agreed that yin-yang and other theories were related to acupuncture "several thousand years ago" but not more recently, and argued that "it is wrong today to use astrologically based theory to explain acupuncture." None of the participants in this National Institutes of Medicine conference showed interest in the relation of acupuncture to other therapies or to conceptions of the body. But these relationships are still central in Chinese teaching of acupuncture, as the *Revised Outline* (chapter 4 below) makes clear. This book was one of several easily available outside China by the time the opinions quoted above were voiced.

depends on a highly abstract view of the body in its environment. Leaders of the medical profession seem to be losing sympathy for righteously ignorant conviction. That, I believe, is why medical anthropology and sociology have become expanding fields of research and widespread topics of instruction.

On the other hand, just how modern medicine may be enriched by broad study of Chinese medicine is not obvious. A full answer can only come as a result of such study, which has barely begun, but some preliminary reflections are clearly in order. Those that follow are concerned with Chinese medicine, but apply to traditional systems of medicine generally, at least to those of the major civilizations.

In summarizing the strengths of modern medicine, I have implied that they are most prominently technical, that it also draws on highly developed bodies of theoretical science, and that it is above all effective for acute, life-threatening disorders. There is much dissatisfaction among thoughtful physicians about its mastery of chronic physical disorder, about its understanding of the interrelations of body and mind in disease, and about its place in the enterprise of public health. Medicine's social arrangements—the roles and responsibilities of those who provide health care, the authority granted them by society, the political and economic aspects of their relations with patients—vary greatly, even across Europe, and are being reexamined everywhere. In other words, there is patently much to be learned about chronic disorders, the psychosomatic aspects of morbidity, and the social matrices of medicine.

Consider the distinction between acute and chronic disorders. The usual dictionary definitions, which state that the first kind move quickly from onset to crisis and the second linger or recur, do not do justice to their significance either for the patient or for society. In acute illnesses time is of the essence. The patient usually experiences what seems literally to be an attack, which must be forestalled without delay. If it cannot be stopped, the patient must withdraw into himself and survive as his vitality and his will allow. His passage through the intense period of danger may leave weakness, permanent scars, or chronic disability, but recovery usually soon follows the crisis.

Some chronic diseases (for instance, brucellosis or undulant fever and certain types of malaria) comprise an endless succession of crises, so that the crucial period loses some of its vividness—

though rarely its pain—through habit. Some chronic illnesses limit activity without crises. Others escalate and kill.

What matters about chronic disorders is that those who have them cannot anticipate recovery. In this sense the ultimate chronic illness is old age, the irreversible loss of physical capacities until none is left. In chronic illness cure is seldom a feasible goal; the physician can at best help the patient to live with the disability, to continue with some approximation to a normal life.

No traditional society, including that of Europe and the United States before the twentieth century, has had powerful means to cure most acute disease. A certain number of people were struck in an epidemic, and a certain proportion survived. By the end of the nineteenth century preventive quarantine, an array of drugs with which to manipulate body processes, and smallpox variolation and vaccination were familiar in Western Europe and societies connected with it, but those infected were still largely thrown back on their own resources. Quinine for malaria was the only widespread "wonder drug."

The advent of asepsis and anesthesia, which made major surgery relatively safe, and the proliferation of powerful specific drugs, moved the focus of clinical medicine away from chronic illness and toward acute disease and trauma. Means to prevent, diagnose, and cure one acute disease after another were uncovered in Europe and the United States by scientific research. In 1900 hospitals were still meant primarily for those not wealthy enough to be cared for at home. They treated mostly chronic disorders, and were prudently avoided by those who could afford to avoid them. By 1925 even the rich were beginning to find them good places to have babies. Diseases that meant a private encounter with death a century ago now mean at worst an uncomfortable but temporary withdrawal from full activity.

The new therapies do not depend on wonder drugs and surgical *tours de force* alone. The passion to subdue acute disease has called into being a medical system that isolates the patient, controls his environment, and provides those who care for him with rapid access to emergency technologies.

As the great capacity to cure acute diseases and overcome dangerous traumas evolved, the roles of doctor and patient evolved to fit the new institutions designed to maximize this capacity. Physicians and their organizations learned to shape this interaction to accord with their views about what was needed to make health care more professional, and how to ensure doctors the authority they needed and the prestige they deserved. Prevention became a matter for national campaigns. The balance tipped away from general practice toward specialization, away from the home and the family doctor's office toward the hospital and the multi-doctor clinic. The physician came to resemble the scientist manipulating an experimental object which had to be kept immobile and passive so as not to hinder operations measured to the millimeter and timed to the split second. The patient's biochemistry and physiology became more crucial than his feelings, which were apt to get in the way of decisions made by the therapist on technical grounds. More often than a generation earlier, technical assessments could make the difference between death and survival. Such assessments justified other narrowly based decisions even when recovery was not in question. The patient's family and friends no longer could be with him except for timed visits after the crisis was past. This new complex of practice and attitude justified itself because it was associated with advancing control over one acute disorder and surgical emergency after another.

Over the past couple of decades many public health physicians have come to believe that this specialization of institutions, despite its remarkable success, has had disastrous side effects in the United States. The direction of most rapid development has been almost diametrically opposed to what meets the needs of the chronically ill. It is difficult for the doctor's help to be available when the patient needs support and unhurried explanation. It is exceptional, except in the upper strata of society, for doctors to have time to know their chronic patients well and to give specific advice about a minimally hampered style of life. It is practically unheard of for doctors to enter patients' homes and form an independent impression of interpersonal factors that may affect physical dependence. It is hard for many patients, especially the poorly educated and the very old, to adapt to the highly routine, stressful procedures of urban hospital clinics, or to feel encouraged when treated impersonally and hurriedly by a succession of doctors.

Not only has medicine largely given up the role of mediator between the patient and those around him who may help or hinder recovery, but society has changed in ways that make it almost impossible for physicians to mediate. The wasting away of communal bonds and common values has meant that a circle of relatives, friends, and neighbors is often unavailable to accept what a chronically ill person has to contribute, and to support his effort to continue a normal life. Only in small, intact communities is useful work available for the old. The social relations of the "senior citizen" with degenerative diseases, shell-shocked by inflation and crime in a large city, may well be beside the point; he may have no relative or friend.

In summary, the transformation of modern medicine—of which I have mentioned only a few manifestations—has been part of, and has been made possible by, the demise of the universal values and usages that define a traditional society. There are indications that more balanced institutions and roles may evolve: a shift of medical students into family practice, the growing importance of family and group psychotherapy, and increased training of paramedical workers who may enhance the quality of human interaction because they have more time than physicians and less psychological distance from patients. But that is the future; the present situation suggests strong contrasts with traditional medicine.

The limitations of classical Chinese medicine were of course formidable. What is more to the point here, they were in many ways opposites of the limits we have just seen in American health care. The framework of classical medicine ordered endless permutations of symptoms. It integrated and explained theoretically an enormous variety of therapeutic measures, including thousands of physiologically active drugs. Most (but not all) were mild. What modern physicians do best for chronic patients—namely, relieve symptoms—traditional doctors could do over a narrower range with fewer side effects and less danger of harm from over-medication.

These remedies were used in a society where access to the patient's social milieu was easy. The curer usually came from the same milieu, and in most cases could be sure what his patients believed, how they saw the world, and what their inner experience of illness might be. He treated the patient at the latter's home. He could make sure that the patient was looked after. He could observe strains between people that might obstruct recovery. He could directly encourage relatives and others to help. This is not a great deal, but it is most of what can be done for much chronic disease. Traditional doctors, simply because they were located in a society where social bonds were still tight, did what could be done better, on the whole, than modern doctors whose institutions and roles are specialized—for other reasons—in ways that make adequate involvement in the care of patients with chronic disorders practically impossible.

The case for an attentive look at traditional medicine rests in part, then, on its ability to let us study the approaches of curers whose holistic views of medical disorder centered on chronic dysfunctions ånd aimed toward effective psychological and social support. The limitations of technology resulted in attitudes toward diagnosis that encouraged unhurried examination before symptoms became serious, and attention to patients' subtle perceptions of body states that overworked physicians today usually consider a waste of time. There is much to be said for understanding how traditional doctors used information of this kind, and to what effect. The point is not to present Chinese practices as the wave of the future, or to hope wistfully for a restoration of traditional social bonds. It is rather to provide those who want to think about the future of medicine with a variety of examples that embody the complexity and concreteness of an actual medical system. Among the other uses of such examples, they remind us that techniques and the social circumstances in which they are used cannot be fully understood without reference to each other.

Particular aspects of Chinese theory and its applications may be suggestive as modern medicine continues to be rethought. One is its holistic character. The body and the emotions are interdependent and influence each other in health and illness. Both are responsive to the physical environment. Diagnosis considers all three realms in a systematic way, and therapy takes advantage of their interaction. The consequences of these ideas for modern psychosomatics have yet to be explored. No one familiar with the ancient Chinese sources will doubt that they bear on such issues as stress. But that is a matter that would take us far afield.

Another promising area of study is the predominantly functional discourse of classical medicine. Early doctors had a rough grasp of the contents and structure of the human body, but their discussions were generally focussed on processes. The body was an organism composed of functional systems that extracted vital substances from air and food, distributed them where they were needed, expelled the residues, and resisted the factors of disease. The normal body was maintained in health by a regular and even circulation of vital pneumata and essences (ch'i 氣) throughout. The great concern in medical disorders was correcting abnormalities—excesses or inadequacies—in this circulation or in other metabolic functions.

The concepts by which function and dysfunction were described are decidedly not of modern type. Some embody striking perceptions; others can hardly be taken seriously by anyone unsympathetic to numerology. Many assumptions of traditional medicine have not been borne out by modern experience. Only research, little of which so far has been conclusive, can decide how much doctrine that invalidates. Researchers outside Asia today are less inclined than fifteen years ago to ignore acupuncture, although its original rationales are difficult to understand and some that have been tested are doubtful from the physical point of view.

The present issue is functional language, not physical description. European medicine, with its early emphasis on anatomy, tended to be greatly concerned with structure; from the Renaissance on, frequent dissection increased its concentration on organs and tissues. But knowledge of anatomy could affect the practice of internal medicine only very gradually, as it became possible to connect disorders in live humans with the lesions that could be observed in corpses and live animals. As medicine began from the seventeenth century on to draw on mechanistic philosophy and then experimental science, thinkers became more inclined to explain the operations of the body by simple physical and chemical processes. This reductionist approach has appeared increasingly unsatisfactory as biology has drawn attention to the cellular basis of vital processes, as biochemistry has begun to explain the complexity of pathological change at the level of the molecule, and as psychology has thrown light on the interaction of emotional and physical processes in every medical disorder.

A medical language to describe the large-scale functions of the body in a holistic way informed by recent scientific insights is gradually being formed. To succeed, those who are forming it will have to find a way round the habit of thought that ignores the body as a whole and concentrates on isolated phenomena that can be reduced to physical, chemical, and biological explanation. Reductionism is perhaps inevitable when beginning to make medicine a science. But it will not carry the quest very far. It is only reasonable to suggest that the sophisticated functional language of Chinese theory should offer useful insights, despite great differences in the questions traditional and modern medicine seek to answer and in what they consider pertinent information. I am not suggesting that modern physicians should adopt traditional discourse, but that there is much to be learned from studying its formation.

There is, in short, ample reason to believe that traditional medicine has more to contribute than a few techniques. One need not overlook its many fundamental differences from modern medicine to recognize that their strengths are to some extent complementary (I have already discussed the instance of acute vs.

chronic illness). Modern medicine in its quest for theoretical and social innovation need not be limited to introspection.

The old Chinese literature is enormous. Roughly ten thousand
medical treatises, some of many volumes, survive from previous
centuries, and additional information abounds in general writing.[7] This trove of sources furnishes case studies of great internal
consistency and rich texture. Once mastered, it can tell us what the
fate of particular ideas was. That is, in the final analysis, what the
integration of old and new medicine in China today is about: using
the past to shape the future.

Traditional Medicine in Twentieth-Century China

Despite the long coexistence of traditional and modern medicine
in China their decisive encounter did not begin until the
1950s.[8] European ideas were written about in China shortly after
1600, but that was not modern medicine. The practical consequences of transmission remained negligible until foreign missionaries
opened a few clinics in the mid-nineteenth century. Since about the
beginning of the twentieth century a set of basic modern institutions
have developed—medical schools, hospitals, professional organizations, systems of licensing, etc.—but in circumstances that at first

---

[7] The estimate of about ten thousand surviving treatises came
   from Li Jingwei 李经纬 (or Ching-wei), Director, The China Institute for the History of Medicine and Medical Literature,
   Academy of Traditional Chinese Medicine, at a conference on the
   history of science, medicine, and technology, University of Pennsylvania, 18 May 1984. Chung-i yen-chiu-yuan & Pei-ching t'u-
   shu-kuan ed. 1961 lists 7,661 titles catalogued in 60 Chinese collections as of 1959. Perhaps 1,500 of these are available in the
   United States and Europe.
[8] There are few reliable sources on the historical encounter of
   Chinese and Western medicine. Among the most useful are
   Ch'üan Han-sheng 全漢聲 1936, Fan Hsing-chun 范行
   準 1944, and Rudolph 1977 for the period of the Jesuit missionaries; for the Republican period, Croizier 1968 and 1976; and
   for the first decade and a half of the People's Republic, Croizier
   1973. An anthropological field study of great value is Francis
   L. K. Hsu 1952.

let them play no direct role in meeting the therapeutic needs of the great majority of the population.[9]

Many legislators in the 1920s and 1930s who supported wholesale modernization considered traditional medicine, like other old institutions, unscientific rubbish to be swept away once and for all. As official support of public medical training programs was undertaken for the first time in a millenium, it was initially reserved for modern medicine. In fact the government was too weak in the first half of the century for its policies to be either steady or effective. By 1937, when the final chaos of war supervened, there were only nine thousand or so registered modern physicians,[10] most of whom would not have been qualified to practice by standards prevalent in Western Europe or the United States.

It was the threat that official rejection might foreclose the future, rather than economic competition from modern physicians, that led traditional practitioners to organize their own societies and schools for the first time in the 1920s. Still, as in the United States in 1870, anyone could hang out his shingle. The usual qualification was to have been the disciple of an experienced master, but if that were lacking, the ability to find patients was qualification enough.

The founding of the People's Republic in 1949 brought an end to more than a century of incessant war and uprising on the Chinese mainland, and provided all its provinces except Taiwan with unified administration for the first time in forty years. Unlike its predecessor the new government was in a position to demand that basic health care be made available to everyone. This was a goal that no large, poor country had yet attained. In most, the health of the rural indigent was ignored aside from rudimentary public health measures.

A centrally directed and subsidized public health program that reaches the whole population has indeed evolved since 1955, its quality high considering the limits of China's national wealth.[11]

---

[9] Particularly illuminating in this regard is Bullock 1980.

[10] The estimate is from Croizier 1968: 55. He considers it high.

[11] The most informative study so far of accomplishments and problems is Jamison et al. 1984; for intellectual patterns see Ågren 1975. On the financing of the health care system up to a decade ago see Hu Teh-wei 1974. Useful policy studies include Lampton 1974 and 1977 and Lucas 1982. Reports on brief trips to China, although seldom well-informed, are occasionally inform-

This could not have happened unless traditional practice had been incorporated. Acupuncture and native herbal medicines are inexpensive; immediate dependence on modern synthetic drugs, whether imported or made in imported factories, would have led to a foreign debt that the government was unprepared to tolerate. Modern medical schools and physicians were so few that there was no prospect of training enough M.D.'s in the immediate future.

But these problems of economic and human resources are only part of the story. What patients knew about their bodies and their health was formed by traditional medicine. Its practitioners were usually skillful at motivating the patient's will to recover, which requires patient and comprehensible explanation; modern doctors were exotics in the eyes of the uneducated, and their explanations (when they had time to give them) practically meaningless.

The health care with which China's new leaders were already familiar, from their work in the countryside in the couple of decades before 1950, was preponderantly traditional. They knew that it was effective within its limits (for instance, that it was more reliable for chronic than for acute disorders, and that the quality of practice varied greatly). It is well to remember that they were comparing it not with the highest world standard but with the work of the undertrained and underequipped modern doctors who constituted the Chinese average. Why it was effective, and for exactly what, were not understood. Unlike the wholesale Westernizers of the 1930s, the planners around Mao Tse-tung saw this as a matter for study rather than as a reason to wipe out traditional medicine. As policymakers used Chinese medicine they reshaped it. They expanded formal medical education on a more uniform standard and required knowledge of modern medicine on the part of all graduates. They founded research institutes in which both theory and practice could be systematically evaluated. Traditional and modern physicians were assigned to the same hospitals, so that patients could choose whom to consult, or so that both types of skill could be brought to bear on the same case. In order to make informed col-

---

ative, especially Committee on Scholarly Communication with the People's Republic of China ed. 1980, Quinn ed. 1974, and Sidel and Sidel 1973 and 1982. Among available bibliographies are Anonymous 1973 (useful only for Chinese articles translated into or abstracted in English), Akhtar 1975 (Western-language sources only), and Kenton 1976 and 1982.

laboration possible, modern physicians were expected to gain a basic knowledge of traditional medicine (the book translated here was compiled for that purpose).

This policy was meant to give both kinds of doctors comparable prestige and some mutual understanding, but did not aim to change fundamentally either type of practice. This "separate but equal" arrangement ended in the late 1960s. One of the explicit aims of the Great Proletarian Cultural Revolution became to produce a synthesis of the two systems that would be fully scientific without being foreign or elitist. The result was an efflorescence of new techniques that combined traditional and modern aspects, such as injection of antibiotics at acupuncture loci (where in classical medicine only solid needles were inserted). The new technique of acupuncture for analgesia in surgical operations was developed until it became practical and fairly common (although never as common as the hyperbole of the Western mass media made it seem). Less superficial were new clinical research projects to combine traditional and modern therapy.[12] Equally significant, the Chinese increased their efforts to use modern science to test every aspect of traditional medicine and separate what is "objectively valid" from "feudal remnants."

There were political outcomes as well, such as more local control of public health by cadres at the expense of the specialists (mostly Western-trained) in the central Ministry of Public Health.[13] The ideological overtones were more ambiguous than public announcements made them appear. Modern doctors, because of the foreign and elitist associations of their profession, had to prove that their political orthodoxy was sincere. An important way to do this was by studying traditional medicine rather than criticizing it as "unscientific." On the other hand, traditional medicine had to be tested by modern research, not the other way around.

The end of the Cultural Revolution in the late 1970s did not simply mark another turn of a cycle. Medical policymaking has once again moved to Beijing, and the juxtaposition of modern and

---

[12] There is a large literature on research of this kind. The most famous monograph is Nan-k'ai i-yuan 南开医院 ed. 1972, on acute abdomen. A conspectus of the trend is provided in Anonymous ed. 1977.

[13] See especially the writings of David M. Lampton on the politics of medical policy.

traditional medicine no longer so greatly resembles a shotgun wedding. But research on traditional medicine, and attempts to create combined therapies, continue, albeit under less pressure than fifteen years ago.

The Ongoing Transition

Traditional medicine has undergone irreversible changes during nearly four centuries of coexistence with the new currents from the West. These alterations were negligible until the end of the nineteenth century. Change has greatly accelerated in the past two decades, when the relation between the two medical systems became intimate and mandatory. In order to assess the transition, it is well to keep in mind several crucial characteristics:

1. The theories of Chinese medicine have borne comparison with those of medicine at the same time in Europe, in point of rationality and sophistication, through most of history, even though their foci of interest have differed. The Chinese theories were large and well-articulated structures that related clinical experience to the underlying reality revealed by what we would call philosophic reasoning.

Theory has been greatly elaborated over the two thousand years of its history, incorporating new ranges of pathological detail and therapies. But its basis has remained concepts such as yin-yang and the Five Phases, defined at its very beginning. Again and again their meanings have been extended and their associations with particular phenomena altered, but, as with the Four Elements and their corresponding qualities in Western medicine, no failure to accord with experience could have proven them invalid. Their rejection could come only with the rejection of classical medicine as a coherent body of knowledge, analogous to the step-by-step rejection of Galenic medicine in Europe completed only in the nineteenth century.

European medicine was transformed by appeals to new sciences and methodologies that called for the systematic and ceaseless testing of hypotheses and theories. Its thinking came to be of an altogether new kind. Its means of accumulating knowledge, methods of reasoning, interplay between theory and practice, and means of therapy underwent accelerated change, which bore its trajectory sharply away from the slow growth (and sometimes stasis) of traditional medical ideas the world over. The habits of thought and conceptions of fact in traditional and modern medicine are now so fundamentally different that understanding between practitioners of the two systems is practically impossible without heroic labors of translation and redefinition. The best physicians in Paris in 1600 had more intellectually in common with their contemporaries in Beijing than with their successors in the Paris of 1900. This point will, I hope, become clearer in the translation of the *Revised Outline*.

2. The care of medical disorders in traditional China was not a profession, or for that matter even a single occupation. Many kinds of therapy, carried out by different kinds of people, coexisted at arm's length: magical and religious curing, treatment by local practitioners who applied a few remedies without elaborate diagnosis, the ministrations of itinerant healers with a little book-learning, the learned practice of hereditary physicians and well-born amateurs, the highly organized services of the palace medical bureaucracy who waited upon the emperor. Ritual remained the therapy of first resort for the majority of Chinese. Over the last millennium, gentlemen who pursued medicine for the sake of learning, self-cultivation, and filial piety had greater prestige than other varieties of healers, including imperial physicians, almost all of whose names have been forgotten. How much prestige the literati doctors (*ju i* 儒 醫) had often depended on their eminence as statesmen, philosophers, or poets. These scholarly physicians did not constitute a profession as the best sociologists define the word. They were not organized, did not think of themselves as a group, and could not set or enforce common standards of medical education, skill, or compensation.[14] The medical civil servants were expected to have certain educational qualifications and at least were subject to penalties for malpractice, but they neither set nor enforced these criteria.

The learned doctors—who rejected the label of technical specialist—would not accept the proposition that they belonged to the same occupational group as the medical bureaucrats, much less that they had anything significant in common with hereditary physicians, rural herbalists, pious laymen who distributed prescriptions as charity, trance-healers, or wonderworkers. They repeatedly expressed contempt for "vulgar healers" (*yung i* 庸 醫 , *su i* 俗 醫), by which they usually designated people working like themselves in the classical tradition who were less learned in medicine,

---

[14] Freidson 1970, 1975; Mechanic 1968.

less erudite in philosophy, less polished in morality, or—what these generally amounted to—lower on the social scale.[15]

Thus "classical medicine" does not refer to the theory and practice of a coherent group, but to the records left by the most literate and scholarly representatives of several traditions (some of whom were compilers or medical philosophers rather than practitioners). Many famous authors were hereditary doctors or minor bureaucrats of the palace medical service rather than amateurs of the scholar-official class, but all belonged to the small upper crust of the population that could read and write.

It is almost exclusively this elite *literary* tradition that has survived in modern China. Large repertories of drug substances and prescriptions have been collected from living local curers over the past two decades to supplement it.[16] But the literary heritage taught in today's colleges of Chinese medicine and summarized in

---

[15] Unschuld (1979, 1980) has muddied this issue by attempting to organize a social history of medicine around putative conflicts between those working within and outside Confucianism—an entity that he does not define clearly in social terms and uses arbitrarily. His analysis does not reflect current understanding of the great changes in Confucianism over the centuries. Nor do these studies take advantage of the recent approaches of sociologists or anthropologists (although the original version refers to *Sozialkonflikte* and the English translation calls itself "a study in historical anthropology"). For solid research in the same area see Hymes 1987, which demonstrates that concerns about careers and prestige are essential to understanding assertions of physicians about each other.

[16] The large literature on local materia medica was mostly published in the early 1970s and received very limited distribution. Fortunately it was largely incorporated in Chiang-su hsin i-hsueh-yuan 江 苏 新 医 学 院 ed. 1977–78. I have not seen any work which collects and digests the prescriptions gathered from local curers who are not traditional physicians in the classical tradition. A number of collections of "folk prescriptions" have appeared in Taiwan, for instance Yen T'ien-shou 顏 添 壽 ed. 1968 and Li Shuo-kuang 李 爍 光 ed. 1976. These tend to be vague about how their materials were collected, and I suspect that some compilers did much of their harvesting in books.

books like this one (the heritage that Chinese call *Chung i* 中 醫
and that I loosely call "traditional medicine" above) is not that of
the "common people," except in the sense that the elite authors of
past centuries have not ignored the experience of the humble practitioners who so outnumbered them. The frequent religious and
magical content of popular curing before modern times has tended
in recent years to throw the latter into the category of feudal superstition, which for decades has not been a respectable topic of study
in China.[17]

The reorganization of medical care in this century, especially
since the 1950s, has greatly changed the traditional constellation I
have described briefly above. Most priests and other operators of
what anthropologists call symbolic therapies have long since been
persuaded to cease their "superstitious" practices. Experienced and
qualified physicians trained in the old master-disciple relationship
have been licensed and are subject, at least in principle, to supervision. Training now takes place in schools with approved curricula
and standard textbooks. As in the case of modern medicine, there
are different levels of medical education. Schools for lower-level
medical workers usually require three years after secondary school.
Chinese physicians enter medical school directly from high school
and receive five or more years of training. On the whole the health
care system is evolving toward well-defined standards of qualification for doctors who will practice as government employees. Private
practice for fees was rare until the early 1980s, but is rapidly expanding. No pattern of regulation or of professional organization
has yet emerged. If neither modern nor traditional medicine is a
profession (since the standards of qualification and conditions of

---

[17] This disapproval extended after 1950 to expunging information
on ritual and other popular therapies from scholarly editions and
reprints of classical medical treatises, although most of these,
printed in old-style orthography, would be studied only by
specialists. This policy of repressing "superstition" has been less
zealously enforced since the end of the Cultural Revolution. For
instance, the most important pre-twentieth-century source for the
repertory of itinerant physicians who did not belong to the classical tradition, *Ch'uan ya* 串 雅 (described in Unschuld 1978),
has been reprinted in three volumes of annotated selections. This
work is exceptionally rich in ritual and magical remedies.

work are set by career policymakers, not by doctors), each has become for all practical purposes an occupation.

3. "Classical" implies a special relation to earlier knowledge, in
which the earliest writings (rather than the most recent, as in
modern science) are considered the most reliable guides to understanding. Thus, in Europe the authority of Galen of Pergamon
(129/130-199/200), and that of Hippocrates and Aristotle before
him, were rarely challenged until the Renaissance.

In China most traditions of science and art were traced from an
initial revelation, incorporating a wisdom so deep that the minds of
a lesser age could only aspire to approximate it. The most
authoritative texts of early medical theory and drug therapy, following this established pattern, were ascribed to semi-divine sovereigns
of a period before history, and were thus known as the *Inner Canon
of the Yellow Lord* (*Huang ti nei ching* 黃 帝 內 經, to which
was joined an *Outer Canon*, now lost) and the *Divine Husbandman's
Materia Medica* (*Shen nung pen-ts'ao* 神 農 本 草, also subsequently called a canon, *ching* 經).[18]

Writers in later ages always knew these books, and often spent
years annotating them line by line; hundreds of commentaries to
the *Inner Canon* are recorded.[19] Other scholars might move off in
quite new directions; for instance, the three-part classification of
simples in the *Divine Husbandman's Canon*, inadequate for
therapeutic needs, was set aside a thousand years ago for less
rudimentary taxonomies (see page 185). Still each new direction
was in principle stepped off not from the last before it, but from the
canons that, in the charter myths of medicine, must be the source of

---

[18] For more plausible dates see note 3 above. Information about
dating, editions used, etc., is given in the bibliography.
Premodern Chinese and other East Asian sources (roughly to
1900) are listed separately by title.

[19] See the incomplete list of 114 versions and commentaries in Kuo
Ai-ch'un 郭 靄 春 1981: 529-35. This list, compiled from
standard histories and gazetteers, does not include independent
works in the same tradition or commentaries on the *Huang ti nei
ching ling shu*. For titles of the Han through T'ang periods it
may be supplemented by Fan Hsing-chun 1965, collected from
citations in early medical books. For detailed information on classical medical sources see *I chi k'ao* 醫 籍 考 (1819) and, for
more complete data on pre-Yuan works, Okanishi 1958.

every innovation. Regardless of the classification of drugs that made up the major headings of each book, the article on each substance noted the rubric under which it had appeared in the *Divine Husbandman's Materia Medica*. This usage was maintained until the end of the classical materia medica tradition in the nineteenth century.

Authors were of course also expected to be familiar with the literature of the centuries that separated the founding works from themselves. Some of these classics were also considered indispensable. The *Treatise on Cold Damage and Miscellaneous Disorders* (*Shang han tsa ping lun* 傷 寒 雜 病 論), attributed to Chang Chi 張 機 (or Chang Chung-ching 張 仲 景 , 196/220), a merely mortal and historical author, was scarcely less influential than the *Yellow Emperor's Inner Canon*, but did not share its hyperbolic reputation for wisdom (partly because the *Treatise* was much more concrete).

Generally speaking, an author's historical predecessors were his colleagues in recapturing what the sagely revelators of the archaic golden age had already understood. Medical education, like general education, meant memorizing or closely studying a large literature, almost all of it written centuries earlier. Some authors were quite aware of the growth in knowledge and in sophistication of method over the centuries; but the current apex of that slow upward curve did not in their minds approach the mastery attained by the sages and lost when the golden age ended. All of a physician's great predecessors coexisted in his mind. The reasoning of Chang Chi might be as familiar as that of his own teacher.

Many elementary introductions and systematic outlines were compiled over the last five hundred years (by which time the accumulated literature was enormous), but they were not considered useful except for beginners. The classics were *meant* to be mastered despite their lack of simple, comprehensive outline, the frequent obscurity of their ancient language and ideas, their lack of consistent terminology, their differences of emphasis, and even their outright disagreement. The neat and unambiguous doctrine of the textbooks simplified this daunting task, but could be dangerous if the healer were unprepared by further study in the canons of medicine and philosophy to grasp the inevitably complicated total situation of a patient—somatic, psychological, and epidemiological— and to reason about it in a way responsive to ambiguity and change. Each doctor was expected to arrive at his own synthesis through the interaction of deep book-learning and practice. The goal was to be fully responsible for his very limited power over life and death, not to become a technician manipulating bodies.

The consequences of this classical character for the present day, seventy years after the end of the last imperial dynasty, are far from straightforward. The curricula of the traditional medical schools still emphasize the study of classical texts. New editions, commentaries, and reprints of premodern sources have continued to pour from the presses from the mid-1950s to the present day.[20]

The classical character of China's general education system has fallen away. Training in social and political morality is no less a basic preparation for civic responsibility than it was two thousand years ago; but now it is provided, not by the books of Confucius and Mencius, but by the canons of Marx and Lenin (in modern Chinese translation), Mao, and contemporary ideologists and educators. With the lessening relevance of the pre-revolutionary past in a socialist state, the perennial ideal of classical training in medicine has had to be maintained by increasing compromise. Few students today can read simple classical prose with the confidence of those who completed their educations before 1966, when the Cultural Revolution threw higher education into turmoil for a decade. The language of the medical classics is anything but simple.

What part can the classics continue to play in forming the intellects of future doctors as classical Chinese dies out in the larger educational system? Even in the early 1960s the most fundamental classics were often studied in modern vernacular translations—

---

[20] Between 1949 and 1976, 27 new editions of, or commentaries on, the *Inner Canon of the Yellow Lord*, for a total of over 900,000 copies; 76 reprints of, republished premodern studies on, or annotations to the *Treatise on Cold Damage Disorders*, four of over 100,000 copies each; 56 reprints or new editions from the literature of classical materia medica; and roughly 350 reprints, editions, and anthologies of other medical treatises that first appeared before 1919 were published in the People's Republic of China. Particulars are given in Kuo-chia ch'u-pan-chü 國 家 出 版 局 1980: 390–492. This flood has shown no sign of abating since 1976, and many studies are substantial aids to research. See, for instance, the excellent critical ed. of *Huang ti nei ching su wen* 黃 帝 內 経 素 問 in Kuo Ai-ch'un 1981 and the well-chosen classical commentaries in Ch'eng Shih-te 程 士 德 1982.

which differ as much from the original as an English translation from a Latin classic—and supplemented with textbooks and outlines. Recently several textbooks of classical Chinese using readings from the medical literature have been published in large editions for use in colleges of Chinese medicine. Some recent authors express hope that most of the important medical classics can eventually be translated into modern Chinese, and a textbook of 1980 provides substantial guidance in making such translations.[21] This will no doubt keep some portion of the medical literature accessible, but there still is no sign of translation on a large scale. It remains an obvious conclusion that traditional medical education, like that of modern medicine, will increasingly depend on the latest textbook, not on the earliest classic.

A further stage in that process is perceptible in the field work of the anthropologist Judith Farquhar at the Guangzhou College of Traditional Chinese Medicine, a leading medical school. Farquhar, observing the education of traditional physicians, finds that the study of integral classical sources is increasingly being replaced by short quotations in textbooks that present modern doctrines of traditional Chinese medicine. These aphoristic citations provide symbolic anchors, asserting the long and stable history of medical doctrine at a time that the tradition is undergoing unprecedentedly rapid change.[22]

---

[21] Liu Chen-min 刘振民 et al. 1980: 219–30, 395–411. This and Shang-hai chung-i hsueh-yuan 上海中医学院 et al. ed. 1978 provide instruction in grammar, diction, use of reference works, etc. Other works of the same sort published in the late 1970s are lower in quality. For instance, Ch'en Chu-yu 陈竹友 1979, although compiled by an experienced teacher for a broad readership of "medical workers," often neglects to gloss the most difficult phrases. Shang-hai Chung-i hsueh-yuan ed. 1980 is a superior collection of annotated selections from medical classics for classroom use.

[22] Personal communications, 1983–86. See also Farquhar 1986. Her conclusions are confirmed by the increase in citations of classical texts in textbooks for the "Foundations of Traditional Medicine" course at medical schools, e.g., Hu-pei Chung-i hsueh-yuan 湖北中医学院 ed. 1978 and Yin Hui-ho 印会河 and Chang Po-no 张伯讷 ed. 1984.

Medical education is more than a matter of textbooks. When it was first being moved out of the households of individual doctors and into government medical schools half a century ago, the teachers remained experienced traditional physicians who, conforming to the old ideal, combined broad general culture with mastery of a large technical literature. Despite the fact that most such instructors were employees or proprietors teaching a curriculum, something of the old master-disciple relationship survived. A half-century later, the schools have been absorbed by a centrally controlled network of colleges of Chinese medicine. The great majority of instructors are by now themselves graduates of such colleges, largely educated with textbooks and conversant with modern medicine. They are much less familiar with the classics than their teachers, and consequently less used to applying elaborate traditional rationales to clinical situations. Western anatomy and pathology often come more readily to their minds. Thus a European scholar who recently examined patient records in two hospitals affiliated with colleges of Chinese medicine reports that although the courses of treatment were traditional the diagnoses were based on modern medical doctrine.[23] This suggests, by analogy with the recent history of chiropractic in the United States, that social change has begun to move medical education toward a synthesis of traditional and modern medicine in which all that remains of the former is elements of technique. This is not the only direction of development, of course, but it calls for thought.

Our present concern is not to determine in what form traditional medicine will survive its decreed modernization, nor indeed to decide whether, contrary to the obvious trend, it ought to remain intact when the values, social relationships, and institutions that nurtured it no longer exist. The advantages that have kept it alive remain. As China becomes wealthier, and once the majority of adults have been given modern educations (so that, for instance, yin-yang

---

[23] Porkert 1982a: 564, confirmed by Fu Xiaoyan 傅 曉 燕 , a traditional physician who practiced 1977–81 in a Beijing hospital (personal communication). For valuable but more hurried impressions see Kleinman 1980a: 64–69. Ågren 1975: 44–47 draws a similar conclusion from study of medical textbooks and handbooks. The medical case histories in the *Revised Outline* bear out this interpretation; see, for instance, 7.5 and 10.6. This matter is taken up again below, pages 176–77.

theory is no longer a basic tool of reasoning), these advantages will no longer remain. Then the question is whether enough of those who use medical services, and those who make decisions about them, have their own reasons to support the traditional system in more or less intact form.

Such support has prevailed in Japan, where Chinese-style medicine has survived in what has become a wealthy and modern nation, with a higher general standard of basic education and a higher rate of literacy than the United States. The traditional art has weathered two centuries of intense competition with Western medicine and a century of governmental preference for the latter.[24] But neither the traditional medicine of Japan nor that of the People's Republic of China has avoided fundamental change through interaction with modern medicine and modern thought. They are not fossils; history is still at work.

These characteristics of contemporary Chinese medicine indicate a state of rapid transition. We have seen that this is the situation, and promises to remain the situation, in administrative policy, education, and the organization of practice.[25]

The remainder of this introductory study will discuss the transition as it can be seen within medical theory and its clinical applications. Anyone who wishes to understand traditional medicine is not

---

[24] Lock 1980a, 1980b.

[25] I am referring to qualitative change, which is not necessarily reflected in numerical trends. There are, of course, no completely reliable data on manpower; the comparatively trustworthy information provided to the World Bank in 1982 by the Chinese government for use in cooperative projects indicates that from 1977 to projections for 1985 the annual percentage of medical college graduates trained to be traditional physicians has fluctuated about a relatively stable average of 16 percent; traditional pharmacologists were about 3 percent of the total projected for 1982 and 1985. Assistant doctors of traditional medicine were expected to fall from 9 percent of all graduates of secondary medical schools in 1982 (an abnormally high figure due to expanded enrollments in 1979) to 3 percent in 1985 and 1990. In 1982 traditional doctors, assistant doctors, and pharmacists made up 30 percent of all medical personnel in these three categories. See Jamison et al. 1984: 143, 146–47, and Evans 1984: table VI.

well advised to think of it as a fixed system that transmits in pristine form two thousand years of clinical experience. It is involved in change so accelerated that two recent descriptions ten years apart would differ considerably, and so turbulent that modern medicine at a given time has influenced very differently rural medical workers and specialists in traditional medicine in urban hospitals.

Selection of the Book Translated Here

It is clear by now, I hope, that anyone concerned with the spectrum of social roles that medicine can play, with the many things that the human body can mean in different cultures, or with the diverse ways in which clinical observation, scientific principles, and therapeutic decisions can be connected, can find food for thought in traditional Chinese medicine. So far very little of the ground has been covered. No general outline of Chinese medicine, no reliable survey of its history, no trustworthy translation of any medical classic, no detailed study of the interaction between Chinese and Western medicine, and no systematic overall analysis of the Chinese health care system is available in any European language.[26] Chinese medicine has often been interpreted to the West

---

[26] Manfred Porkert has contributed a useful introduction to one classical tradition of medical thought and practice, which is not meant to reflect practice in the second half of the twentieth century (1982b), as well as an exposition of certain basic theoretical concepts (1974) and clinically oriented handbooks of pharmacy (1978) and diagnostics (1983). Kaptchuk 1983 is clear and insightful in some respects. Ōtsuka 1976 introduces Chinese medicine as practiced in Japan by a very eminent physician; this differs greatly from contemporary practice in China and Chinese communities outside the People's Republic. For historical orientation to general topics in medical thought and practice little can be recommended besides the history of acupuncture (1980) and several articles (gathered in Needham et al. 1970) by Lu and Needham. Early Chinese materia medica is introduced and attractively illustrated in Unschuld 1973; for contemporary pharmacognosy in the P.R.C. see C. P. Li 1974; in Taiwan, Yen K'un-ying 1980a and 1980b. Nakayama and Sivin ed. 1973: 302–8

from one point of view or another, but most of the flood of such publications has not been sufficiently informed to convey a clear sense of what concrete Chinese experiences and ideas are being interpreted.

Making an authoritative Chinese outline of medical ideas available in English is only one priority among many, but surely it does not need additional justification. I will therefore proceed to explain why I chose to translate a portion of the *Revised Outline of Chinese Medicine (Hsin pien Chung-i-hsueh kai yao* 新 编 中 医 学 概 要).[27]

A few substantial introductory writings of well-trained and experienced traditional Chinese physicians are already available in Western languages. But their central concern is therapy, and most of their space is devoted to inventories of medicinal plants and acupuncture loci.[28] These publications would be well complemented by one that emphasizes the general, conceptual, and strategic aspects of contemporary Chinese medicine. I looked for a relatively full and systematic outline of medical ideas, one that does not presuppose a great deal of knowledge that only readers educated in China would possess. I also wanted to include information on the social organization of medical care, but no Chinese textbook or handbook addresses this topic. That hope abandoned, there were many introductory texts to consider.

The representative selection that I evaluated (appendix A) covers several levels of practice. At the lowest level are the barefoot doctors' manuals (*ch'ih-chiao i-sheng shou-ts'e* 赤 脚 医 生 手 册 , etc.), used to train part-time medical workers whose main responsibilities were providing care for simple ailments and emergencies, teaching hygiene, organizing environmental sanitation, and referring patients to more specialized facilities as needed.

---

provide a critical bibliography, now obsolescent. Supplements will appear in *Chinese Science.*

[27] Kuang-chou pu-tui 广 州 部 队 et al. ed. 1972.

[28] Revolutionary Health Committee of Hunan Province ed. 1977, a barefoot doctor's manual, is a broad introduction to this eclectic low-level therapy. The other works of adequate quality all translate manuals of acupuncture and moxibustion: Academy of Traditional Chinese Medicine ed. 1975, Beijing College of Traditional Chinese Medicine et al. 1980, and O'Connor and Bensky 1981.

Barefoot Doctors, Red Medical Workers, and similar minimally trained practitioners were the base of the rural health care pyramid in the 1970s. They were not paramedics as the word is understood in the Occident. They did not practice under the case-by-case supervision of a qualified physician, but were empowered to dispense drugs and authorize admission to hospitals. A substantial training manual of this kind has been translated into English.[29]

At an intermediate level are such handbooks as the *Village Physician's Handbook* (*Nung-ts'un i-sheng shou-ts'e* 农 村 医 生 手 册), meant for the more fully trained independent workers and staff members of production brigade clinics and similar facilities. At both this and the lower level the introduction to the traditional principles of medicine is understandably superficial. Diagnosis is predominantly based on modern medicine, and therapy uses both traditional materia medica and modern synthetic drugs without regard for the difference in their origins. Neither the barefoot doctor nor village physician literature represents current practice, since the primary care system is now being fundamentally revised.[30]

For thorough discussion of traditional medical principles and their application one must go to more specialized books, the contents of which differ according to whether they are meant as supplementary reading for lower-level personnel, as orientations for modern physicians, or as textbooks for the training of traditional doctors in colleges of Chinese medicine (purpose is noted for each title in appendix A). The most comprehensive and informative introductory books are those written for the last two of these audiences, most of whom have at least the equivalent of a high-school education by the time their medical training begins.

Four books stand out. The *Outline of Chinese Medicine* of 1958 (*Chung-i-hsueh kai-lun* 中 医 学 概 論) was compiled by the Nanjing College of Chinese Medicine, one of the leading institutions of its kind, for use as a textbook. The authors were little influenced by modern medicine; their exposition of traditional theory is relatively full, systematic, and pristine.[31]

---

[29] See note 28.

[30] Hu-nan i-hsueh-yuan 湖 南 医 学 院 ed. 1971; Ågren 1972; Sidel and Sidel 1982.

[31] This is truer of the first ed. (Nan-ching Chung-i hsueh-yuan 南 京 中 医 学 院 ed. 1958) than of the second (1959). See

The *Revised Outline of Chinese Medicine* of 1972 was written and edited by a consortium of medical, military, and political units in Guangdong, Guangxi, and Hunan provinces.[32] The purpose of this book is to acquaint modern physicians with traditional medicine. Because of this purpose, and no doubt because its authors realized that most readers would depend on it exclusively for their knowledge of the topic, it does not presuppose much knowledge of traditional ideas. Attempting to make the most of its readers' modern medical educations, it tends, unlike the earlier and later books, to provide comparisons. These are not the muddled explanations of traditional concepts in modern terminology so frequent in European and American writing, but tell in detail how traditional and modern interpretations of the same term differ (for example, see section 2.3 in the translation below). Ideas of Western origin have influenced this book's general interpretations in ways, general and specific, that are examined below. This influence is visible in all later handbooks and textbooks, albeit in different ways. Such changes in content reflect changes in educational philosophy.[33]

---

the examination of these two editions and the *Outline* of 1978 in Porkert 1979.

[32] See the title page for a list of compiling organizations. This style of designating authorship marks the heyday of the Cultural Revolution, as does the prominence of the People's Liberation Army in the book's sponsorship.

[33] Porkert (1979) expresses regret at what he considers the Chinese abandonment of classical strengths that differ from those of modern medicine; see also 1982a: 563–70. Porkert's aim is to maintain traditional practice at the highest possible level. He argues that traditional medicine can make the greatest possible contribution to health care only if its own standards are maintained without compromise and Western influence is integrated in a rational and systematic way, as is now patently not the case. Whether a pristine classical medicine can meet the needs of the modern society that China has set out to become is not at all clear; in any case traditional medicine is no longer pristinely classical. The dilution of educational standards, and the increasing incoherence of theory on which I remark below (for instance, pages 114–15, 129, and 146), may or may not signal an irreversible process. My immediate aim, unlike that of Porkert, is to provide a first step toward understanding current doctrine and its

Among the outstanding textbooks still widely used in medical colleges in the mid-1980s were the *Outline of Chinese Medicine* of 1978, meant for students of pharmacy, and the *Foundations of Chinese Medicine* (*Chung-i-hsueh chi-ch'u* 中 医 学 基 础) of the same year, meant for medical students. In many respects they are similar, except that the former includes a large section on diseases and the drugs used for them, and the latter's exposition of theory is more than twice as long as that in the *Revised Outline*. Both, unlike the 1972 book, include many quotations from the *Inner Canon*, and a few from other classics. But despite the quotations both present a much less traditional account of classical medicine, an account much more influenced by modern medicine, than the 1958 textbook.

Like the *Revised Outline*, the two 1978 publications compare Chinese concepts with those of Western medicine, but their discussions of differences are less detailed and less emphatic. For instance, they point out that the traditional visceral systems of function do not correspond to the Western internal organs of the same names, and state the basic difference concisely, but they do not compare the individual visceral systems individually with organ functions. Such comparisons are a useful feature of the *Revised Outline* (2.1). On other issues the comparison yields inconsistent results. For example, the discussion in the later books about what entities in modern medicine correspond to the circulation tracts ("meridians," *ching-lo* 经 络) are derived from that in the *Revised Outline* (4.4.3). The *Outline* of 1978 provides its pharmacy students with a summary in one sentence flanked by two sentences of vague generalities; the *Foundations* recasts the 1972 account, expanding it by almost a quarter of its length, to incorporate the results of studies made in the interim.

The overall impression is that between 1972 and 1978 understanding of conceptual differences between Chinese and Western medicine as reflected in these textbooks became increasingly blurred.

This blurring accelerates in two other current textbooks, which in this and other respects are less useful for our purpose than the four books just mentioned. *Internal Medicine (Nei-k'o-hsueh* 内 科

---

use in practice. For this modest purpose a handbook that clearly reflects change is preferable to one that presents an idealized picture of an unchanging art.

学 , 1979–80) is mainly concerned with clinical medicine (using both traditional and modern nosologies), and gives scant attention to foundations. Neither viscera in the modern sense nor the circulation tracts are discussed. *Basic Theories of Chinese Medicine* (*Chung-i chi-ch'u li-lun* 中 医 基 础 理 论 , 1984), a shorter book, is entirely devoted to foundations. It avoids comparing the traditional visceral systems and the modern viscera, and quotes a wide variety of classical sources.

Its exposition of classical theory is, however, anything but pristine. The authors freely ignore the weight of the evidence to read modern knowledge into ancient texts. For example, they claim (without documentation) that in the *Inner Canon* and other early sources "human mental affect and the conscious activity of thought are functions of the cerebrum." They acknowledge that the ancient classic (in fact, the import of all sources) divides mental activity among the five yin visceral systems under the control of the cardiac system. They do not see this as a challenge to their extravagantly unlikely thesis: "This is not a failure to recognize the physical function of the cerebrum. [The *Inner Canon* merely] has gone a step further and applied a scientific classification of mental affect and conscious mental activity in order to explore their relation to the physiological activities of the visceral systems."[34]

This book is not speaking openly to the challenge of modern medicine as the textbooks of 1958–78 met it. Instead it is shaping its argument in a most unclassical way to make traditional medicine seem respectable from the otherwise unacknowledged modern point of view. How this looks to Chinese medical students I cannot say. It cannot meet the needs of Western readers in search of orientation, impartial discussions, and open, specific comparisons of traditional and modern concepts. In my judgment this need is best met, despite its limitations, by the *Revised Outline*.

Ten out of fourteen chapters of the 1972 book are translated in this volume. This is the portion concerned with diagnostic and therapeutic strategy. The remaining chapters deal with principles

---

[34] On the circulation tracts, see the *Outline* (Hu-pei Chung-i hsueh-yuan ed. 1978), page 15, and the *Foundations* (Pei-ching Chung-i hsueh-yuan ed. 1978), page 9. On the circulation tracts refer to pages 43 and 50–51 respectively. The passage on the function of the cerebrum occurs in Yin Hui-ho 印 会 河 and Chang Po-no 张 伯 讷 ed. 1984: 29.

of pharmacy (11); therapeutic tactics, primarily the use of drugs and composite prescriptions (12); prevention and pest control, mainly using traditional drugs (13); and diagnosis and therapy for modern, not traditional, diseases, mainly using traditional prescriptions, with indications for surgery and other emergency treatment (14; see appendix B for detailed contents). A complete translation would be desirable—mainly for those already qualified to practice Chinese medicine—but chapters 11-14 are altogether over four times as long as those translated in this volume. A better choice for a translation oriented toward therapy would be the corresponding chapters of both the 1958 and 1978 versions of the *Outline*. They are more concise, and discuss traditional rather than modern diagnostic entities.

Evaluating Change in Traditional Medicine

The book translated in part here is a document of a particular time and particular circumstances. It was written at the height of the Great Proletarian Cultural Revolution to convey a general picture of contemporary reasoning and resources to modern physicians, who were expected to inform themselves about traditional medicine. Although it is the product of a tragic era, and although— like every other handbook of traditional medicine known to me—it is obsolescent, this book still has its uses.

Some will read this translation for practical orientation, and will not care that, like a still photograph made from moving picture film, it records a moment of transition. In order to use it wisely, it is well to keep its transitional character in mind, to ask what aspects of medicine are glimpsed on the wing.

Every live art is always changing. There are as many puzzles about the earliest phases of Chinese medicine as about the latest. But the early development, which took place while China was a traditional society—one that valued stability, not change—was gradual and conservative. No previous epoch can compare in pace of change with the twentieth century, as an imperial order passed and a socialist state was created. The pressure of events and conscious decisions have aligned traditional and modern medicine in a competition that both cannot survive intact. Their occasional cooperation may only speed the assimilation.

We have seen that the demands on the two medicines for mutual adjustment accelerated in the 1950s, when old-style and new-style physicians found themselves working in the same hospitals, and the new medicine began to be taught on a large scale in schools of traditional medicine. They accelerated again when, for a decade beginning in the late 1960s, many innovations were shaped by an intent that the two types of practice ultimately become one. The abrupt redirection of policy in the early 1980s has only added to the flux. New convictions about the place of traditional medicine in health care, and the increasingly direct influence of modern medicine, have produced greater changes in the use of medical knowledge over the last thirty years than in the thousand years preceding.

How is the character of change to be judged? It is possible, in fact it is usual, to evaluate a medical system by some combination of norms that have little to do with each other:

1. how well it cures disease
2. how well it prevents disease
3. how it affects the death rate
4. how accurately it describes the body's structures
5. how accurately it describes the body's vital functions
6. how accurately it describes pathological processes
7. how comprehensively it views the body in health and illness; that is, whether it is holistic
8. whether it remains internally consistent as knowledge becomes more extensive—a basic characteristic of natural science—or whether eventually it becomes snarled in its own complexity.

These tests seem straightforward, but using them to evaluate a medical tradition is not at all simple. One can, of course, compare morbidity and mortality figures—if perchance they exist—for two countries or for the clients of two types of practice. But what do the figures mean? Are the diagnostic procedures that determine morbidity rates actually commensurate? One does not even find the same diseases in two systems (not even in European medicine a hundred years apart). How much of the difference in death rate is in fact due to differences in medical practice, how much to differences in public sanitation, and how much to differences in nutrition and the standard of living generally? This is a matter of debate even in countries where statistics are plentiful.[35]

It seems that if a medical system accurately describes the body and its ills, it should be good at curing them. Neat though that relation may seem, it does not necessarily hold in the real world. American medicine in the early nineteenth century embodied a knowledge of anatomy and physiology that was not bettered in many respects by 1900. It was also holistic. But the endless purging, bleeding, and dosing with calomel—due to the need doctors felt to produce perceptible changes in patients' secretions—amounted to an orthodoxy that worked to weaken and defeat patients' own powers of recovery.[36]

It is merely honest, then, to admit that students of cross-cultural medicine are unprepared to evaluate conclusively any medical system before modern times by any of the above criteria, except conceivably the seventh. That we lack the comprehensive data needed to assess clinical results across the spectrum—even for present-day modern medicine—is obvious enough. We are equally unready on the basis of present knowledge to weigh criteria related to learning rather than practice. There is no doubt that twentieth-century European doctors are immensely more knowledgeable about anatomy than their traditional Chinese contemporaries, for whom anatomy has never guided therapy (see below, pages 139–46). But who understands physiological functions more adequately for the purpose of preventing and treating medical disorders across the board, mild and serious, acute and chronic? Few of those familiar with both systems would be naive enough to answer this question. Criteria of accuracy which do not depend on the particular concepts of either system have yet to be defined. It would thus be premature to foreclose the future of any reasonably successful medical tradition—to judge that it has nothing substantial to contribute to the health of its accustomed public that modern medicine could not better provide—on the basis of uninformed rankings by the criteria I

---

[35] Much of this discussion has centered around the work of Thomas McKeown (see especially 1971, 1979).

[36] Rosenberg 1977, especially pages 488–89. Rosenberg is writing about allopathic medicine. This essay includes an invaluable discussion of holistic tendencies in the medicine of the time. Holism is by no means incompatible with draconian and ineffective therapy.

have listed. It is no doubt time to give some thought to how, singly or in combination, they might eventually yield meaningful conclusions. This requires understanding the implications of each criterion, patiently amassing pertinent information, and paying attention to clues offered by the values found within each medical system.

The criterion of internal consistency in particular calls for reflection. It means little or nothing to the contemporary practitioner of European medicine, which for more than two hundred years has moved away from a unitary understanding of illness. The prevalent doctrine of therapeutic nihilism finds room for any therapy that works, regardless of whether its action is understood. Furthermore, as modern medicine increasingly draws upon bacteriological and biochemical knowledge, the specific effects of many drugs are understood to an extent inconceivable in any traditional system. When it is knowledge of particulars that leads to breakthroughs, general theory seems a waste of time.

In traditional medicine, many drugs and other therapeutic resources affect specific symptoms or functions. Acupuncture at the site of the pain may be used in emergencies when analgesia is needed.[37] Nevertheless the systemic activity of any therapeutic agent is never overlooked. The cure of the underlying condition, in the eyes of the Chinese physician, mandates treatment of the whole organism. In order for the doctor to think about the organism as a whole, all the available information must be tightly related. That is why in traditional medicine theory is expected to be well articulated and, within limits, internally consistent.

This internal consistency was a central ideal of medicine, but it could never be entirely realized, as I will show by examples below. Classical physicians saw the *Inner Canon* as a single revelation that began the evolution of their art. They were thus inclined to overlook its many internal contradictions, and contradictions between it and other early treatises such as the *Treatise on Cold Damage Disorders*. The most serious of these contradictions had been reconciled

---

[37] Such sites if irregular are called "'that's it' loci" (*a shih hsueh* 阿 是 穴). For examples of their use see Academy of Traditional Chinese Medicine ed. 1975: 230, 235, 241, and, for discussion, Shang-hai Chung-i hsueh-yuan ed. 1965: 7–8.

in early works of synthesis.[38] The new understandings created by their juxtapositions of old texts and redefinitions of old ideas did not, however, entirely supplant the old ones. The Chinese tradition was cumulative in the old sense, like that of medieval Europe. Diversity was additive; only the positively false or impracticable became entirely obsolete. The main effect of the syntheses was to strengthen the prevalent notion that the early canons did not differ with respect to essentials. But the divergences were still in the record, and thus part of the doctor's knowledge. As the *Canon of Problems* (*Huang ti pa-shih-i nan ching* 黃帝 八十一 難 經) and other works of reconciliation in time became "ancient classics" themselves, their own syntheses, because they differed from the diverse views of the books they drew on, were seen by the most critical scholars of medicine as just that much more divergence. But no one doubted that underlying all the variety was unitary bedrock. That conviction motivated the unending quest for synthesis.

Over the centuries the syntheses accumulated, moving gradually in the direction of a common view, but never quite reaching it in the absence of institutions empowered to establish a single version of theory.

The imperial government saw the establishment of orthodoxy as its own responsibility, in medicine as in morals. Occasionally, from the seventh century on, it issued textbooks or re-edited and printed selected classics for this purpose. Such publications bore enough prestige to ensure widespread use, but neither the palace medical service nor imperial patrons of medicine had the intellectual authority to acknowledge old divergences and to resolve them once and for all.

The revolutions of 1911 and 1949 that mark decisive breaks between the empire and the present day opened the possibility of a fresh beginning in medicine. The result has been an entirely new system of medical education and qualification, drawing on the old tradition and on modern science. Some of the consequent shifts in medical theory have been in the direction of standardization. But still no institution effectively mediates between the research institutes and medical colleges to reach a common understanding of doctrinal details. Some of the old divergences can still be seen in the new textbooks. Because accommodation with modern medicine is proceeding independently along many fronts, with imperfect com-

---

[38] These are discussed below. See especially pages 89–90.

munication among them, we also see fresh inconsistencies as authors accept piecemeal facts established by scientific research. These are copied from one textbook to another. Authors do not pause to assess the relation of each new fact to its context and its repercussions for the traditional system as a whole. The result is a rapid decrease in the coherence of theory, especially over the decade in which the Cultural Revolution overcame the earlier separation of traditional and modern medicine.

The growing combination of old and new inconsistencies is not hard to see, as examples below show, but it has not been publicly acknowledged. It does not bode well for a tradition that over the centuries has striven for coherence, and trained its doctors to presuppose it. There is no reason to believe that a coherent theory which draws fruitfully on modern knowledge cannot finally be realized by a body appointed to set national standards. China has, after all, already evolved a national pharmacopoeia incorporating traditional materia medica and chemical drugs—an easier but not utterly dissimilar task.[39]

So far, however, the net result of Western influence on traditional medicine has been to weaken the theoretical structure of the latter. The incoherence that I have just mentioned is not balanced by efforts toward synthesis. Attempts to combine traditional and modern approaches are very much in evidence. So far, however, they are more concerned with therapy than with reasoning, and their results are fed back only to claim that traditional medicine is "scientific," not to renovate it.

The spread of modern medicine has undoubtedly contributed to a general improvement in rates of morbidity and mortality in China. This has been possible because, through practice alongside and in combination with traditional medicine, modern medicine has begun to reach everyone. Modern physicians are far too few to provide universal primary care. The survival of traditional medicine and of eclectic "assistant doctors" has magnified the benefits of modern medicine.

The effect of modern medicine on less obvious aspects of public health is not so easy to estimate. Unless care is taken to make the modern contribution to Chinese medicine systematic and constructive, the cost may be the loss of some of traditional medicine's

---

[39] Chung-hua jen-min kung-ho-kuo Wei-sheng pu 中华人民共和国卫生部 ed. 1978–79. See also Unschuld 1981.

strengths, ultimately lessening the latter's contributions. I will return to this question, after surveying the evidence, in the conclusion of this introductory study.

First, it is necessary to understand the matrix out of which twentieth-century Chinese medicine has grown, and how social change is subtly altering the inner texture of medical thought. The topics of this inquiry will illuminate the systematic discussions in the *Revised Outline*: basic philosophic concepts and their adaptation to medicine; ideas of health and medical disorder; the visceral systems of function, circulation tracts, and metabolic substances; basic approaches to diagnosis; and certain ideas that underlie therapy.

Chapter II

THEORETICAL CONCEPTS

In the first sustained flowering of philosophy from the fourth century to roughly 100 B.C., theoretical accounts of Nature and its processes appeared and proliferated (always as part of philosophical teachings concerned with right conduct and political legitimacy). The schools of thought that evolved naturalistic theories generally shared such fundamental concepts as yin-yang 陰 陽, the Five Phases (*wu-hsing* 五 行), and *ch'i* 氣 , but differed in how concretely or abstractly they used them. Between roughly 200 B.C. and A.D. 200, medicine and other specialized realms of knowledge broke out of the philosophy books and evolved distinct literatures (as their practitioners had long been distinct).[1] The physicians, mathematicians, astronomers, alchemists, and so on each created new concepts and narrowed the definitions of old concepts to fit their own discourse.

As in Europe before modern science, much Chinese medical language was borrowed from common speech. In the most technical discussions by highly educated doctors, everyday words moved decisively away from everyday usage, with its vagueness and irrelevant associations. Common words were joined to form technical compounds. Even so, precise usages of different authors accumulated side by side in the minds of the learned, with no professional mechanism to force the choice of one of them as standard. There was no single doctrine in medicine, but rather a spectrum from the most sophisticated (with much variation of detail among schools) to the explanations of illiterate practitioners whose language did not differ from that of laymen.

---

[1] Berger and Luckmann 1966: 122–46.

Certain assumptions and basic ideas, such as yin-yang, were universal. It is impossible to understand any kind of Chinese curing, or the medical notions of patients, without grasping this common basis; but as its components ranged up and down the social scale, connotations varied within remarkably wide limits.

The discussion in the remainder of this introductory study draws on the high tradition, the one we know most about because, in its mature phase, it accumulated in the writings of one eminent physician after another. The knowledge of early doctors closer to popular curing is no less interesting, but it is less pertinent to traditional medical theory in contemporary China, which is entirely adapted from the high classical tradition. That may seem unlikely in a society that puts so much stress on the creativity of the poor and uneducated, but recent concern with gathering peasant knowledge has visibly influenced only materia medica and—to a much smaller extent—therapeutic methods. Classical theory, despite its inner diversity, is at least coherent and self-critical in ways that resemble premodern sciences elsewhere. Much of the hodge-podge we call popular curing has been officially classified as superstition for the past thirty years, and has been little studied as it continues to die out.

At its origin, in all the great ancient civilizations, scientific thought was part of philosophy—that part concerned with Nature and with man as part of Nature. It was seldom a distinct part. Philosophy at first separated itself from religious thought not so much by the issues it raised as by where it looked for the answers. Among the Greeks its motivation was not simply knowledge for its own sake, as a glance at the famous Pythagorean simile might suggest: "In this life there are three kinds of men, just as there are three sorts of people who come to the Olympic Games. The lowest class is made up of those who come to buy and sell, and the next above them are those who come to compete. Best of all, however, are those who come to look on (*theorein*)." John Burnet, in a famous discussion of the connections between Greek religion and natural philosophy, saw a deeper significance: "The greatest purification of all is, therefore, science, and it is the man who devotes himself to that, the true philosopher, who has most effectually released himself from the 'wheel of birth.'"[2]

---

[2] Burnet 1930: 98.

A single question, when answered in one way, led to communal liturgy, and, when pondered in a different way, to abstract physical concepts not patterned after manifestations of divine will: Why is it that, despite the incessant flux and change of everything in the world we experience, the overall order or pattern seems in the long run to remain the same? What accounts for the underlying constancy of a world in which no individual person or thing remains the same or endures—what the poet Richard Eberhart calls "the fixed form in the massive fluxion"? What ties the individual to the living cosmos, and the moment to the continuum of time?

The most characteristic early Greek philosophic answers to these questions were phrased in terms of a basic substance. What appears to be a change of one material into something entirely different—wood going up in flame and smoke, metal rusting—is just a change in qualities. Decay and dissolution are not something turning into nothing at all (which is very difficult to think rigorously about). For Anaximenes, for instance, dissolution was simply a change in the state of basic stuff from solid to imperceptible air. This line of thought led eventually to the idea of four complementary basic substances, the Four Elements. No matter how diverse the materials in the world, if you divided one of them often enough you would sooner or later find bits of earth, air, fire, or water, which could not be subdivided into anything more basic. What made them complementary was the qualities that pairs of them shared. Water, for example, is cold and moist; it shares cold with earth and moisture with air. If the elements in a material could not be directly observed, their qualities could at least be sensed. As Aristotle gave the notion of the Four Elements finished form, all four coexisted in every perceptible substance, so that what seemed to be chance transformation from one element to another was explainable as a shift in predominance—an instance of regularity, not chaos.

There were of course other approaches. Closest to the yin-yang idea was Heraclitus' attempt to change the issue from stuff to process, to see changes in relation to the cycles of which they were part, to trace the dynamics of "the way upward and the way downward" to the tension between opposites. But this was far from the main trend in Greek speculation.

Ch'i

In China as well, the first long outburst of philosophical thought explored practically all the options for thought about Nature, including many that did not continue to be taken up. One of these explained change as alterations in the state of a basic stuff, *ch'i* 氣. This substance, like Anaximenes's *aer*, could range in density from imperceptible air to hard solid.

Early associations of the word *ch'i* are diverse, but tend to cluster: the mists, fogs, and moving forms of clouds that are what we see of the atmosphere; the air we inhale, and the breath we expire; the vitality in us. By the time of Confucius (551–479 B.C.), *hsueh-ch'i* 血 氣 (literally, "blood and air") meant "the physical vitalities" or "the physical powers."[3]

Along another early line of thought, *ch'i* came to be used for anything perceptible but intangible—smokes, aromas, vapors, mists, even perceptible but intangible beings such as ghosts.

Another line, which first appears in anecdotes dated 540 and 516 B.C., uses *ch'i* to denote a set of fundamental cosmic influences (light, weather, and yin-yang) that affect other phenomena such as the procession of the seasons, the flavors of foods, colors, and the musical modes. These influences, we are told, must be moderate

---

[3] See the *Confucian Analects* (*Lun yü* 論 語), 16.7. For an extended study of early meanings of *ch'i* see Kuroda Genji 黑 田 源 次 1977: 3–221 and Onozawa Seiichi 小 野 沢 精 一 et al. 1978. My analysis draws on a wide range of materials, including those collected in both books, but is not identical with that of either source. The understanding of the essays in Onozawa et al. is generally inferior to that of Kuroda in areas taken up by both, notably with respect to medicine. Onozawa's work is also greatly vitiated by anthropological speculation based on obsolete methodology. For archaic senses see Maekawa Shōzō 前 川 捷 三 1978, which is not up to date, but does not conflict with information in other recent publications. Maekawa concludes that, although a graph corresponding to the modern *ch'i* can be found in oracle documents and early bronze inscriptions, it is used for phonetic loans, and expresses ideas unrelated to the philosophical senses emergent from the time of Confucius; the meanings of *ch'i* described here do not appear. In medical books *ch'i-hsueh* usually appears rather than *hsueh-ch'i*.

and balanced, or the result will be confusion in Nature and illness in man. Ritual (and Confucian government through ritual), seeking a similar moderation and balance, is to be patterned after this inter-play of *ch'i*.[4]

Thus by 350, when philosophy began to be systematic, *ch'i* meant air, breath, vapor, and other pneumatic stuff. It might be congealed or compacted in liquids or solids. *Ch'i* also referred to the balanced and ordered vitalities or energies, partly derived from the air we breathe, that cause physical change and maintain life.

These are not distinct meanings. Before modern times there was no separate conception of energy in Chinese thought. This is not a sign of deficient curiosity, but of a tendency (like that of the Stoics in the West) to think of stuff and its transformations in a uni-tary way. We might define *ch'i*—or at least sum up its use in Chinese writing about Nature by about 350—as simultaneously "what makes things happen in stuff" and (depending on context) "stuff that makes things happen" or "stuff in which things hap-pen."[5]

---

[4] *Tso chuan* 左 傳 , Duke Chao 昭 公 , year 1.8, addendum, translated below, page 55, and year 25.2.

[5] This lack of separate concepts to distinguish energies from their carriers (which has nothing to do with the complementarity of distinct matter and energy in modern physics) is reflected in Manfred Porkert's more technical discussion, in which he Englishes *ch'i* as both "energetic configuration" and "configura-tive energy" (1974: 167). For an analysis of *ch'i* in early texts see Moran 1983, chapter VII, and, for underlying assumptions in late Chou thought, Hansen 1983.

I do not translate *ch'i*, but sometimes I describe certain aspects of it as "vitalities" or "energies." These words refer to the everyday, purely qualitative acceptances of "energy" (*OED* sen-ses 4 and 5), not to the nineteenth- and twentieth-century use of the term in science (*OED* sense 6). Neither "vitality," "energy," nor "pneuma" (as the Stoics used the word) can be used consis-tently as English equivalents of *ch'i*. Other current translations of *ch'i*, such as "matter-energy," "ether," "vapor," and "breath," cover only a small part of the word's meaning. Most of these usages are based on superficial parallels in Western natural philosophy.

Just as philosophy was not at first an autonomous department of thought, medical conceptions did not develop independently from the start. Ideas about the body and vital functions continued for a couple of centuries after 350 to be explored, so far as we know, only in general philosophic writings. In the interim a coherent understanding of these functions began to emerge.

The physical vitality of the newborn child is drawn before birth from the *ch'i* that fills the cosmos. This point is well put in a late chapter (second century B.C.?) of the *Chuang-tzu* 莊子 , arguing for the relativity of life and death: "Life itself is a companion of death, just as death is the beginning of life; who can fully comprehend their relationship? The birth of a human being amounts to an accumulation of *ch'i*. When it has accumulated birth takes place, and when it has dissipated death takes place. If death and life are companions, what have we to be concerned about?" The concern of this passage is not the material substance of the body, which does not dissipate by the time death takes place, but the energies that make the vital functions possible.[6]

During life, vitality was drawn not only from air but from food. In Mo-tzu's 墨子 (ca. 350 B.C.) ideal social order people ate "no more than enough to augment their *ch'i* and make up for its depletion, to strengthen their bodies and ease their bellies." The *Annals of Lü Pu-wei (Lü shih ch'un ch'iu* 吕氏春秋 , 241/235 B.C.) writes of the body's vitalities not as "blood/*ch'i*" but as "seminal essence/*ch'i*" (*ching-ch'i* 精氣, 3.3 below). This implies that these vitalities are, at least in part, food essences: "One wants the skin to be tight, the blood vessels (*hsueh-mai* 血 脈) to allow unimpeded motion, the sinews to be firm and the bones hard, the heart, mind, and will to be concordant, the vital energies (*ching-ch'i*) to flow. When this is happening, agents of disorder (*ping* 病) have nowhere to abide, and pathology (*o* 惡) has nowhere to be produced. The abiding of agents of disorder is the origin of pathology, blocking the flow of vital energies."[7]

---

[6] *Chuang-tzu*, 22.10–12.

[7] *Mo-tzu*, 6.22; *Lü shih ch'un ch'iu, 20* (5): 1373; cf. R. Wilhelm 1928: 358. Note that the channels in which the flow takes place are called "blood vessels," but what flows in them is described in a more general way as vital energies, with no mention of blood (*hsueh*). The point of this passage is avoiding a corresponding

Here we find stated in one place what remained in the eyes of physicians the basic somatic conditions of health: the surface of the body sealing vital substances inside and pathological factors (that is, anything that does not belong in the body) outside; vital energies admitted and distributed in a free flow without anything foreign to interfere with or block them. Inseparable from this process that today would be regarded as straightforwardly physical is balance in the mental and emotional sphere. Self-cultivation must begin with "using the fresh and casting out the old, so that there is a free flow within the interstices of the flesh (*ts'ou-li* 腠理). The vitalities (*ching-ch'i*) are renewed daily, heteropathic *ch'i* (*hsieh-ch'i* 邪氣) is completely expelled, and a full span of life is attained." Health and longevity are the results of daily renewal.

Both the vital resources of the body's internal order and the agents of disorder opposed to them are *ch'i*, dynamic agents of change. Porkert neatly refers to these two types as "orthopathic *ch'i*" and "heteropathic *ch'i*," using Greek roots that mean "proper to" and "different from." The orthopathic *ch'i* maintains and renews the measured, orderly changes that comprise the body's normal processes; the heteropathic *ch'i* causes change that violates this normal order, that is disorderly and dysfunctional.[8]

But these are only two among myriad labels that can be applied to *ch'i*. They do not state the composition of a certain variety of *ch'i*, a matter of rare concern in Chinese discourse, but rather what the *ch'i* relates to or what it does. They specify not quality but function. Definitions involving *ch'i* are therefore more faithful to the Chinese mode of thought if they are turned the other way round, such as: what maintains and renews the measured, orderly changes that comprise the body's normal processes is called "orthopathic *ch'i*"; what causes change that violates this normal order is called "heteropathic *ch'i*."

When medical writers theorized that excesses of emotion can cause physical disorders without external stimuli, positing het-

---

"blockage" in political circulation—the flow of the ruler's virtue downward and the yearnings of his people upward.

[8] P52–54, 172. The quotation is from *Lü shih ch'un ch'iu*, 3 (3): 144.

eropathic *ch'i* that originate within the body (5.4),[9] they did not suggest that a new material substance was created or transformed from orthopathic *ch'i*. Since their concern was *ch'i* as pathological *activity*, it did not have to be accounted for, as the body's physical constituents might, by a principle that kept the amount of matter constant. Nor did they have reason to think of it chemically, as a unique substance transformed by reaction with other substances. *Ch'i* is often the material basis of activity, but the activity itself is often also described as *ch'i*. "Fire *ch'i*" may be thought of as a stuff responsible for the transmission of heat; but it more often refers to the process of burning or of generating heat. These must be explained in English—or even in modern Chinese—as different senses, but in ancient medicine they add up to one concept.

When Fire heteropathy (a pathogenic Fire *ch'i*) appears in the hepatic system instead of the Wood *ch'i* that normally characterizes hepatic functions (5.1.6), has one substance or element somehow replaced another? No; what has changed is the predominant kind of physiological activity. When the body is suffering from *ch'i* depletion, has the volume or density of *ch'i* decreased? No; *ch'i* is not a quantitative notion. It is neither the matter nor the energy of modern physics. The volume of *ch'i*, apart from the volume of the body that contains it, was never measured or calculated. Even a famous early estimate of fifty complete circulations per day of constructive *ch'i* (3.1) in the human body and a discussion of the relative proportions of *ch'i* and *hsueh* in various circulation tracts do not consider the volume of the *ch'i*.[10]

A yin or yang *ch'i* depletion, when we read the old descriptions carefully, consistently turns out to be a lower-than-normal level of vital function or a lower-than-normal *concentration* of *ch'i* in one or more of the body's systems. In neither case was it a quantitative idea. This is not an easy idea for moderns, with their clear distinction between substance and function, to grasp. The ambiguity is impossible to overlook, but discourse was adapted to it, and the

---

[9] On the relation of *ch'i* to emotions and perception see Moran 1983: 211–13.

[10] These passages in the *Inner Canon* are discussed below, pages 152, 153, and 154, note 48. I cannot agree with the assertion in CL30–32 that the estimate of fifty circulations refers to those of blood.

readers for whom it was intended did not complain that it is confusing.

By the time a medical literature developed, its authors tended to use *ch'i* predominantly in the functional sense. As good an example as any occurs in the discussion of acupuncture loci near the beginning of the Divine Pivot: "At the articulations within the body there are 365 points of communication. . . . 'Articulations' refers to where the divine *ch'i* travels freely and moves outward and inward, not to skin, flesh, sinews, and bones." A modern Westerner expects these points of communication, where the physician's needles can affect the circulation, to be places in tissue, but here we find them related instead to processes.[11]

The vital energies follow regular cycles of activity, for proper activity in the cosmos, the body, and society is cyclical. This point is made elsewhere in the *Annals of Lü Pu-wei*, where avoiding catastrophe in the state depends on incorporating in the political hierarchy this characteristic of change. "The vital energies (*ching-ch'i*) rise and fall in alternation, cycling and recycling, never falling behind." These are the vital energies of the cosmos.[12]

In the medical literature the need to describe intricately related subsystems of activity within the economy of the body led to many subdivisions of *ch'i* function. The vitalities that maintain health and growth were divided in several ways. These energies were the finer and more active part of the pneumata and blood that carried them through the body; the pneumata and blood, thought about in connection with the circulation and its ensemble of vital processes, became types of *ch'i* themselves (even Confucius used the term *hsueh-ch'i* in this sense, as I have noted). At this general level all orthopathic *ch'i* could remain undifferentiated in thought. They could also be separated in thought into yin and yang aspects, the reactive and active parts, among other things the grosser and subtler essences extracted from food and drink.

The yin part of the general *ch'i*, the yin vitalities and the blood that carried them, was called *hsueh*   (cf. 3.1.2). It is not that physicians could not tell the difference between vitality and blood,

---

[11] TS, *21* (1): 11, in TIZ only = LS, *1* (1): 3. I have omitted two sentences of questionable authenticity and no relevance. "Divine *ch'i*" is *shen ch'i* 神氣 , the active, transforming *ch'i* (P173, 181).

[12] *Lü shih ch'un-ch'iu, 3* (5): 171–72.

but that they saw them as aspects of the same stuff. When they wished to refer to one rather than the other, context could resolve ambiguity easily enough.

The yang fraction of *ch'i* complementary to *hsueh* was called *ch'i*. This double meaning of *ch'i* frequently confuses recent Western writers on Chinese medicine, but it did not confuse classical authors. Such double usages are not rare in Chinese; *erh* 兒 on one level means any child, male or female, and on another, a son. The word may be ambiguous, but sentences by native speakers using it are not.

If one wished to distinguish not the carrier but the part of the body in which circulation was taking place, the *ch'i* essences would be divided instead into constructive and defensive *ch'i* (*ying ch'i* and *wei ch'i*, or *ying wei* 營 衛 , 3.1.3). The former, the purer (relatively yang) fraction extracted from air and aliment, circulates within the tract system (4.2); the latter, less pure, makes the round of the body outside the tracts, and defends its periphery. If one wished instead to explain the role of *ch'i* in the creation of new body substance or in sexual reproduction, the part that carried out such functions, relatively yang by definition, would be distinguished as *ching* 精 (in its fluid aspect, "semen," 3.3), and the rest, relatively yin, would be called *ch'i*.[13]

These paired concepts of *ch'i hsueh*, *ying-wei*, and *ching-ch'i*—do not refer to chemically distinct substances, but to different ways of dividing the body's *ch'i* into two functional types (other examples are given below). Any such division will yield a yin-yang pair, since one member will be yang in relation to the other. The book translated here sees these three pairs as four (or five) substances—*hsueh* simply as blood, for instance—but that is due mainly to the very recent influence of modern medicine. Because this influence remains limited, inconsistencies are not hard to find. Most of what the book says about these three pairs reflects the traditional, largely functional understanding outlined here.

The picture sketched above of *ch'i* as substance, activity, and vitality represents how the word would have been understood in

---

[13] This is only one meaning of the *ching-ch'i* pair, on which see P179-80. I do not translate *ching* except when its meaning is clearly material. In classical medicine *hsueh* is also usually not identical with blood, but in the *Revised Outline* it is not distinguished from blood, so I translate accordingly.

relation to Nature and the human body for the past two millennia by any educated Chinese with no special knowledge of medicine. We will return to its more technical usages in medicine. We can already see that *ch'i* provides a language for thinking about the stuff involved in change, as well as the energies that make change possible. This concept cannot tell us how overall patterns of change remain constant. What changes, after all, is *ch'i*. In order to understand what is unchanging about it, we will do well to ponder the character of cyclic process.

Cycles

The regularity that Chinese physical theories were built upon was that of the biological cycle, the inevitable succession of birth, growth, maturity, decay, and death. This regularity, because it was universal, was a key to thinking about change. Chinese thinkers explored ideas of progressive time, especially with reference to technological achievement, and regressive time, above all in thought about social decline.[14] Interesting though these explorations were, the most influential systems of thought at every level of society were built on the notion that all natural phenomena followed periodically repetitive patterns.

The growing and declining shape of the mayfly's fleeting life is the same as that of the great tree in which change can be noticed only in the course of a human lifetime or even of generations. The Chinese were convinced, as were other peoples, that the same pattern, broadly interpreted, applies to the mineral world as to the animal and vegetable realms. Miners in China as well as Europe commonly believed that an exhausted deposit will regenerate itself if left untouched for some time. Alchemists in several civilizations believed that earths gradually mature in the terrestrial womb along a scale of perfection to become minerals and metals.[15] In China one such line of maturation led to gold, another to crystalline translucent cinnabar of a size, shape, and medicinal efficacy with which even the most valuable commercial cinnabar could not compare. This ripening was analogous to biological growth—the weathering of

---

[14] Needham 1965; on the connections of these ideas with conceptions of cyclical time see Sivin 1966.
[15] Eliade 1962, 1968; Sivin 1966, 1976, 1980.

exposed minerals and the corrosion of ordinary metals (unlike im-
mortal gold) corresponded to the downslope of the life curve. The
imperishable gold and cinnabar were natural metaphors for immortality.

What seems superficially to be a chaos of birth and death was
thus resolved into a vast concert of changes rung on a single pattern. The outcome was a vision of all the activity in the cosmos as
meshed and interdependent, what Joseph Needham has called an
"organic view of the universe."[16]

Another major formative insight explains what enforces this
universal pattern. The innumerable individual life rhythms are affected and indeed paced by a small set of cycles that do not vary in
the long run—those seen in the sky. The eternal daily and annual
rotations of the sun and the equally regular revolutions of the moon
and planets tie together by their resonance all the cycles of individual transformation. The *Annals of Lü Pu-wei* speaks of the
Round Way (*yuan tao* 圜 道), the cyclic processes that unite sky
and earth: "Day and night make up a cycle: this is the Round Way.
The threading of the moon through the twenty-eight divisions of its
path, from Horn (roughly Virgo) through Axletree (roughly Corvus),
belongs to the Round Way. The luminaries alternate through the
four seasons, encountering each other [in due course]: this is the
Round Way. [On earth] something stirs and burgeons; burgeoning,
it is born; born, it grows; growing, it matures; mature, it declines;
declining, it dies; dead, it becomes latent [preceding another birth].
This is the Round Way."[17]

Macrocosm and Microcosms

This resonant cyclic cosmos is reflected in every perspective on
health and illness. One of the most recurrent themes in classical
medicine is that the body's activity is analogous to that of the
natural order, and is in that sense a microcosm. Cosmos and body
correspond part to part and function to function; this is not at all
like the idea of European astrological medicine, which made the
stars, near the top of the hierarchy of being, radiate influence
toward the human body further down. In China the body was not

---

[16] Needham et al. 1954- : II, 412.

[17] *Lü shih ch'un ch'iu, 3* (5): 172.

the only microcosm; the state was a second mirror of the universe. Both the political order and the physiological order could maintain a spontaneous dynamic integrity only so long as they were in concord with the cosmic order. The resonance of the universe, the state, an'l the body affected all three.

Here is the oldest surviving description of the body as mi ·ocosm, in an account dated 540 B.C., of a physician's advice to a n. arquess ill because he had been too fond of his palace ladies. This discourse is older than any extant medical book, but is typical of t e later technical literature in its concern with activity and chan ·e:

> In Nature there are Six *Ch'i*. Embodied [in growing things] they give rise to the Five Flavors. They appear in the Five Colors and are manifested in the Five Modes of music. When they are in excess they produce the Six Illnesses. These Six *Ch'i* are yin and yang, wind and rain, dark and light. In their divisions they form the four seasons; in their order they form the Five Nodal Points [of the round of the year]. Their imbalance is responsible for natural calamities. Excessive yin activity is associated with cold illnesses; excessive yang with hot illnesses; excessive wind with disorders of the extremities; excessive rain with disorders in the belly; excessive dark with disorders involving mental confusion; and excessive light with disorders of the heart and mind.[18]

In this passage six kinds of activity in Nature, originally embodied in three polar pairs, provide a basis for what the senses perceive (rain and wind are yin-yang as the wet and dry extremes of

---

[18] *Tso chuan*, Duke Chao, year 1.8, addendum. See the discussion above, pages 46–47. The Six *Ch'i* enumerated here are not the same six that were later incorporated in medical theory (5.1; cf. CL142–44). The former resemble the Eight Rubrics (*pa kang* ﾉ丶 綱), the set of four polarities that much later were used in a somewhat similar way (7.1–7.4). The Six *Ch'i* of the *Tso chuan* were not made obsolete by the medical concept; see, for instance, *Wu hsing ta i* 五 行 大 義 (shortly after 581), chapter 18, pages 148–52.

weather). When unbalanced, the Six *ch'i* are themselves responsible for medical disorders. In the macrocosm their dynamics are responsible for orderly seasonal change (typified by the four seasons and a set of five important festivals) as well as for floods, fires caused by lightning, and other signs of disorder.

The point is clear: long before any extant medical book, polar couples were being used to analyze wholes into two complementary parts, whether the objects of analysis were in the physical universe, within the body, or intermediate and concerned with relations between the two. Such couples were combined into systems of concepts, not yet elaborate, that could be used, as in this instance, to argue that moral discipline is essential to health.

When a medical literature emerged, analogies between the cosmos and the body were even more elaborately developed. Here is a representative portion of a large set of correspondences given in the *Inner Canon*:

> The sky is round, the earth rectangular;[19] the heads of human beings are round and their feet rectangular to correspond. In the sky there are the sun and moon; human beings have two eyes. On earth there are the nine [archaic] provinces; human beings have nine orifices. In the sky there are wind and rain; human beings have their joy and anger. In the sky there are thunder and lightning; human beings have their sounds and speech. In the sky there are the four seasons; human beings have their four extremities. In the sky there are the Five Sounds [i.e., the musical modes that correspond to the Five Phases]; human beings have their five yin visceral systems (2.1). In the sky there are the Six Pitches; human beings have their six yang visceral systems. In the sky there are winter and summer; human beings have their chills and fevers. In the sky there are the ten-day "weeks"; human beings have ten fingers on their hands. . . . On earth there are towns and villages in which people gather; human beings have their bulges of [or thickened] flesh (*chiung jou*

---

[19] That is, locations in the sky are measured by degrees, those on earth by the four directions.

腘 肉). In the year there are twelve months;
human beings have their twelve major joints. On
earth there are times when no vegetation grows;
some human beings are childless. These are the correspondences between human beings and sky and
earth.[20]

This is not meant to be a rigorous or systematic set of
metaphors. Passages of this kind became a staple of the medical
literature, found in one introductory or general work after another,
sometimes dwelling on such trivialities as whether the poles of the
sky have a somatic counterpart.[21] Such discussions did not multi-
ply because additional proof was necessary to carry the point that
man is a microcosm. To the contrary, anyone who looks at them
together can only conclude that any analogy was acceptable. They
aimed not to accumulate empirical fact but to drive home symboli-
cally two underlying points. The first is that the individual, to
remain healthy, must attend to the relations among the body, the
moral order, and the physical environment. The other is that the
doctor's success in therapy depends on deeply understanding the
bond between cosmos and man. The challenge to the physician is as
much philosophical as technical.

Both themes can be seen in this passage from the *Inner Canon*.
The image of the physician blends into that of the sage, familiar
from philosophical classics. The physician, mediating between the
cosmic and somatic orders, is likened to the emperor, who mediates

---

[20] LS, *10* (71): 104–5 = TS, *5*: 53–54. TS is incomplete; I follow
its text in translating the next-to-last sentence. Note that here
as elsewhere "sky" is often used to mean "Nature" generally.
Ten days was the classical Chinese equivalent of the week.
Many of the themes in this passage appear, almost certainly earlier, in *Huai-nan-tzu* 淮 南 子 (compiled 164–139 B.C.), 7: 1a-
4a. This source, which draws upon the *Lao-tzu* 老 子 and
Chuang-tzu 莊 子 as well as upon Confucian sources, argues in
chüan 7 that the correspondences make the body integral with
the order of Nature, and that sageliness depends upon emulating
Nature's husbandry of its powers and resources.

[21] See the essay on this latter topic by the Suzhou physician Shen
Ch'ien 沈 謙 (1671?–1732), in *Wu i hui chiang* 吳 醫 滙
講, 4: 43–44.

between the cosmic and political orders. The doctor's sagely self-cultivation makes it possible to cure others:

> Man is born on earth, but his destiny depends on heaven. Heaven and earth blend their *ch'i* [and the result] is called man. If man is able to remain responsive to the four seasons, heaven and earth are father and mother to him, as when he who shoulders the burden of dominion over the myriad things is called the Son of Heaven. In the sky there are yin and yang; human beings have their twelve major joints [which allow the limbs to move in alternation]. The sky has its hot and cold weather; human beings have their depletions and repletions. He who can model himself on the transformations of sky and earth, yin and yang, will not fail to be attuned to the four seasons. He who can know the pattern underlying the [motions of the] twelve joints will not be surpassed in wisdom even by a sage. He who can visualize the metamorphoses of the winds of the eight directions, and the changes in ascendancies of the Five Phases as they overcome each other, who can master the regularities underlying depletions and repletions, goes in and out alone [i.e., has no peer among mortals, and will survive as an immortal]. No matter how faint the moan [of the patient], nor how subtle the symptom, nothing escapes his eye.[22]

The analogy between body and state implies that the conditions necessary for normality are the same in both. Among the many statements on that theme one can hardly do better than a beautifully balanced passage from the physician, occultist, and enthusiast of alchemy, Ko Hung 葛 洪 (ca. A.D. 320):

> A human body is the counterpart of a state. The placement of the [organs within the] thorax and ab-

---

[22] TS, *19* (6): 326–27 = SW, *8* (25): 141. This translation mainly follows TS. It is tentative, since the last three sentences are not clear and may be corrupt.

domen is like that of buildings [in a compound]. The
arrangement of the limbs is like that of suburbs and
outlying districts. The articulation of the bones and
joints is like [the organization of] officials in the civil
service. The spirit [i.e., the body's governing
vitalities, *shen* 神] is like the monarch; the *hsueh* is
like the ministers; the *ch'i* is like the people. Thus
we know that one who keeps his own body in order
can keep a state in order. Loving care for one's
people is what makes it possible for a state to be
secure; nurturing one's *ch'i* is what makes it possible
to keep the body intact. When the people are dispersed the state perishes; when the *ch'i* vitalities are
exhausted the body dies. What is dead cannot be
brought to life; what has perished cannot be
preserved. Because all this is so, the perfected man
allays catastrophe before it happens, and cures illness before it has developed. He treats it in advance
rather than chasing to catch up after it has passed
him by. One's subjects are hard to nurture, easy to
endanger; one's *ch'i* is difficult to keep pure, easily
sullied. That is why one cultivates a majestic virtue
in order to protect one's lands, and gets rid of desires
in order to preserve one's vitalities [that would be
dissipated by sensuality]. . .[23]

One can hardly mistake these assertions for magical thinking.
Nor are they concerned with the objective understanding of Nature.
They are didactic through and through. Their aim is to persuade
readers that self-cultivation and self-discipline are the foundation of
sound governance, no less than of good therapy.

Yin and Yang

We have seen that cycles of natural change were resolved into
two aspects that are opposite in quality but whose interaction was
always understood by Chinese thinkers to be complementary and

---

[23] *Pao-p'u-tzu nei p'ien, 18*: 4b-5a. "Lands" is literally "the Altars
of the Land and Grain."

harmonious. These pairs could describe sequences of change within a constant framework, and thus define the framework.

Take the regular and predictable daily cycle of the sun. One might describe it in terms of the rise and fall of a single quality, light, maximal at noon and minimal at midnight. The Chinese chose another option, which was to apply two opposed concepts, one of which was minimal (or nonexistent) when the other was maximal. Thus they spoke of a phase of light that peaks at noon and a phase of darkness that peaks at midnight.

The moment that light is brightest also marks the beginning of its decline. As it declines, it continues to predominate over darkness for a while, for the latter is only slowly increasing from its low point at noon. Light's predominance lasts half the day, from 6 to 6 (at the equinoxes, but less than half the day in winter, and more than half in summer). As light is declining, darkness (considered in an abstract way) continues to gain strength, until at 6 P.M. it overtakes its opposite and becomes predominant. Its rise in power goes on as light's power falls, until at midnight darkness reaches its height and light its minimal strength. At midnight light is extinct momentarily, but only momentarily, for midnight is also the moment of its rebirth, the beginning of its regrowth. The inverse of all this is true for the other half of the day, until darkness dies and is reborn at noon.

The cycle of the year can be analyzed into two phases in the same way. One might choose as the variables heat and cold. It happens that the Chinese, who were primarily concerned with the agricultural seasons, chose increasing activity of growth to define what becomes predominant at the vernal equinox, reaches its height with the fecundity of vegetable life around the summer solstice, and loses its predominance at the autumnal equinox. The opposite function, quiescence or latency, has its greatest dominion in midwinter, around the winter solstice, when plant life is dormant and animal activity is at its most torpid.

Configurations of phenomena in space rather than in time could also be analyzed to make sense of their internal relationships (1.1). In order to comprehend change within a constant overall pattern one might resolve spatial phenomena into such pairs as upper part and lower part, outer part and inner part, outward and inward orientation, or front and back. In the body such pairs as medial/lateral and dorsal/ventral might be used to describe relationships. Other oppositions neither temporal nor spatial might be incorporated: light and heavy, light and dark color, stimulation and restraint or inhibition, and so forth.

Every new application reinforced the universality of the basic pattern and made possible a wider range of generalization from experience. Any number of paired qualities or opposed functions could be applied to almost any continuum in Nature to demarcate significant aspects and explore their interaction. We might think of all these pairs as instances of a completely general pair, an opposed but complementary x and y for which any pair could be substituted in its appropriate concrete situation.

Yang and yin as scientific and medical concepts were precisely that x and y. They were the abstract foundation upon which a metaphysics could be distilled out of the multiplicity of physical situations, a metaphysics that remained applicable to all of them. In the course of a day yang predominates from 6 to 6, peaking at noon; in the course of a year it predominates from the vernal to the autumnal equinox, peaking at the summer solstice, and so on. Halfway between the extremes, at the equinoxes in the annual cycle and at 6 and 6 in the diurnal cycle, yin and yang are momentarily balanced. Any statement that involves complementary opposites can be translated into the language of yin and yang.

Yang and yin are best considered the active and latent phases of any process in space and time. "Latent," "reactive" and "responsive" are better English counterparts of yin than "passive," since yin not only accepts yang stimuli but responds to them. This response is as important as the stimulus in bringing about change. Porkert, who coins the word "structive" (Latin *structio*) for yin, points out that a yang stimulus (what he calls in his very careful argument an "active effect") is perceptible only when it acts upon something else and calls forth a response.[24]

The scope of yin-yang as applied to medicine may be seen in a classic statement from one of the influential tractates (1624) of Chang Chieh-pin 張 介 賓 . Its many yin-yang correspondences

---

[24] P14. "Structive" is a more rigorous solution to the translation problem than "latent." For the present purpose, when rigor is needed I prefer to retain the original "yin" rather than translate into Latin or newly coined words. For a historical and comparative discussion of yin-yang theory see Needham et al. 1954- : II, 273–91.

are only a small fraction of those that physicians used in their reasoning (and still use, as this book will make clear):

> In diagnosis and therapy it is essential to consider yin-yang first; it is the organizing principle of the medical art. If there is no error with regard to yin and yang, how can therapy be deficient? Only one term can cover the whole art of medicine, manifold though it is—yin-yang. Thus yin and yang are distinguished in manifestation type determination (pages 109–11 and section 7.0), in pulse examination (6.4.1), and in pharmacy.
>
> In manifestation type determination, outer manifestations are yang and inner are yin (7.4); hot manifestations are yang and cold are yin; manifestations in the upper part of the body are yang and those in the lower are yin; ch'i [here, yang vitalities] is yang and hsueh [yin vitalities] is yin; activity is yang and quiescence is yin; loquacity in patients is yang and taciturnity is yin; a preference for light is yang, and a desire for darkness is yin. Those whose yang vitalities are weak exhale with difficulty, and those whose yin vitalities are weak inhale with difficulty. Those with disorders of the yang type are unable to gaze downward, and those with disorders of the yin type are unable to gaze upward.
>
> With reference to the pulse, the floating, large, smooth, and accelerated types are yang, and the sunken, subtle, small, and rough types are yin (6.4.1.2). With reference to drugs, those that send [ch'i and nutriment] upward and those of diffusing tendency are yang, and those of concentrating tendency and those that send them downward are yin; pungent, heating drugs are yang, and bitter, chilling drugs are yin; drugs that act in the active ch'i sector are yang, and those that act in the hsueh sector are yin (9.1); drugs of dynamic and motile character are yang, and those of latent and reactive character are

yin. These taken together compose the grand arcanum of medicine.[25]

Here "yin-yang" refers, as is usual in medical discourse, to a
number of polarities, to a dynamic balance of vitality (maintained
by both *ch'i* and *hsueh*, P11–31), and to signs and symptoms that
indicate an imbalance, to be corrected by drugs whose activity is of
opposing character. Some of these yin-yang correspondences, long
familiar by Chang Chieh-pin's time, are based on clinical experience
(for instance, the classifications of drug activity); others are certainly deduced from theory and connected with experience by an arbitrary analogy (for instance, inability to gaze upward or downward,
which reflects the association of yang with up and yin with down in
spatial configurations). Most yin-yang correspondences originate in
the middle ground between pure empiricism and analogical reasoning. In medicine's "grand arcanum," yin and yang connect theory
and practice, with about the same mixture of rigor and speculation
that we find in the humors and temperaments of European medicine
at the time when Chang was writing.

"Yin-yang" as a compound usually stands for the idea of opposed but complementary pairs into which phenomena can be
analyzed, and out of which a unitary understanding of phenomena
can be formed. Yin and yang as aspects of particular phenomena
are not, as some Western popularizers have tried to make them,
constituents, forces, or pure abstractions. Abstract they are, but
they remain rooted in concrete experience. They are not things or
materials, but qualities, kinds, or phases of something else.

Yin is always defined with respect to yang, and vice versa. An
old man is yin with respect to a young man, but yang with respect
to a woman. The idea that yin or yang is a property—for instance,
that all men are always yang, or conversely that yang is masculine—is not a Chinese idea. A relationship, if not stated, is always implied. To say that masculine is yang implies the masculine-
feminine relationship. It is not necessarily true when the young-old
relation is involved.

Sometimes yin and yang describe not people, substances, or
things, but the energies that maintain them or the processes that

---

[25] *Ching-yueh chüan shu, 1*: 18b ("Ch'uan chung lu," *1*). On the active *ch'i* and *hsueh* sectors see the Translation, section 9.1, where
hsueh is translated "blood" to reflect the authors' understanding.

change them. In other words, they identify aspects of *ch'i*, the term
for those vitalities. Chu Hsi 朱熹 (1130–1200), the most comprehensive of Chinese thinkers, phrased it to his disciples: "Yin and
yang are one and the same *ch'i*. The retreat of yang *is* the birth of
yin; it is not that once yang has retreated a yin separate from it is
born. . . . You can look at yin-yang as single or as twofold. Seen as
twofold it divides into yin and yang; seen as single, it is simply a
waxing and waning."[26]

Although yin and yang classify, it should be clear by now that
their point is not taxonomy. They do not simply sort phenomena
into fixed categories, or compare inherent qualities or properties.
Yin-yang reasoning is usually applied to explain dynamic processes.
Calling something yang describes its relations to something else, or
to itself in another developmental phase. This emphasis on process
and change is typically illustrated by a passage from the *Inner
Canon of the Yellow Lord* that richly describes correspondences between the macrocosm and the somatic microcosm:

> Yin and yang are the Way of sky and earth, the
> network that supports the myriad phenomena, the
> parents of transformation and change, root and
> starting point of giving life and taking life, seat of
> the divinity [within man]. In treating medical disor-
> ders it is essential to search back to the root.
> Accumulating yang formed the sky; accumulat-
> ing yin formed the earth. Yin is quiescent, yang ac-
> tive. Yang gives life; yin sustains growth. Yang

---

[26] *Chu-tzu yü lei* 朱子語類 , 65: 1a (V, 3367). The text contains four additional graphs, which if included would make the
last sentence read "divides into yin and yang, and thereby the bi-
modal pair is established" (using F. W. Mote's translation of
liang i 兩儀 in Hsiao Kung-ch'üan 1979- : I, 651, note 97).
This rather literary phrase, which breaks the rhythm of speech,
appears to be a parenthetical allusion to the *Book of Changes*
(Chou i 周易 , "Hsi tz'u 繫辭 ," A.11) by the disciple who
recorded Chu's discourse.

kills, yin sustains latency. Yang changes *ch'i*; yin forms shape. . . .[27]

The pure, yang portion [of *ch'i*] formed the sky; the turbid, yin portion formed the earth. The *ch'i* of earth ascends to form clouds; the *ch'i* of the sky descends to make rain. But the rain is brought out by the *ch'i* of earth, and the clouds by the *ch'i* of sky. Thus pure, yang [fluids—mucus, tears, etc.] are excreted through the upper orifices of the body and turbid, yin [wastes] through the lower. The pure, yang [defensive *ch'i*, 3.1.3] moves forth through the interstices of the flesh; the turbid, yin [constructive *ch'i*] passes through the yin visceral systems. The pure and yang [*ch'i*] fills out the extremities; the turbid and yin reverts to the yang visceral systems.[28]

Contemporary readers would have been aware of the simple associations on which this schema is built. The sky and its *ch'i* are ordinarily considered yang because the normal standard of comparison is the relatively yin earth. Such prosaic correspondences are intertwined here to explain how cosmic yin and yang *ch'i* form clouds and rain, themselves a conventional pair. This interaction, we are told, is analogous to the cooperation of the body's yin and yang *ch'i*, separated fractionally from breath and nutriment, in maintaining life and health.

For the medical thinker even prosaic and seemingly fixed associations are only relatively stable points in a network of unceasing process. To return to the yin-yang pair "feminine-masculine," the yang character of a male child becomes more marked as he grows to maturity, and less so from then until he dies. In medicine, the growth of yin or yang may proceed past normal limits until it becomes unstable and changes spontaneously into its opposite. Thus a heteropathy of cold type, if its development in the body is unchecked, becomes hot in type and penetrates inward (1.1.1.3).

---

[27] I.e., yang is primarily responsible for the vital aspect of life processes, and yin for their visible, tangible, substantial aspects, P22.

[28] SW, *2* (5): 27–28 = TS, *3* (1): 25. The latter source is incomplete.

Subdivisions of Yin and Yang

We have seen that yin and yang provide a conceptual language for understanding things, events, or processes by examining the interaction of two complementary aspects. Within cycles described by yin and yang, students of change saw five or six kinds of qualitatively distinct activity.

Both yin and yang could be subdivided into two phases. In the spring of the year, for instance, the yang *ch'i* is growing in strength, quickening growth in living things. But the predominance of yang over yin can continue for only so long. Eventually the days no longer become hotter and longer. The luxuriance of plant growth levels off as the time for harvest approaches. In the days around the summer solstice, the growth of yang, having reached its maximum, must give way to the rebirth and revived power of yin. The other half of the year provides a mirror image of this progression, in which the slowing and quieting action of yin *ch'i* proceeds to the point of pure latency at the winter solstice. From that time on yang once again proceeds to grow.

The phase of growth and increase in the yin character of *ch'i* was called *shao yin* 少 陰 , which might be translated as "immature yin," "young yin," or "minor yin," and the maximal phase, *t'ai yin* 太 陰 , "mature yin," "old yin," or "major yin." *Shao yin* represents the upslope, and *t'ai yin* the part of the curve near the point of zero slope and reversal of direction (figure 1). The terminology for the yang phase was similar. A cycle passes once through each of the yin and yang phases.

In the cycle of the day, yang *ch'i* is reborn at midnight, the point of greatest yin intensity. We have already seen that it remains incipient, as "immature yang," until its strength has grown equal to that of the declining yin *ch'i* that characterizes night. The active function, now called "mature yang," continues to grow until its maximum at noon. The dominion of yin, which has shrunk through the morning to vanish momentarily at noon, then reasserts itself as the other half of the cycle begins.

The terminology of maturity was not the only one used for the natural subdivisions of yin and yang. In the *Inner Canon of the Yellow Lord* we find the same quartering of the diurnal cycle in different but equally prevalent language. Here, as we would expect in a medical classic, the same subdivisions are extended to the human body:

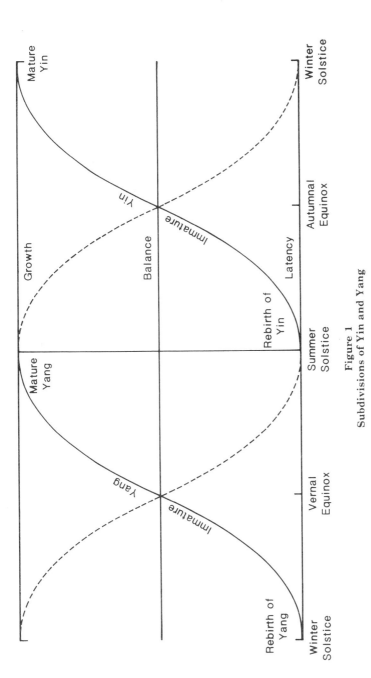

Figure 1
Subdivisions of Yin and Yang

These sinusoidal wave forms suggest the alternation of yin and yang. The latter are not quantitative concepts and cannot be rigorously represented by a graph. Chinese thinkers give primary attention to the growing phases of yin and yang, represented here by solid lines. The declining phases are shown by dotted lines to indicate the momentary balance of yin and yang at the equinoxes, where the solid and dotted lines cross.

Within yin there is yin, and within yang, yang.
From sunrise to noon is Nature's yang, the yang
within yang. From noon to dusk is Nature's yang,
the yin within yang. From the onset of night to
cockcrow [evidently, midnight] is Nature's yin, the
yin within yin. From cockcrow to sunrise is Nature's yin, the yang within yin.

In man there are corresponding relationships.
When we discuss yin and yang in man, the exterior
part is yang and the interior part is yin. When we
discuss yin and yang in the human body, the dorsal
aspect is yang and the ventral aspect yin. When we
discuss yin and yang in the visceral systems of the
human body, the five *tsang* 藏 —the pulmonary,
hepatic, cardiac, splenetic, and renal systems of
function—are yin and the six *fu* 府 —the gall bladder, stomach, large intestine, small intestine, triple
chiao, and urinary bladder systems—are yang (2.1).

If we want to understand from this [what aspects
of the body correspond to] the yin within yin and the
yang within yang, how do we proceed?

. . . We have seen that the back [as the dorsal
aspect] is yang; the yang within this yang is the cardiac system, and the yin within the yang is the pulmonary system. The belly is yin; the yin within the
yin is the renal system, the yang within the yin is
the hepatic system, and the extreme yin within yin
is the splenetic system. These [and all the other
somatic] allegiances to yin and yang accord with the
relations of outer and inner aspect (*piao-li* 表 裡 ,
1.1.1, 7.1, P204), exterior and interior [of the body,
nei wai 內 外], left and right, female and male,
and above and below, so we use them to respond to
the yin-yang relationships of Nature.[29]

---

[29] TS, *3* (3): 43–44 = SW, *1* (4): 22–23. "The extreme yin within
yin" is obviously not the balance point between yin and yang. As
the compiler of TS, Yang Shang-shan 楊 上 善 (ca. 600), explains, "the spleen occupies the most yin position in the belly,"
presumably because it is inmost (page 44). Most later commentators follow Wang Ping's 王 冰 commentary to SW (762),

The two gradations of yin and yang are not mere headings for use in classification. Certain functions are characteristic of each, in the diurnal cycle or any other: for immature yang (yang within yin), incipience and germination; for mature yang (yang within yang), activity, growth, and maturation; for immature yin (yin within yang), yield of fruit and the beginning of decline; for mature yin (yin within yin) quiescence, latency, and the formation of a ground upon which future action will take place. In the agricultural cycle these are the functions associated with spring, summer, autumn, and winter. Spatial correspondences are determined by the sun's location in the sky (that is, along the ecliptic) in the four seasons: east, south, west, and north.

Although in principle mature yin and yang might be considered mere moments at which their corresponding activities die at the solstices and immediately begin to quicken again, in practice they define whole seasons. Flexibility and a recognizable account of experience was what people were looking for. Yin and yang were coherent concepts. They provided the abstractions needed for theoretical explanation over the whole range of culture, but logical rigor was not expected of them, much less quantifiability. There was no need for scholastic debates about whether mature yang ended at the summer solstice (considered midsummer by the Chinese) or six weeks later when autumn began.

The four symmetrical states of yin or yang predominance do not provide a full account of change. A fifth aspect of yin-yang appears at the balance points where the two tendencies are equal. These points are not defined by numerical equality, of course, but by transitory states of dynamic balance as yin and yang pass, one rising and the other declining. The function associated with this phase is the neutralizing of opposites, in preparation for new relations between active yang and responsive yin. This phase was often described by the metaphor of "central house" (*chung kung* 中 宮). "House," among other meanings, was the central of the five

---

which argues instead that the splenetic system corresponds to mature yin relative to the other yin systems, and furthermore is in a yin position (page 23). Both commentators are assuming that two similar effects add, so to speak. *T'ien* 天 , literally "sky," often has the broader sense "Nature" or "the natural order" in cosmological writing. The translation omits one sentence that interrupts the argument and may be an interpolation.

musical modes and of the sound-cosmos that they defined. Another term for what this fifth phase described was "harmony" (*ho* 和 , 合).[30]

Yin-yang and the five subphases defined by the relations between yin and yang are certainly abstract analytic concepts. There is no denying that they were used in every department of scientific thought to resolve complicated phenomena and processes into parts. At the same time Chinese thinkers took care not to lose sight of the whole, so that analysis always serves a synthesizing approach to the understanding of nature. Analysis or synthesis may predominate in a given frame of explanation, but the essential point if we want to understand yin-yang thought is the regular association of analysis and synthesis, dissecting out of a whole its basic components and learning how they work together.

Because the yin-yang concept was so broadly useful, the overall vision of change that it implied was ever more firmly imposed on the perception of physical reality. This vision is, to recapitulate, cyclical. The pace and quality of a given change reflect the shifting predominance of opposed characteristics of things or of their *ch'i*. In opposition these qualities are complementary rather than antagonistic. Overwhelming primacy of one over the other, as well as perfect balance between the two, are never more than momentary passages in the oscillatory growth of one at the expense of the other. This regular oscillation defines the good order of the whole.

Five Phases

Yin-yang was not the only combination of entities used in medicine, and indeed throughout the realm of Chinese thought, to identify the complementary aspects of change. An idea of comparable importance was *wu hsing* 五 行 , translated by most students of Chinese science as the "Five Phases."

---

[30] This is, I believe, the most sensible interpretation of *ho* (first form) in *Lao-tzu*, 42. See the unambiguous occurrences of *ho* (first form) in *Ch'un-ch'iu fan lu* 春 秋 繁 露 , 16 (77): 19a and elsewhere in *chüan* 16 and 17, and the similar use of *chung ho* 中 和 (centrality and harmony) in *16*: 17a-17b. On "house" see Needham 1954- : IV.1: 157–71.

In the formative centuries of Chinese natural philosophy (roughly the last four centuries B.C.), when every possibility of thought was being tried out, a tendency to break natural phenomena and human activities into several complementary types was much in evidence—often three, four, six, or nine categories, most often two or five. The early books in which the term *wu-hsing* appears are mostly difficult to date, or turn out under critical scrutiny to be much later than their traditional dates. In what is possibly the earliest appearance of *wu-hsing*—in the "Declaration at Kan" preserved in the *Book of Documents* (*Shang shu* 尚 書)—the word refers not to aspects of the physical world but to five moral qualities. Hsun-tzu 荀 子 (ca. 350 B.C.) uses the term in the same sense. The "Declaration" is probably earlier, but dates proposed for it are widely scattered and all are problematic.

The "Great Norms" of the *Book of Documents*, a discussion of the nine norms revealed by heaven to the monarch as the basis of an enduring political order, is now considered by many scholars to be a late addition to the collection of documents, but was extremely influential for two thousand years because of its supposed archaic origin. Four of its norms are expressed in fivefold categories, among them the canonical *wu hsing*: "The *wu hsing* are, first, water, second, fire, third, wood, fourth, metal, and fifth, earth. Of water it is said that it soaks and goes downward; of fire it is said that it flames and goes upward; of wood it is said that it bends and straightens; of metal it is said that it conforms and can change [its shape]; of earth it is said that it accepts seeds and gives forth crops."[31]

Over a long period, in thought about nature in general, and particularly in numerology and astrology, these five categories were linked in various combinations with each other and with other categories. Some fivefold combinations, including the group of five just listed, were associated by writers in the period of philosophic exploration not only with moral qualities but with material constituents.

When the centuries of experimentation with categories of thought were over, the Five Phases as they appear in the "Great

---

[31] *Shang shu*, 7.0027, 24.0155; *Hsun-tzu*, 20.48. On the use of *wu hsing* for moral qualities see P'ang P'u 庞 朴 1977.

All of these are functional explanations. They say not what their subject is made of, but what it does.

Norms" had become an enduring combination. What was initially a simple set of ideas was greatly elaborated in the second and first centuries B.C. to provide the foundation for a cosmological theory of monarchy, which justified the imperial political order as a reflection of the order of Nature. In the process a sophisticated view of natural phenomena emerged.[32] It was then gradually adapted to the emerging needs of particular sciences. As functional approaches to explanation became the norm in the sciences, the Five Phases were used preponderantly to analyze types of activity. Wood had become, and remained in scientific writings, not a material but a characteristic of change. Sometimes, as in the "Great Norms," it implies flexibility, but more usually it suggests accelerating activity and growth.

The notion of wood, fire, metal, water, and earth as material constituents faded to insignificance for the systematic study of nature as recorded in the literature of the sciences. The gradual delineation of the Five Phases and their specialization in technical discourse are historical topics of great interest, but this is not the place to explore them. My present concern is only with the mature understandings of the Five Phases as found in scientific discourse of the last two thousand years, particularly their special meanings in medicine—the meanings that this book draws on and transforms (1.2.1).

Why "Five Phases" as a translation for *wu hsing*? Answering this question is as good a way as any to clarify the concept. Until

---

[32] I see no reason to accept as history the legend that makes Tsou Yen 騶 行 (ca. 305-ca. 240 B.C.) the inventor of the mature Five Phases theory or the founder of a school of "Naturalists." The sources generally adduced to support these claims are so vague and contradictory that his responsibility even for a *wu hsing* theory of history and morality (which is all that the soundest sources imply) is greatly uncertain. Settling this confusion would require more space than the question merits in the present connection. Pending a full discussion, see the historical doubts registered in Ch'ien Mu 錢 穆 1956: 441-43.

I capitalize the names of the phases to distinguish them from the materials—if fire can be called a material—of the same names. "Five Phases" and translations of certain other traditional scientific terms are capitalized as a reminder that they are not drawn from or directly related to modern science.

about twenty years ago, *wu hsing* was regularly translated "five elements." In the formative period of philosophy, we have seen, the term was indeed applied to material constituents, among other things. This sense became unimportant in the sciences, but never entirely died out in general philosophy. Even so, material constituents in Chinese physical thought are not elements. The *wu hsing* were never described as ultimate, irreducible "roots" like the Greek four elements of Empedocles, which were always intermixed in natural things. These four elements (earth, air, fire, and water) could be revealed in pure form not by any operation, only by a thought experiment in which they were the ultimate result of division repeated to a point far below the threshhold of visibility. A sample of water in nature contained all four elements. In the Chinese conception, the link between a piece of wood in Nature and the *hsing* Wood was not through the ultimate fine texture of the former, but through processes, such as flexing and growing, characteristic of wood. Material wood need not be present so long as these processes were involved. The Greek elements, in their Aristotelian and medieval European form, were connected with qualities (hot, cold, moist, dry), but the Chinese were primarily concerned with process and change. The similarities between the Greek elements and the Chinese *wu hsing* do not extend past the surface of the ideas.

The confusion originated nearly four hundred years ago, when the earliest Catholic missionaries in China identified *wu hsing* with the European four elements in order to persuade the Chinese that the latter were superior and ought to replace the former in scientific explanation. Thus Matteo Ricci, in the first Jesuit treatise on cosmology (1608), argued that "since a *hsing* is what produces all things and phenomena, it must be an element, perfectly pure. It must be that nothing is intermixed with it, nothing contained in it except itself." He proceeded to demonstrate that by this definition Chinese discourse about five "elements" is inconsistent and illogical. *Wu hsing*, he concluded, is plainly inferior to the European four elements.[33] Whether this was a polemical trick or the result of misunderstanding is difficult to judge. In any case Chinese writers had not claimed that *hsing* are pure substances, or that they produce all things and phenomena. Ricci's argument is roughly equivalent to pointing out that Peking Duck, considered as a type of

---

[33] *Ch'ien k'un t'i i* 乾 坤 體 義, *1*: 11a-13a.

fried chicken, is an inferior kind, and concluding that we ought to eat true fried chicken instead. Such an argument convinces only those who already prefer fried chicken. It is not surprising that this part of Ricci's book did not arouse Chinese interest.

Ricci's confusing view of *wu hsing* as five elements, and sloppily conceived elements at that, long outlasted the scholastic four elements, which were beginning to die out in Europe in Ricci's time, and were laid to rest as modern chemistry was born. But a mistranslation is not easily discarded after 350 years of use. A quarter-century ago Joseph Needham noted that "the conception of the elements was not so much one of a series of five sorts of fundmental matter (particles do not come into the question), as of five sorts of fundamental processes. Chinese thought here characteristically avoided substance and clung to relation." But although it "has never been satisfactory for *hsing*, . . . the term 'element' has for so long been used of the Wu Hsing that it is hardly possible to discard it." Partly as a result of Needham's clarification, an increasing number of those investigating the history of Chinese science over the past couple of decades have found it imperative for the sake of clarity to discard it.[34]

Why is "Five Phases" the only widely accepted replacement for "Five Elements"?

Wu means "five"; the pertinent meanings of *hsing* are "to do, to act, to move, to set in motion; action, activity, motion," etc. If the idea that *wu hsing* was first applied to moral discourse turns out to be true once the tangle of dates is unravelled, the word *hsing* must almost certainly refer to types of action based on such qualities.

We have two especially clear definitions from the end of the first century A.D., by which time the cosmological sense of *wu hsing* was fully formed. In a chapter on the Five Phases in the *Comprehensive Discussions in the White Tiger Hall* (*Pai hu t'ung* 白虎通 , ca. A.D. 80), we find: "When we say *hsing* the meaning we wish to express is that it is the activity of *ch'i* [as maintained] by the natural order." The dictionary *Explanations of Names* (*Shih ming* 釋名), about twenty years later, also asserts that *hsing* is what *ch'i* does: "*Wu hsing* means what is carried out by the five *ch'i*, each

---

[34] Needham et al. 1954- : II, 243–44; Major 1976, 1977; Kunst 1977.

in its own domain."[35] In this understanding "Wood," "Earth," and so on are labels for five types of *ch'i* characterized by their activity. These definitions agree with the purport of many discussions from the second century B.C. on. They suggest that the most accurate definition based purely on literal translation of *wu hsing* would be "Five Agents."

This translation has not been generally adopted because it encourages new misunderstandings in place of the old ones. Such a misunderstanding is not surprising in the conclusion that the great philologist Ch'en Meng-chia 陳夢家 drew when forty-five years ago he studied the early significance of the Five Phases: "'Wu hsing' is the relative cyclic flow of five kinds of force, not five static elements."[36] This definition pioneered in speaking of relative cyclic change in a system of entities. It slightly misses the mark when it moves beyond the evidence to call the *wu hsing* forces. That is understandable in a trailblazing study. What is remarkable is that Ch'en's insight has been so consistently ignored.

As the Han definitions above make clear, in the mature form of the concept—as we see it in countless sources, including medical literature as a whole—a *hsing* is not a force, not even an agent, capable itself of performing actions. What brings about the activity described by the *wu hsing* is the force of *ch'i*.

The *wu hsing* name five types of *ch'i* that interact in an ordered way to make up spatial or temporal configurations (that is, complex phenomena extended in space or time). The process to which they are most usually applied is, as Ch'en's emphasis indicates, the temporal cycle, whether of body functions, celestial motions, or political changes.

Jen Ying-ch'iu 任應秋 , the leading contemporary author on traditional medical theories, paraphrases *wu hsing* with precision: "*Wu hsing* simply means the cyclical activity (*yun-hsing* 運行) of five *ch'i*."[37] *Ch'i* acts; *wu hsing* categorizes the types of activity so that they may be related to each other. "Five *ch'i*" are not five chemically or physically distinct substances, but five aspects of a

---

[35] *Pai hu t'ung, 4:* 24b; *Shih ming* in *T'ai-p'ing yü lan* 太平御 覽 , *17:* 85a. The crucial phrases are *wei t'ien hsing ch'i* 為天 行氣 and *wu ch'i yü ch'i fang ko shih-hsing che* 五氣於其 方各施行者 respectively.

[36] Ch'en 1938: 52.

[37] Jen 1960: 23.

process, the activity that drives it, or the substance that changes character in it. Jen's definition reflects the use of the Five Phases to describe how vital energies are distributed and adjusted in medical disorder and therapy. This dynamic aspect explains the emphasis in medical writings on the developmental successions of phases—mutual production, mutual conquest, and several others—that can interact in subtle ways, as described with examples below (1.2.1). But there is only one agent responsible for their interaction, namely *ch'i*.

With this in mind, we can see the point of "Five Phases" as a translation for *wu hsing*. It lacks philological elegance because it is not etymological; but it justifies itself by conveying what the term meant to scientific authors and readers. "Phase" reminds us that above all each *hsing* describes a complementary part of a process or configuration in which *ch'i* is the agent of both change and stable identity. "Phase" is used here in a common English sense that goes back to the seventeenth century: "Any one aspect of a thing of varying aspects; a state or stage of change or development."[38] The more technical meanings in modern physics and chemistry also apply to relations within both spatial and temporal configurations, but are irrelevant to this discussion.

To sum up, *wu hsing* theory provides a language for analysis of configurations into five functionally distinct parts or aspects. The names of the phases refer both to these spatial and cyclic relations and to the energies, the *ch'i*, that make them possible, maintain them, and guide their change. In other words, the Five Phases do what yin-yang does, but with finer divisions, analyzing into five aspects instead of two. Both are sets of labels for *ch'i*.

The phases, in fact, correspond to the five types of yin-yang activity described in the last subsection. Wood is the name of the phase of growth and increase, or immature yang; Fire, of the maximal phase of activity, or mature yang; Metal and Water, the reactive counterparts, correspond to immature and mature yin; and Earth is the phase of balance and neutralization, the "central house" (see Table 1, page 77).

Tung Chung-shu's 董仲舒 *"Abundant Dew" Interpretation of the Spring and Autumn Annals (Ch'un-ch'iu fan lu* 春秋繁露 , ca. 135 B.C.), which developed an influential cosmological ideology

---

[38] *OED* sense 2; spelled "phasis," from Latin, until the mid-nineteenth century.

of government, recapitulates the main characteristics of the Five Phases. The relevant passage begins a chapter that sets out at length the correspondences between the phases and the responsibilities of high officials. The argument begins by relating yin-yang and the Five Phases, as two among several equivalent ways of marking out aspects of *ch'i*: "The *ch'i* of sky and earth unite to become one. Divided they become yin and yang; subdivided, the four seasons; set out in order (*lieh* 列), the Five Phases. *Hsing* means 'activity' (*hsing-che, hsing yeh* 行者行也). Their activities differ; that is why they are called *wu hsing*. The *wu hsing* are [i.e., correspond to] the Five Officials [, those phases responsible] for correct, timely activity. The phases next to each other make up the mutual production sequence; those two apart make up the mutual overcoming sequence. Thus they provide order (*chih* 治). If [the pertinent Five Phases relations are] violated the result is disorder; if followed, order."

Table 1
Equivalences between Yin-yang and Five Phases

Wood	Immature yang	Yang within yin
Fire	Mature yang	Yang within yang
Earth	Central house, harmony	
Metal	Immature yin	Yin within yang
Water	Mature yin	Yin within yin

The normal succession of phases (the mutual production order) is that by which one activity naturally produces the next (*hsiang sheng* 相生), namely Wood, Fire, Earth, Metal, Water, Wood, in an endless chain. We will see that in the body this is the order of physiological processes. The order by which one phase overcomes (*hsiang sheng* 相勝) or conquers another (*hsiang k'o* 相克) is Wood, Earth, Water, Fire, Metal, Wood. This sequence corresponds to every other phase ("two apart") in the production order. In the body this is the order by which pathological processes are transmitted (1.2.1; see figure 2).[39]

Another tradition in general philosophy, which was not influential in scientific writing, put *ch'i* and yin-yang at a higher level of abstraction than the Five Phases, which belonged to the level of substance (*chih* 質). Still, Chu Hsi in the twelfth century, who carried on this tradition, emphasized that the distinction held for discussions of the formation of the cosmos, not for physical reasoning about its regular workings: "Yin and yang are *ch'i*, and the *wu hsing* are substance. It is through the existence of this substance that phenomenal things were made. Although the *wu hsing* are substance, they also have their *ch'i*; only by virtue of [these five *ch'i*] could things be made. The two *ch'i* of yin and yang are divided into these five. It is not true that in addition to yin and yang there are Five Phases. . . ."[40]

In relation to things and events in the world of experience—such as bodies and illness—yin-yang and the Five Phases are not two kinds of activity, but two ways of thinking about the same process and the vitality or force that drives it.

The Five Phases provided the scientific thinker's everyday labels for these five types of activity (which ordinarily have nothing to do with the materials of which the things examined are made). In analyzing processes or configurations into five aspects— particularly when reflecting on sequences of change—the names of the Five Phases are more common than mature yang, "central house," and the other yin-yang terms. The latter appear when reference to complementary opposites is particularly important.[41]

This discussion would be misleading if it gave the impression that yin-yang and the Five Phases were perfectly articulated with each other and were used with entire consistency. These concepts

---

[39] *Ch'un-ch'iu fan lu*, 13 (58): 7a-7b. See the discussion in Needham 1954- : II, 247–59. Needham's mutual conquest sequence is the converse of that given in most Chinese sources, but they are equivalent.

[40] *Chu tzu yü lei, 1*: 9a (page 155), discussed in Yamada Keiji 山 田 慶 兒 1978: 109.

[41] It is not unusual for medical writings to mix or interchange Five Phases and yin-yang terminology. See, for instance, the variety of sources cited in the sections on "yin-yang" and "Water and Fire" of the anthology *I shu* 醫 述 (1826), *1*: 17–30.

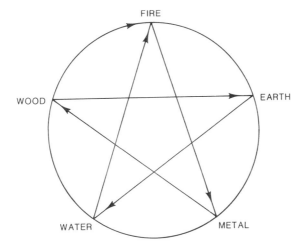

Figure 2
Relationship of the Mutual Production and
Mutual Conquest Sequences of the Five Phases†

†The former follows the arcs of the circle, the latter the straight lines. Each phase overcomes the second one after it in the mutual production order. In medicine the production sequence is characteristic of physiological processes, and the conquest sequence marks the order of pathological change.

have provided a basis for two thousand years of systematic technical discourse. But the consistency that made this role possible was achieved only gradually and within limits, as attention to the roles of yin-yang and the Five Phases in medicine will illustrate. But first it is necessary to be aware of another important conception, found only in medicine, with which these two overlap.

Six Warps

The Six Warps (*liu ching* 六 經 , named after the lengthwise threads in weaving) represent a threefold division of yin and yang. *Ching* also implies regularity (see page 138). Just as yin and yang relate two kinds of activity to each other, each can be subdivided, as we have seen, into types that are yin or yang in relation to each other. We have already noted a fourfold subdivision into immature and mature aspects, and a fivefold subdivision which includes the point of balance between opposites. In principle any number of subdivisions may be justified, as a dialogue in the *Inner Canon of the Yellow Lord* asserts. The royal counselor Ch'i-po 歧 伯 has just pointed out that yin-yang and the Five Phases can be associated with the circulation tracts in discrepant ways, depending on whether one considers the correspondences of cosmic yin-yang theory as manifested in the body, or those of the Six Warps theory that refer to the body in particular. The Yellow Lord, ever the obliging interlocutor, asks: "I have heard that the sky is yang and the earth yin, the sun yang and the moon yin. (Their cyclic alternation through long and short months for) three hundred sixty-five days forms a year; [the processes within] the human being correspond to this. Now I hear that the threefold yin and threefold yang [within man] does not correspond [exactly] to yin-yang [in the cosmos]. Why is this?" Ch'i-po replies: "Yin and yang [in their cosmic aspects] may be counted by tens, divided into hundreds, subdivided into thousands, carried further into myriads, and the myriads may be multiplied beyond counting. Still essentially they make up one whole. . . . The transformations of yin and yang within the human being may also be subdivided by numerical categories."[42] Various sets of concepts that describe the parts of

---

[42] TS, *5* (2): 57–58 = SW, *2* (6): 40. The words in parentheses occur in SW only.

the body or the phases of a vital process, in other words, do not describe different things. They are ways of looking at different aspects of the body or process, which remains one. When the results of two such analyses differ, the discrepancy does not lie in the reality described, but in the aspects chosen to characterize it. Each analysis is true for the aspects analyzed. Each is one way (sometimes one of several ways) to understand the whole. This is not an "either/or" mentality at work.

The six "warp" subdivisions include immature and mature yang and yin. The meaning of these familiar concepts is altered somewhat to make room for two additional yin-yang types, "yang brightness" (*yang ming* 陽 明) and "attenuated yin" (*chueh-yin* 厥 陰). In the chapter of the *Inner Canon* just cited, the latter two, as indicated by their correspondences to months of the year, fall in the middle of the periods that yang and yin govern. They represent phases in which the yang or yin *ch'i* that precede and succeed them converge. Unlike the other subdivisions, as figure 3 shows, the two months that mark the temporal order of yang brightness (months 3–4) and attenuated yin (months 9–10) are consecutive (although, for instance, the mature yang months are 2 and 5). The *Inner Canon* remarks "these two yang [*ch'i*] add in the front [that is, the corresponding circulation vessels join in the ventral aspect of the body]; thus it is called 'yang brightness' . . . these two yin [*ch'i*] join and reach the lowest intensity [possible for yin]; thus it is called 'attenuated yin.'"[43] The overall image is not quantitative; the figure

---

[43] TS, *5* (2): 54–55 = LS, *7* (41): 68. The statements on which the figure is based are from the same section. Later on page 55 the first sentence is rephrased: "These two Fires add; thus it becomes 'yang brightness.'" Elsewhere in the *Inner Canon* the two circulation tracts associated with each of the Six Warps differ according to whether they pass through the arms or legs, but in this chapter of TS all the tracts correlated with the Six Warps correspond to foot tracts. The two in each pair differ according to whether the tract traverses the right or left half of the body. The right-foot tracts correspond to months 4 through 9, the downslope in figure 3. The hand tracts are discussed separately. They are associated with both conventional yin-yang and Five Phases, combined to give a total of only ten possibilities. For the classical enumeration (on which table 4.1 below is based) see LS, *3* (10), missing from TS.

renders time and sequence, but the vertical axis does not represent numerical measures. The sequence shown is only one of three that frequently occur. The other two are shown in table 4.1 (page 252). One is the order in which the tracts are usually listed, as in that table; the other is the order of circulation within them, as noted in the right-hand column. Figure 3 can represent neither of these orders. I will discuss still another order below.

The Six Warps is not, in other words, a single concept in the *Inner Canon*, but a variety of sixfold schemata related in various ways to the circulation tracts by way of yin-yang theory.

The most obvious way to look at the two new phases is that, as in figure 3, they represent the high and low points of a cycle that begins with the immature phase and in which the mature phase is intermediate. The points of balance between yin and yang are not named, because they are of no consequence in this particular connection. When they are important, conventional yin-yang and Five Phases concepts can be used to express them.

To sum up, in the *Inner Canon* the Six Warps are aspects of a cyclic process, that of the *ch'i* circulation. The book names the twelve cardinal (literally, "warp") circulation tracts after these six divisions of yin and yang, each "warp" designating two branches of the circulation (see table 4.1 for one set of associations with the circulation tracts; cf. CL40–46). The main purpose of the Six Warps, in other words, is to describe the order and symmetries of normal energy distribution through the body. By extension this concept becomes a basic tool of therapeutic reasoning. Since the *Inner Canon* is little concerned with any therapy except acupuncture, the use of Six Warps reasoning in regulating the flow of vitality is reflected mainly in chapter 4 of the *Revised Outline*, on the circulation tract system and its application to needling.

The term "Six Warps" has an entirely different meaning in the other main tradition of medical reasoning, concerned with the transmission of cold heteropathy from one tract to the next. It posits as the normal sequence for this process:

1. mature yang
2. yang brightness
3. immature yang
4. mature yin
5. immature yin
6. attenuated yin.

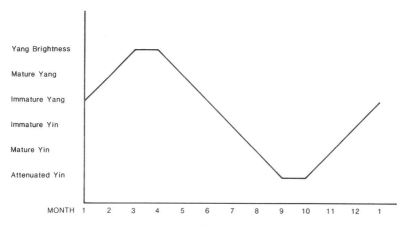

Figure 3
Correspondences of Six Warps to Months

This tradition begins with a very simple schema in the *Basic Questions* of the *Inner Canon*, but it is developed in great detail in the *Treatise on Cold Damage Disorders* (*Shang han lun* 傷 寒 論), which may be as little as half a century or as much as a couple of centuries later.[44] Unlike the all-encompassing dialogues about the body, health, and the most general aspects of medical disorder in the *Inner Canon*, the *Treatise* restricts itself to information that points toward a concrete therapeutic goal. It is concerned only with treating one broad class of disorders, all acute at onset, caused by external factors, and with hot sensations as a prominent symptom. This class is roughly equivalent to the acute infectious febrile disorders of modern medicine, although the grouping of symptoms to define particular diseases differs from that of modern medicine here as elsewhere in the traditional art. The name of the class, Cold Damage, is taken from one of the disorders in it, caused by cold factors. The particular disorder Cold Damage, in its early stages, is defined by so vague a collection of symptoms that it may correspond to anything from the common cold to typhoid.

The point of the book is not so much diagnosis as demarcating the stages of development, from initial infection to death, that the Cold Damage Disorders share. Each disease has its own manifestations that appear at their own pace; but these were fitfully analyzed and treated as variants on a common pattern rather than as the courses of individual disorders. According to the generalized pattern, the infecting agent (or heteropathy, 5.1) enters the periphery of the body, mainly through the pores, and works its way gradually inward, if not stopped by prompt, appropriate therapy, to interfere mortally with the central control of metabolic functions. The *Treatise* is not interested in particular visceral systems, or for that

---

[44] TS, *25* (1): 423–25 = SW, *9* (31): 163–64, where the heteropathy in normal circumstances passes through one tract per day, making two rounds in the course of the disorder. In the *Treatise* normal and abnormal sequences are discussed in a flexible but clearly delineated framework for a great variety of periods and febrile syndromes.

Shang han lun (or "the *Treatise*") was originally part of *Shang han tsa ping lun* 傷 寒 雜 病 論 , evidently written between A.D. 196 and 220. For the history of the latter work see bibliography A.

matter in the abdomen. It merely speaks of a progression from the outer to the inner aspect (7.1, 9.5).[45]

At each step of penetration the heteropathy's interaction with the body's health-maintaining vitalities (orthopathy) differs. Each stage is thus defined by a cluster of intermittent hot or cold sensations and other symptoms. For instance, at the first, most superficial level of penetration typical symptoms for the whole Cold Damage group of disorders are floating pulse (6.4.1.2), stiffness and pain in the head and neck, and in most cases aversion to cold (the patient may not yet complain of hot sensations). In various disorders in the Cold Damage group these symptoms differ, but the book concentrates on identifying the manifestation type (9.5) that indicates the depth of the heteropathy. Each manifestation type— several for each stage, to accommodate varying symptoms, not different diseases—is associated directly with a drug prescription, which may be modified as circumstances require. The physician is encouraged to use therapy flexibly to cope not only with the rapid changes of acute febrile disorders but with the inevitability of human error in such fluid circumstances, calling for prompt correction. Throughout the book these lessons are driven home by lists of

---

[45] The viscera and circulation tracts figure only in the "miscellaneous disorders" portion of the old *Shang han tsa ping lun*. Nevertheless, Chinese medical scholars have pointed out a variety of implicit connections between the circulation tracts and the Six Warps in the *Shang han lun*. Symptoms of a Six Warps stage sometimes are associated with parts of the body on or near the circulation tract of the same name, or are related to the visceral system corresponding to the circulation tract. See, for instance, Nan-ching Chung-i hsueh-yuan ed. 1958: 507–8, and Hao Yin-ch'ing 郝 印 卿 1982. D. C. Epler has also remarked on these affinities in an unpublished paper on the concept of disease in the *Shang han lun*. For differences between the Six Warps of the *Treatise* and the visceral and tract systems, see Ho Chih-hsiung 何 志 雄 1983. The differences are substantial. They indicate the extent to which the *Treatise* has abstracted and elaborated on the Inner Canon's schema. Because of the difference in the character of the two books, the formative influence of the *Inner Canon*, acknowledged by Chang Chi in his preface, is seldom so obvious.

symptoms and ingredients, not by an overarching explanatory framework.

Here as an example is the first disorder for which detailed symptoms are given in the *Treatise on Cold Damage Disorders*:

> In the mature yang stage of disorder, the pulse is floating, the head aches, the neck is stiff, and the patient is abnormally sensitive to cold. Mature yang disorder in which there are also hot sensations [*or* fever, *fa je* 發 熱], perspiration, abnormal sensitivity to wind, and a moderate [floating] pulse is called Wind Attack disorder. . . . In mature yang Wind Attack disorder, when the yang pulse [i.e., the pulse taken with light finger pressure] is floating and the yin pulse [under heavy pressure] is weak, the sensitivity to cold and wind extend to the slightest exposure, the fever is intense, and there are wheezing in the nasal passages and dry heaves, it will be controlled by Cassia Twig Infusion.

This infusion is made from cassia twig (*kuei chih* 桂 枝 , Cinnamomum cassia), peony root (*shao yao* 芍 藥 , Paeonia lactiflora), licorice root (*kan-ts'ao* 甘 草 , Glycyrrhiza uralensis), fresh ginger root (*sheng chiang* 生 姜 , Zingiber officinale), and jujube fruit (*ta-tsao* 大 棗 , Zizyphus jujuba). In contemporary medicine this set of symptoms would correspond to a variety of the Wind Cold Outer manifestation type (9.1.1.5).[46]

In current practice the *Treatise's* approach to therapeutic reasoning for acute febrile diseases has largely been supplanted by the later Heat Factor Disorder approach. The latter distinguishes only four levels of penetration but analyzes more complicated progressions of development than the Six Warps theory does. Heat Factor Disorder theory is explicit about its theoretical underpinnings and relatively simple in its approach to therapy.[47] The historical

---

[46] *Shang han lun*, sections 1–2, 4 (prescription in 5), 134–49. The adjectives that describe cold and wind sensitivity and fever in section 4 are uncertain in meaning, so this translation is tentative.

[47] This tradition began in the twelfth century with attempts to distinguish more clearly than in *Shang han lun* the differences between disorders of different etiology (with special attention to

authority of the six-step Cold Damage Disorder approach is still sufficient to earn mention for it below (9.5); in Japanese practice its importance is undiminished.[48]

Differences in Early Concepts

Nor was the use of the Six Warps the only basic divergence between the *Inner Canon* and the *Treatise on Cold Damage Disorders*. As Ōtsuka Keisetsu 大 塚 敬 節, who has studied the *Treatise* deeply, has pointed out, the latter not only ignores the circulation tracts and the visceral systems of function, but does not even refer to the Five Phases.

The point is easily overlooked. The early commentators, aware that the author in his preface includes the *Basic Questions* among the works he used and refers to the Five Phases as an important notion, assumed that the basic ideas of the two books were identical. They then freely read the *Treatise as though it drew on* the Five Phases and other ideas from the *Inner Canon*, and incorporated this understanding into their annotations.[49] But when we set their ex-

---

epidemic diseases) and to simplify their treatment. *Shang han lun* is not concerned with etiology. Heat Factor theory was developed into a conscious four-stage manifestation type determination, the basis for chapter 9 of the *Revised Outline*, by Yeh Kuei 葉 桂 in his *Wen je lun* 溫 熱 論 (ca. 1740?). Yeh's use of the triple *chiao* system to classify manifestation types was then elaborated by Wu T'ang 吳 瑭 in his *Wen ping t'iao pien* 溫 病 條 辨 (completed 1798) to form another system based on the Six Warps. Both systems are described briefly below (9.5).

[48] Ōtsuka Keisetsu 大 冢 敬 節 1956.

[49] The notion that the *Treatise* drew on the same conceptual stock as the *Inner Canon* was established in the *Mai ching* 脉 經 of Wang Shu-ho 王 叔 和 (ca. 280). Wang freely read into the *Treatise* the theoretical structure of its predecessor. This monolithic view of early doctrine was authoritative for centuries. The reassessment of the *Shang han tsa ping lun* as a work based on conceptions different in many ways from those of the *Inner Canon* began with the *Shang han lun t'iao pien* 傷 寒 論 條 辨 of Fang Yu-chih 方 有 執 (author's preface 1589) and the

planations aside and look at the *Treatise* in its earliest surviving form, we see (even though the extant text is not at all pristine) that its ideas are indeed much simpler than those of the Inner Canon, and that the Five Phases are not found among them. For that matter, yin-yang does not appear as a concept; it occurs only in names of diseases and disease phases.

Various recent historians who became aware of this difference have overlooked the evidence in the preface. Assuming that the author of the *Treatise* was ignorant of the Five Phases, they have explained his ignorance by geographic isolation or by the unimportance of the Five Phases concept at the time compared to that of yin-yang. Thus the confusion of centuries has been replaced by new confusion.

Ōtsuka, who largely deserves credit for clearing up the first confusion, leaves no room for the second. He emphasizes the specific aim of the *Treatise*, which Chang Chi's preface tells us was to collect and set in order prescriptions for a group of diseases that had taken a heavy toll of his clan. Chang's compilation was organized according to a theoretical schema, in which changes in symptoms mark six stages in the inward penetration of the disease process, but he had no reason to pause for abstract reflections. After studying all the surviving fragments of the author's other writings, Ōtsuka concludes "Chang was a physician in the tradition of the *Inner Canon* who acknowledges [in his preface] the importance he accorded to the world-view—absent from the text of the *Treatise*—of which the Five Phases theory, the visceral systems of function, and the circulation tract system form parts."[50]

Shang lun p'ien 尚 論 篇 of Yü Ch'ang 喻 昌 (printed 1648), but is largely the achievement of the last couple of decades.

[50] Ōtsuka 1966: 24–25. See also Wu K'ao-p'an 吳 考 槃 1984 on specific theoretical assumptions in *Shang han lun*. The reader would do well to be aware that my discussion of the relations between early sources is not only greatly simplified but tentative. Recent research by the Japanese scholars mentioned below and by Wu (1983) and others in China has cast into doubt many conventional opinions about the earliest medical literature, including the very conviction that the surviving *Basic Questions* and *Divine Pivot* are the ancient *Inner Canon of the Yellow Lord* (see also note 3, pages 5–6 above).

For that matter, the *Inner Canon* itself does not relate yin-yang and the Five Phases in a consistent way, nor are its various Five Phases correspondences internally consistent. There is so much variation in the correspondence of such entities as the five sapors (governed by the Five Phases, 1.2.2, 11.1.1) to visceral systems and body parts that it is impossible to think of the *Inner Canon* as one book. This lack of unanimity has been documented in detail, especially by Japanese medical historians, for a quarter of a century.[51]

No less significant than these theoretical differences are practical, therapeutic ones. As D. C. Epler has recently demonstrated, the *Inner Canon's* discussions of acupuncture can be divided into chapters in which the technique involves drawing blood and those in which it merely regulates the flow of *ch'i* vitalities.[52]

Akahori Akira 赤 堀 昭 and Yamada Keiji 山 田 慶 児 have provided a compelling analysis in which certain chapters of the *Inner Canon* are understood to be commenting upon others, two sometimes differing in their interpretation of a third.[53] The book as a whole is conceptually more elaborate than several manuscripts recently excavated from a tomb of ca. 168 B.C. They clearly prefigure it (see below, page 135). Still the *Inner Canon* now can be seen as a collection of theories in the making, theories that did not reach more or less standard form until they were digested in the *Canon of Eighty-one Problems* [in the *Inner Canon*] *of the Yellow Lord* (*Huang ti pa-shih-i nan ching* 黄 帝 八 十 一 難 經 , probably second century A.D.).[54]

---

[51] Maruyama Masao 丸 山 昌 朗 1977: 238–75 (originally published 1958–62); Maruyama Toshiaki 丸 山 敏 秋 1979, 1980. The sapors are discussed in the *Revised Outline* as flavors, but see below, pages 182–83.

[52] Epler 1980.

[53] Akahori 1978a, 1979b; Yamada 1979a, 1979b, 1980.

[54] This statement assumes that the current version of this book, usually called *Nan ching* (*Canon of Problems*) for short, is reasonably faithful to the work as it first appeared. Quotations in early sources support this assumption in a general way, but we know that like its predecessors the *Nan ching* was considerably altered by later editors; see Okanishi 1974: 14–18.

Yamada has attempted to associate the diverse views found in the *Inner Canon* with different schools, which he identifies with

This process of reconciliation continued for a long time. Late in the third century the *"A-B" Canon* (*Huang ti chia i ching* 黄帝甲乙經 , 256/282) assembled from three extant works in the Yellow Lord tradition a consistent anthology of doctrine underlying acupuncture therapy. At about the same time the *Canon of the Pulse* (*Mai ching* 脈經 , ca. 280) drew upon the *Inner Canon of the Yellow Lord*, the *Canon of Problems*, the *Treatise on Cold Damage Disorders*, and other early works to provide a comprehensive handbook of diagnosis and therapeutics. From this point on, one can indeed speak of one set of basic medical doctrines. Students still learned the earliest classics, but came to rely on commentaries that explained away or ignored the divergences within and between them (as most commentaries and explanations being published today still do).

This is not to say that concepts remained unchanged from the fourth century on. They were incessantly re-explained and re-understood. New understandings often led to new discrepancies, since doctors were expected to master old books as well as new; but they saw what they studied as a single consistent body of doctrine, with certain differences due to the corruption of ancient texts, and other seeming divergences that would disappear when one comprehended the classics deeply enough.

Use of Concepts in Medicine

Yin-yang, the Five Phases, and the Six Warps made possible discourse about patterns of health, illness, and therapy compatible with patterned views of Nature. Therapeutic tasks could perhaps have been carried out without such reference to the world outside the body, as indeed most are carried out by modern clinicians. But because Chinese doctors were convinced that the body is a

---

Ch'i-po and the other five spokesmen who engage in dialogue with the Yellow Lord. The case for this identification is not persuasive. Whether the competition between schools, by any meaningful definition of the word "school," is responsible for the dissonance of ideas remains to be seen. Yamada, nevertheless, leaves no room for doubt that the *Inner Canon of the Yellow Lord* is an unintegrated compendium of writings by various hands.

microcosm and the environment a chief factor in health, abstract concepts of natural philosophy were important to them.

It will be obvious to attentive readers of the *Revised Outline* that theoretical discussions are not carried out for their own sake. Basic concepts are elaborated because they are fundamental to diagnostic and therapeutic reasoning—the overall subject of the chapters I have chosen to translate. References to diagnosis and manifestation type determination are found throughout the *Revised Outline*. References to therapy are nearly as frequent. They may appear as mentions of acupuncture loci, or in the form of phrases such as "cultivating Earth to produce Metal" (1.2.2) and "warming the splenetic system to dry up the moisture" (2.1.3.3) that sum up common therapeutic strategies in unobtrusively technical language.

As we have seen, yin-yang, the Five Phases, and the Six Warps are largely equivalent ways to divide body processes into their various aspects or phases. They were names for the types of *ch'i* responsible for change. Looking at it the other way round, the usefulness of these concepts encouraged physicians to think of the body as an ensemble of processes carried out in functional systems by *ch'i*, rather than as a structure of tissues that grow and maintain themselves and are susceptible to lesions. They encouraged doctors to see the agents of medical disorder not as things that penetrate the body and cause lesions but as external or internal agencies identified by morbid functions (heteropathic *ch'i*) that interfere with the body's vital functions (maintained by orthopathic *ch'i*). Because this relationship, like those of normal processes, was dialectical, yin-yang remained the central explanatory notion. The Five Phases and Six Warps were necessary only when a finer division was necessary. They made it easy to relate several aspects, as when discussing processes that involve the circulation tracts or the visceral systems, or the levels of penetration by heteropathy.

Use of these concepts is not mandated by the functional character of Chinese medicine. We have seen that the *Treatise on Cold Damage Disorders* restricted itself to a Six Warps explanation used with restraint, relying on lists of symptoms that directly specified the prescriptions required to treat them. By the time of the *Treatise* there had also grown up in China a literature that simply listed symptoms and prescriptions with little or no theoretical discussion.[55] For this earliest period we do not know whether the compilers of prescriptions were innocent of abstraction, or simply saw no need to use it in that connection. It is clear that later authors of this literature were considered competent in large part because they had mastered the fundamentals of theory, whether or not they imposed it on their clinical formula-books. Some did; others made the point in their prefaces or introductory chapters.

The prescription literature is inherently limited in its usefulness. Among well-trained classical physicians diagnosis in the sense of categorizing and naming the disorder was not a central task, nor even a necessary one. To proceed directly from a list of signs and symptoms to a disease and from there to a course of treatment, usual though it is in modern medicine, ignores areas of concern that become central in a holistic system of therapy.

Syndromes vary too greatly from one patient to another to be adequately described by clear-cut disease categories based on signs and symptoms. In the day-to-day work of bedside diagnosis these categories blur and flow into each other. One might of course seek precision by defining more diseases, each with a more clear-cut set of symptoms within its narrower borders. This was bound to happen as clinical experience accumulated, but the multiplication of entities made the work of the doctor no more manageable, as Yü Chen 俞震 explained in his famous collection of medical case histories (1778):

> From antiquity to the present there have been more
> books on medicine than one can keep track of. For

---

[55] Two such MSS, found in recent excavations, have only the titles given by their discoverers. *Wu-shih-erh ping fang* 五十二病方, found in 1973 at Mawangdui, Hunan, was written before 168 B.C. It has been excellently studied from a philological point of view, and a translation of the very imperfect text attempted, in Harper 1982, with full bibliography. For discussions more concerned with issues in medical history see Ma Chi-hsing 馬繼興 and Li Hsueh-ch'in 李学勤 1975 and Shang Chih-chün 尚志鈞 1981. *Wu-wei Han tai i chien* 武威漢代醫簡, unearthed in Gansu in 1972, is provisionally dated on epigraphic grounds in the mid-first century A.D. See Lo Fu-i 羅福頤 1973, Chung-i yen-chiu-yuan 中医研究院 1973, and Akahori 1978b.

each medical disorder a special category has been established, and for each category, numerous techniques. In the final reckoning, although the number of techniques may be limited, there is no limit to [the variety of] disorders. Even the variations in a single disorder are limitless. If several disorders converge in the body of one patient the variations are all the more endless. The techniques of medicine are thus bound to be inadequate. It would seem, therefore, that a preoccupation with technique will take one no further than the carpenter's or wheelwright's square and compass [would take him without ingenuity in their use]. Medical disorders do not manifest themselves according to square and compass. If the doctor simply tries to treat them according to square and compass, the cases that fit the rule will survive, and those that vary from it will die. [People who do not see the fallacy of this rigid approach], casting about, will finally blame the doctor for the insufficiency of his techniques, not realizing that it is impossible for techniques to suffice. What is crucial is the ingenuity of the one using the techniques.[56]

Yü goes on to recommend the study of cases treated by great physicians as a guide to the needed flexibility in the use of techniques.

Classical physicians were also aware that disease processes in a given patient are not static. They alter vital functions in ways that are unpredictable but not unpatterned. Their pattern is knowable only when the underlying pathological process is understood. This pathology is affected by the interaction of all the body's systems and by the interaction in time and space of the body with the macrocosm. The doctor continually gathers information—signs, symptoms, and the direct reflection of whole-body energetic states in the pulses. He digests, interprets, and reinterprets this information by applying yin-yang and the other concepts. The tool he uses for this purpose is manifestation type determination (chapters 7–9),

---

[56] *Ku chin i an an* 古今醫案按 , preface. In the second sentence Yü is referring to the classification of disorders in medical books, not to specialized fields of practice.

which will be discussed shortly in connection with diagnosis (pages 173–77 below).

The understanding and use of classical concepts have been changing rapidly in recent decades. For instance, the interpretation of the Five Phases in classical thought offered above is plainly at odds with the definition of this concept in the *Revised Outline*. According to the latter's depiction of ancient thought, the "fundamental materials out of which the universe was constructed" provided a classification system for all things and events (1.2.1); this was "a simple materialist theory" (1.0). This is a defensible way to understand the earliest speculations about *wu-hsing*, but the emphasis on materialist character and static classification ignores the sophisticated form of the theory that shaped early medical thought. The emphasis is understandable when we recall that the book is written for physicians trained in modern Western science and (like every educated Chinese) in dialectical materialism. Such readers are not likely to take seriously ideas that do not look respectable from at least one of these viewpoints. One can understand the authors' desire to meet the understanding of their public halfway. In any case this view of origins does not deter the authors from describing the Five Phases as a system of thought used to investigate "the mutual relations between phenomena" (1.2.1) rather than the material composition of things.

Chapter III

HEALTH AND DISORDER

Health

The *Revised Outline of Chinese Medicine* does not define either health or sickness, nor do its predecessors or more recent publications. There is in fact no single word in traditional medicine that corresponds exactly to "health."[1] Health has come to mean a great many things in Western European languages, from the mere absence of disease or injury to well-being in the broadest sense. If we consider the conservative lexicographer's understanding, "soundness of body; that condition in which its functions are duly and efficiently discharged,"[2] we find in Chinese a number of everyday words—words that mean "normal," "harmonious," "relaxed"—used by physicians to describe just that condition of the body or its

---

[1] The term for health in everyday language, *chien-k'ang* 健康 , is a recent borrowing from modern Japanese.

[2] *OED*, sense 1, going back to the beginnings of the English language. It is interesting that a few decades earlier medical lexicographers were less concerned with efficiency than harmony: "a state in which all the functions are exerted with regularity and harmony" (Dunglison 1874: 921, s.v. *sanitas*). The World Health Organization gives health a scope that lies far beyond the physician's power to affect it fundamentally: "a state of complete physical, mental, or social well-being and not merely the absence of disease or infirmity" (Clayton L. Thomas ed. 1973: H-9). Dunglison, by contrast, considers a blind man healthy when all his functions except sight are regular. Deane C. Epler is preparing for publication a study of health concepts in Chinese medical sources to ca. A.D. 300; see also Chiu 1986.

functional systems. For instance, in the *Divine Pivot* of the *Inner Canon, p'ing jen* 平 人 means "a person whose body functions normally."

We have seen in connection with the discussion of *ch'i* above that some of the aspects of normal body function had been defined by the third century B.C. (see page 48). Recapitulating these aspects along with others that became important later gives us a general outline of what for the past thousand years has constituted health in classical medicine:

1. Energies are continuously extracted from food and breath and the residues are expelled. According to the capacity of the stomach and intestines computed in the *Inner Canon*, the body normally processes fixed amounts of solid and liquid nutriment determined by the capacity of the stomach and intestines.[3]

---

[3] In order to understand these passages, it is necessary first to determine what metrological standard is used—assuming, as one must at the outset, that there is one consistent standard. The choice lies between the measures of the Western Han period, when the early *Inner Canon* texts were probably written, and those of the Chou, which would not be out of place in texts seeking to create an impression of archaic origins. A criterion for choice is offered by two passages. TS, *13* (2): 228 = LS, *4* (14): 39 speaks of a commoner (*chung jen* 眾 人) as 7.5 *ch'ih* 尺 tall; TS, *5* (4): 65 = LS, *3* (12): 34 speaks of a gentleman (*shih* 士) as 8 *ch'ih* tall. By the Western Han standard of 27.65 cm/ *ch'ih* these would amount to 2.1 m (6 feet 10 inches) and 2.2 m (7 feet 3 inches); by the Chou standard (19.91 cm/*ch'ih*), 1.5 m (4 feet 11 inches) and 1.6 (5 feet 3 inches) respectively. The latter heights are typical of excavated male human remains, so an obvious working hypothesis is that the Chou system was used.

According to TS, *13* (3): 231–35, the combined capacity of the stomach and intestines for solid and liquid nutriment is 66.68 *sheng* (in Chou volume measure, equivalent to 12.92 liters). Because these organs are not simultaneously full in a normal person (*p'ing jen*), the amount of nutriment they regularly contain is 24 *sheng* (5 1) of solid food and 11 *sheng* (2 1) of liquid. The corresponding texts in LS, *6* (32): 131, give different figures, 92.13 *sheng* (17.85 1), 20 *sheng* (4 1), and 15 *sheng* (3 1). The sum of

2. Vital energies penetrate throughout the body in an equitable, unimpeded circulation. This metabolic circulation maintains not only life but order and invulnerability to invasion.

3. Vital substances are sealed within the body and heteropathy sealed out, without interrupting normal ingestion and excretion.

4. The mind is centered and free of inappropriate, immoderate emotions.

5. A dynamic balance maintains itself among somatic functions, among emotional functions, and between the two aspects.

6. This endless process of renewal is spontaneous and ordered, cyclical in character, its daily and seasonal rhythms in accord with those of the environment.[4]

7. The orderly character of this process depends on an orderly life. The understanding of order came to include

---

the last two values, 35 *sheng*, is the same in both books (an earlier mention of 30 *sheng* total content is obviously a rounded figure). Quotations in later writings give still different figures, so there is no basis for choosing between the TS and LS versions.

The two books agree that the normal body excretes 5 *sheng* (1 l) of solid waste per day. The further statement that a person who fasts will die after seven days (when the 35 *sheng* of food is used up) implies that a normal diet is also 5 *sheng* of solid food per day. Yang Shang-shan and other commentators make this point explicit. No volume is assigned to the part of the food that is extracted as vital essences, so there is no difference in intake and outflow on that account. The figures given above are not said to be averages, nor is there any discussion of variations in body size.

[4] It is difficult to choose between texts that illustrate these six points, but one of the most compendious is TS, *6* (2): 76 = LS, *74* (47): 75. The central importance of yin-yang balance in health is emphasized in TS, *3* (2): 34–41 = SW, *1* (3): 13–20.

not only physical and mental hygiene, but moral discipline, spiritual purity, and a life lived in harmony
with the physical environment, governed in turn by the
cosmic order.

This last point, read into the archaic Golden Age and contrasted
with the degenerate present, is set out in the opening chapter of the
Inner Canon's Basic Questions:

> The people of archaic times who understood the
> Way modeled [their lives] on [the rhythms of] yin
> and yang, and accorded with the regularities im-
> posed by disciplines [of self-cultivation]. Their eating
> and drinking were controlled, their activity and rest
> were regular, and they did not exhaust themselves
> capriciously. Thus it was possible for their bodies
> and their consciousnesses to be at one, so that they
> lived out their natural spans of life, passing away
> when their hundred years had been measured out.
> People of our times are not like that. Wine is
> their drink, caprice their norm. Drunken they enter
> the chamber of love, through lust using up their
> seminal essence (*ching* 精 , 3.3), through desire dis-
> persing their inborn vitality (*chen* [*ch'i*] 真 氣 ,
> 3.1.1). They do not know how to "hold up the full
> [vessel"; that is, avoid "spilling" their energies], nor
> how to control their consciousness (?*shen* 神).
> Devoted to the pleasures of the heart and mind, they
> reject the bliss that accompanies cultivation of the vi-
> tal forces. Without self-control in their activity or
> rest, they are worn out at half a hundred.[5]

These notions became general among laymen as well as doctors,
although the latter could of course express them more technically.
They still underlie traditional medical thought, and are abundantly
reflected in this book. We need not expect them to be stated. Some

---

[5] SW, *1* (1): 2. I have consulted emendations in Ch'eng Shih-te
程 士 德 ed. 1982: 2. This is a comprehensive but often careless digest of textual variations and pertinent commentaries. Un-
fortunately its basic text is in simplified characters.

medical books before modern times discuss them explicitly, especially in connection with hygiene and longevity, and often with reference to the passage just translated—but most do not.[6]

The most obvious recent change has affected the final characteristic of health. Although many ideals of imperial times have been decisively rejected in the twentieth century, respect for a disciplined life has hardly lessened; but it is no longer defined with reference to spiritual and cosmic dimensions. The conditions of health as taught today hardly go beyond physical and mental hygiene, although it is understood that morality, especially political morality, affects the state of mind.[7]

Medical Disorders

Medical disorders are interruptions of the normal functions outlined above. These interruptions, called *ping* 病 , correspond not only to what are now called systemic diseases or syndromes but also to localized lesions. There is remarkably little difference in the way these two types are discussed. In principle even wounds and skin disorders are treated holistically. Since "disease" is too narrow, I translate *ping* as "medical disorder."[8] Although *ping* is the

---

[6] Two of the best-known discussions that take the *Inner Canon* chapter as a starting point are in the introductory works *I hsueh ju men* 醫 學 入 門 (1575), prefatory chapter: 77, and *Ching-yueh ch'üan shu* (1624), "Ch'uan chung lu," 2: 46a-48b.

[7] The *Village Physician's Handbook*, a product of the Cultural Revolution, instructs medical workers treating mental disorders to "help the patient use Chairman Mao's dialectical materialist viewpoint to analyze and recognize the abnormal condition and . . . establish a correct ideological viewpoint, a correct attitude toward the masses, and a reformed world view," a procedure more than slightly parallel—despite great terminological differences—to the use of Freudian theory in some traditions of American psychotherapy. See Hu-nan i-hsueh-yuan ed. 1971: 454b.

[8] This conveys a fundamental connotation of *ping*, the antonym of which in classical medical writings is *chih* 治 , or "order." When used verbally, *chih* is often translated "treat" or "cure," but the basic sense is "to overcome disorder." A common antonym of

most common word for disorders, there were other words for narrower uses (see below, pages 106–7).

Causes

Physicians generally thought about the causes of medical disorders in two ways. The first was concerned with what irregularity
in hygiene or orderly life (point 7 above) created an internal imbalance or broke the accord with the environment (point 6), weakening the ability of the orthopathic *ch'i* to maintain internal order
(point 5) and keep the body invulnerable to invasion (point 3). The
second way of thinking about etiology considered the character of
the heteropathy and, more centrally, its activities within the body
that oppose the body's regular functions. Exhaustion, defective diet,
or inappropriate expression of emotion may lead to an abnormal
level—depletion or repletion (*hsu shih* 虛 實 , 7.3 below)—of the
body's vital resources (5.4–5.6). The influence of unseasonal
weather, which overwhelms the body's ability to adapt to its surroundings, may then be reified and invade as a heteropathic *ch'i*
(5.1–5.3). These irregularities of internal and external origin interact to bring about disorder, as in the *Inner Canon*:

> If wind, rain, cold, or heat do not encounter a deple-
> tion [of bodily vitality], their heteropathic *ch'i* alone
> is unable to harm people. When one unexpectedly
> experiences a windstorm or rainstorm and does not
> become ill, the reason must be that there is no deple-
> tion, and the heteropathy alone is unable to harm
> people. It must be that only when a depleting,
> heteropathic wind encounters within the body a
> second depletion that it can possess the body. When
> the two repletions meet, [as when the wind and rain,
> etc., are normal seasonal phenomena, and] the flesh
> is firm as in the majority of people [and thus a sign
> of repletion, the body does not become possessed by
> heteropathy and no disorder results]. When one is
> attacked by depletion heteropathy, when Nature's

---

chih in political rather than medical contexts is *luan* 亂 : "disorder, chaos."

> season and the body interact in circumstances in
> which [the latter is] depleted and [the former]
> replete, a serious disorder will result.[9]

Although the importance of interaction is clear in this passage, the basis for determining what is depletion and what is repletion is not. In the *Inner Canon* depletion and repletion, as yin and yang aspects of energetic imbalance, are always relational to each other or to a norm, but the relation is usually vague. They refer, among other things, to relative strength of orthopathic versus heteropathic *ch'i*, to strength of the disorder, to cold or hot character, and to whether the disordered function is downward and diffusing (depletion) or upward and congealing (repletion).[10]

Systematizers of medicine over the centuries attempted to define depletion and repletion with reference to symptoms, for instance the dictum of Ch'eng Kuo-p'eng 程 國 彭 (1732): "Whether a given disorder is of repletion or depletion type is distinguished entirely by whether or not there is perspiration, whether there are distention and pain in the abdomen, whether the distention abates, whether the pain is aggravated or diminished by pressure, whether the symptoms are old or new, whether the patient's constitution is delicate or robust, and whether the pulse is empty or full (i.e., depleted or replete, *hsu shih*; 6.4.1.2.3)."[11]

This still ignores the substantial question of exactly what states one is distinguishing. It could have been settled only by rigorous and comprehensive definitions of depletion and repletion, which have yet to appear. The account of the relations of these two entities in

---

[9] TS, *27* (5): 512–13 = LS, *10* (66): 100. In the first three sentences the two texts differ sufficiently to call for quite different punctuations, and would thus require different translations. I follow the wording of LS, since, read according to TS, the argument is internally contradictory; a depletion heteropathy (*hsu hsieh* 虛 邪) *in addition to* the climatic factors is placed both outside and within the body. The penultimate sentence is defective, and is not improved by the free rewording in *Chia i ching*, *8* (2): 9a-9b. I have filled out the sense by inserting the words in brackets to reflect Yang Shang-shan's commentary (666/683?); this cannot be considered better than a reasonable guess.

[10] See the discussion in Jen Ying-ch'iu 1978: 70–71.

[11] *I hsueh hsin wu* 醫 學 心 悟 , *1*: 18b.

the *Revised Outline* (7.3) is typical of modern doctrine, which tends to equate depletion with a deficit in the orthopathic energies and repletion with invasion by a heteropathic *ch'i*. But that is, as the last quotation from the *Inner Canon* makes clear, a simplification of the classical understanding.[12]

The language of possession

In the citation from the *Inner Canon*, it may be surprising to find language reminiscent of spirit possession. The terminology for agents of medical disorder considered as a class is in fact derived from an ancient stratum of popular thought that sees disease as invasion by malevolent spiritual forces. The terms translated "heteropathy" or "heteropathic" (*hsieh* 邪) and "possess" (*k'o* 客) above reflect this popular view, in which *hsieh* (lit., "malignancy") is the general term for beings that enter and take over control of the body. Despite this origin, in medical writings *hsieh* has such animistic connotations only when possession is being explicitly discussed as one cause of illness among many. The word has simply become a technical term, suggestive to the student of history but matter-of-fact to the doctor, just as the word "evil" was used in English until the late nineteenth century for certain diseases.[13]

"Heteropathy" in this classical understanding was as featureless a term as "infectious agent." Even broader, *hsieh* referred to anything responsible for a breach of the body's order. Disease was an invasion, normally commencing through the pores and interstices of the flesh, and—unless halted by strong orthopathic forces or time-

---

[12] The explanation in section 7.3 below is less reductive than those given in many recent publications, for instance Pei-ching Chung-i hsueh-yuan ed. 1974: 117 and Chung-i yen-chiu-yuan et al., ed. 1982: 275, s.v.

[13] *OED*, substantive sense 7. See for instance, the "King's evil," scrofula; the "Aleppo evil," cutaneous leishmaniasis; the "foul evil," various eruptive disorders; the "falling evil," epilepsy. Other Chinese medical terms for invasion by a heteropathy that were borrowed from the popular language of spirit possession, in addition to *hsieh* and *k'o*, include *kan* 干 and *chu* 注 (see below).

ly therapy—advancing inexorably inward.[14] The movement from periphery to center could be analyzed in several ways: from the skin (outer aspect, 7.1) toward the visceral systems (inner aspect); through the Six Warps, or the circulation tracts associated with them (9.5); or through the sectors named for four vital fluids (9.1). These schemes originated in different writings, and are chosen according to the diagnostic and therapeutic approach the physician wishes to take.

Not only did doctors of the classical tradition tend to abstract the meanings of popular terms as they adapted them, but even when discussing possession as a source of medical pathology they were more concerned with its propagation through the body's functional systems than with the character of the spiritual agencies responsible. Here, for instance, is part of the general discussion of possession disorders from *Origins and Symptoms of Medical Disorders* (610), the first comprehensive handbook of etiology and symptomatology, which remained the main source of information on its two topics for more than five hundred years:

> When we say that "possession" (*chu* 注) means "to stay" (*chu* 住), we mean that a heteropathic *ch'i* (*hsieh ch'i*) takes up residence within the patient's body. That is why these disorders are called "possession." They are brought about by wind, cold, hot, or moist factors or by exhaustion (5.1, 5.6) when yin and yang [orthopathic *ch'i*] fail to maintain their division of responsibility and the circulation tracts (4.1) have become depleted. When in Cold Damage Disorders perspiration is not induced in time [to flush out the heteropathy] or, although it is induced, one does not obtain "genuine perspiration"; when the

---

[14] The "interstices of the flesh" (*ts'ou-li* 腠理 , a terms that includes the pores) refers to the space in the boundaries within the flesh, between flesh and skin, and sometimes between flesh and internal organs. These provide avenues through the body's periphery. One passage in the *Inner Canon* speaks of the spaces in the twelve main joints of the extremities and 354 minor junctions, in which, when the circulation of defensive *ch'i* is interrupted, heteropathy may settle. See TS, *17* (1): 313 = SW, *3* (10): 63.

heteropathy is transmitted from the three yang
tracts to the yin tracts and, entering the five yin visceral systems of function (2.1), is not promptly expelled and becomes static; when a [hot or cold]
heteropathic *ch'i* due to Overnight Food Accumulation Disorder (6.3.2) or an imbalance of cooling and
heating food enters the circulation and possesses
[some part of the body]; or when one unbeknownst
provokes [invasion by a contaminating] *ch'i* consequent upon childbirth or death, or disturbs demonic
beings, these possession disorders may be the outcome.[15]

The topic is treated in highly rational language, and the emphasis on predisposing depletion of the body's vitality ties it into the
main body of classical theory (as do the many diagnostic terms).
We can see plain traces of popular spiritualistic beliefs such as
taboos connected with birth and death near the end of this quotation, but for many classical authors demonic *ch'i* have come to
represent only a subgroup in a large class of entrenched
heteropathies which may "possess" part or all of the body, and in
many cases may be communicated to other people. The book
describes individually thirty-three types of possession disorder.

Possession disorders have generally been cast out of traditional
medicine as it is now taught in China. Ideologists identify anything
connected with popular religious belief as "superstition"; a great
deal of administrative effort has gone into eradicating belief in spirit
possession.[16] Belief in possession is now obviously rare among

---

[15] *Chu ping yuan hou lun* 諸病源候論, 24: 130a. The first
sentence is an instance of definition by homophone, frequent in
Chinese lexicography. "Genuine perspiration" (*chen han* 真汗)
is perspiration capable of expelling the heteropathy while it is in
the outer aspect of the body (9.0, 9.5).

[16] Even some new editions of classical medical books excise "superstitious" content, although only the highly educated can read
their classical Chinese. This censorship is prevalent particularly
in early sources on obstetrics and gynecology, which tend to richly reflect popular beliefs. See, for instance, the 1958 ed. of *Fu
k'o yü ch'ih* 婦科玉尺 (1774; reprinted 1983), and the
1982 ed. of *Ch'an chien* 産鑑 (1618). Most unfortunate is the

people who have grown up since 1949, although not at all hard to find in Asian Chinese communities outside the mainland.

Someone who wants to understand how healing works may doubt that shades of the dead can enter the bodies of the living, without denying that a set of experiences that people in many parts of the world interpret as possession was a social fact in traditional Chinese communities, often felt and witnessed by their members. Despite the rejection of spiritualism in China, it is not difficult to find traces of possession disorders in recent pedagogical writings if we follow the principle that the most conservative elements tend to be retained in the most specialized materials. In a series of lectures on manifestation type determination for graduate students at the Academy of Traditional Chinese Medicine, the highest research organization in the field, for instance, we find a list of about a hundred and fifty traditional *ping*-syndromes, diseases, and disease groups. Eight of these fall clearly into classical possession categories. Four

---

removal of "superstitious and irrational material" from the 1959–62 reprint of the section on medicine from the great universal encyclopedia of 1725, *Ku chin t'u shu chi ch'eng*, "I pu" 古 今 圖 書 集 成 醫 部 . This source, which quotes over a hundred books in full or at length, is often used by sinologists to locate original sources.

Some new editions that are not censored still treat the ideas of popular religion as dangerous. For instance, Nan-ching Chung-i hsueh-yuan ed. 1980, an annotated critical edition of *Chu ping yuan hou lun* with translation into modern Chinese, does not translate the Chinese phrase corresponding to "or disturbs demonic beings" above (1, 689–90). In an introductory note to the 1983 reprint of the pediatric textbook *Ying-t'ung lei ts'ui* 嬰 童 類 萃 (1622), the editors find it necessary to "point out that in premodern Chinese medical books there are problems that modern science cannot yet explain and, due to limitations of historical circumstance, some improper content may be interspersed. We hope that readers will respond in a correct manner from a dialectical materialist point of view, seriously studying the theories and experiences recorded in these books, using scientific method to sort them out and enhance them, in order to 'excavate their treasures and absorb their essences.'" Warnings of this kind are not lightly disregarded by anyone who has lived through the Cultural Revolution.

are varieties of *chu*. Although the approach is rationalistic and spirit possession is not mentioned, in some cases the implication remains clear. Cardiac system *chu* pain, for instance, is "brought on by fright when one goes into old shrines in mountains or forests and sees unusual things."[17]

Symptom, syndrome, disease

We have seen that medical disorders can be explained not only as regular bodily functions gone awry but also as abnormal functions that take over the body's systems. Pain is usually explained as a by-product of the struggle between abnormal and normal functions, reified as heteropathic and orthopathic *ch'i* (e.g., 8.4.7). But disorders were not merely dysfunctions; they were also phenomena.

Modern physicians distinguish the ideas of symptom, syndrome, and disease. The symptom is the smallest unit employed in diagnosis. It is sometimes divided into symptoms reported by the patient and signs observed by the physician, in this century increasingly supplemented by laboratory findings. The syndrome is a recurring set of symptoms that characterize a pathological process but may be associated with more than one disease. The disease is a group of symptoms with a coherent and recurring etiology and developmental history. There is considerable blurring at the borders between these concepts.

In traditional Chinese nosology, as in European medicine as late as the nineteenth century, there is much more blurring between categories. I have already noted that the universal term *ping*, translated "medical disorder" or "disorder" here, includes the modern categories of traumas as well as diseases. It often refers to symptoms, syndromes, and groups of related syndromes or diseases as well. Traditional doctors are perfectly able to make distinctions close to that between symptom, syndrome, and disease when it is important to do so. The terms *hou* 候 and *cheng* 症 correspond roughly to "symptom," and *chi* 疾 to "disease."[18]

---

[17] Fang Yao-chung 方藥中 1979: 79.

[18] In late writings we can find lucid discussions of the differences between these categories, e.g., in *I hsueh yuan-liu lun* 醫學源流論 (1757), *1*: 68. *I hsueh hsin wu* (1732) prints symbols alongside the text when its author wishes to distinguish dis-

More often than in modern medicine, however, given diagnostic entities can belong to more than one category. Jaundice (*huang tan* 黄疸 , *fu huang* 膚黄 , etc.) is often, as in modern medicine, a symptom, but it can also be a group of diseases that share a collection of symptoms. *Huang tan* is sometimes a subclass of the larger jaundice group *huang ping* 黄病 . *Origins and Symptoms of Medical Disorders*, for instance, lists more than forty kinds of *huang ping*, in all of which the skin is yellow. This group of disorders as described in the seventh century has in common not only jaundice, but generalized body pains, aching in the eyes and the bridge of the nose, feelings of tension in the belly and elsewhere, and hot sensations intensifying after a week or so. They also share certain aspects of causation, notably hot or moist heteropathy, often due to incorrect diet, building up in the splenetic and stomach systems (2.1.3).[19]

This looseness of distinction between disease and symptom is not unique to Chinese medicine, but was common in other advanced systems before very recent times. As an example, take Robert Thomas' *The Modern Practice of Physic, Exhibiting the Characters, Causes, Symptoms, Prognostics, Morbid Appearances, and Improved Method of Treating the Diseases of All Climates* (first published in 1801), one of the first treatises to describe worldwide diseases and at the same time one of many contemporary attempts to produce a taxonomy of disease as exact as that of Linnaeus in botany. Jaundice appears as Order III of Class III, "cachexiae" (wasting diseases connected with chronic conditions). It is clearly a disease, with complex symptoms, caused by bile stones, tumors, "passions of the mind," and so on, but "jaundice is often an attendant symptom on an inflammation or schirrhosity of the liver, pancreas, &c., and frequently likewise on pregnancy."[20]

Cases are easy to find in which premodern European nosology was as ambiguous as Chinese classification of the same period. Fever was not an entity in traditional Chinese medicine. The word

---

orders (*ping*) from symptoms (*cheng*), a vertical rectangle for the former and small triangles for the latter.

[19] *Chu ping yuan hou lun, 12*: 70–72. Some important later sources call this large class *huang tan* (for instance, *Sheng chi tsung lu* 聖濟總錄 of 1117, *60*: 1100–61: 1123) or simply *tan* (*Ku chin t'u shu chi ch'eng,* "I pu," ch. 285–87).

[20] Robert Thomas 1817: 599–609, especially page 600.

used in modern medical discourse for fever, *je* 熱 , when used alone by traditional doctors referred unambiguously to a symptom, hot sensations reported by the patient, and was the opposite of *han* 寒 , "chills." Only in certain compounds, such as *fa je* 發熱 , does it sometimes (not consistently) refer to elevated skin temperature.

Either *je* or *han* might indicate fever to the modern physician. He would confirm this interpretation with a thermometer, for he thinks of fever as elevated body temperature—not primarily a sensation of the patient, but a state determined by the doctor. But until the fever thermometer came into general use in the twentieth century, fever was a disease of which "increased heat of skin" was only one of many symptoms. As the American *Medical Lexicon* (1874) of Robley Dunglison puts it, "A person has an attack of fever, when is is affected with rigors [i.e., sensation of cold with involuntary shivering], followed by increased heat of skin, quick pulse, languor, and lassitude. Rigors, increased heat, and frequency of pulse have each been assumed as the essential character of fever. It is not characterized, however, by any *one*, but depends upon the coexistence of *many* symptoms." Savill's *System of Clinical Medicine,* the great English diagnostic handbook revised and reissued over a generation from 1903 on, was still, in its 1930 edition, using the clinical thermometer only to confirm a diagnosis based on an even longer list of signs and symptoms than Dunglison's.[21]

The catalogue of disorders in Chinese medicine became enormous. The massive *Imperial Grace Formulary* (*T'ai-p'ing sheng hui fang* 太平聖惠方   , completed 992), for instance, provides prescriptions for roughly a thousand distinct disorders (not counting those listed separately for women and children). In the prescription literature and the materia medica tradition, bites of different animals, poisoning from different foods, growths of different shapes on different parts of the body, abscesses of different etiology, hemorrhoids of different shape, similar syndromes that affect different visceral systems, and so on, are listed separately. This is not surprising in a tradition attempting to organize an enormous accumulation of prescriptions, especially when these prescriptions originally identify their object in ways that were systematized only so far. Such a detailed catalogue of suffering is useful to physicians

---

[21] Dunglison 1874: 416; Savill 1930: 498. The *Revised Outline,* like other recent texts, tends to use *je* in the modern rather than the traditional sense. I translate accordingly.

seeking a specific formula (specific by traditional, not modern, criteria). It is hardly a satisfactory basis for diagnosis, which depends not on accumulation but on classification. As diseases multiplied, the effort to find a rational arrangement for them did not intensify.

Manifestation types

Chinese physicians were nevertheless cutting through the plethora of diseases as quickly as these diseases multiplied. They concerned themselves less with diagnosis in the sense that modern doctors use the word than with manifestation type determination (*pien cheng* 辨 證).[22]

Several systems for typing manifestations—making the necessary distinctions—are described in chapters 7-9 of the *Revised Outline*. Each yields a simple, schematic characterization of the patient's condition, in which a great many symptoms have been translated into a small number of dynamic characteristics (*ch'i* level, visceral functions involved, penetration of the heteropathy, etc.). In the most popular system (chapter 7), based on the *Inner Canon*, the type was expressed in up to four terms each chosen from a binary pair (outer/inner, hot/cold, etc.). Once the physician

---

[22] For this translation I am grateful to the ingenuity of Hans Ågren, M.D. A literal translation, "making distinctions on the basis of evidence," misses the technical meaning. *Cheng* alone may refer to particular manifestations, signs, or symptoms, that serve as the basis for typing, to the analytic process that leads to determination of type, or to the outcome of the determination. *Cheng* are basically interpretations of symptoms, "processed pieces of information that are utilized in correlating disease with a proper therapy" (Ågren 1975: 39). Fang Yao-chung (1979: 86–89) argues in an extended discussion of the meaning of *pien cheng* that in medicine *cheng* means primarily "evidence" (the most common sense of the word). His argument makes it clear that *cheng* is evidence after it has been processed—assimilated to a dialectical framework so that it determines a type. "Manifestation" (*OED* sense 1) is superior to "evidence" for conveying the scope of *cheng*. Kaptchuk's "distinguishing patterns" for *pien cheng* is also satisfactory (1983: 179).

has determined that the disorder is of the outer cold type, the therapeutic approach is settled (7.2.1).

In the Six Warps system of the *Treatise on Cold Damage Disorders* (9.5), the types were originally referred to by the name of the prescription recommended in the *Treatise* for each. For instance, the Mature Yang stage, the first stage of penetration of febrile disease, is also called the Cassia Twig Infusion manifestation type.[23] The Six Warps system was the least abstractly organized of the typing systems widely used through history. What we find under each of the six rubrics—themselves abstract enough—is elaborate lists of variant symptoms and complications, each example with its own therapy. The connection is so direct that there is no need for intermediate concepts. But implicit in all this detail is an idea of deviant process which the physician seeks to control and overcome.

The preference of highly trained doctors for manifestation type determination over disease classification—and the prominence given manifestation type determination in this book—amounts to an insistence on thinking about medical disorder as a dynamic process. Instead of choosing one pigeonhole in a large, rigid structure, the doctor assesses the multivariate relations of a small number of characteristics that apply to every clinical picture. Chu Chen-heng 朱 震 亨 , one of the major theorists of the last millennium, stresses in his *Supplementary Discussions for the Perfection of Understanding through Investigation of Phenomena* (1347) the need to track the penetration of heteropathy if therapy is to root it out:

> In medical disorder there is a root aspect (10.4.1), just as a plant has a root. If you get rid of the leaves but not the root, the plant is still there. Treating illness is like getting rid of a plant. If the disorder is in the yin visceral systems and you treat the yang systems ["outer" with respect to yin systems, 2.1, 2.1.1.3], or if it is in the outer aspect and you use attack therapy in the inner aspect, not only will you do violence to the *ch'i* [i.e., vitality extracted

---

[23] See above, page 86.

from nutriment] in the stomach system but you will actually aid the heteropathy in its work.[24]

Therapy depends much less on the specific character of the heteropathy than on what functions it is affecting at the moment. Have we come upon a neat opposition between Chinese holistic, process-oriented pathology and a European tendency to isolate distinct species—whether diseases, lesions, or microorganisms? Like many such neat distinctions, this one disappears when we compare like with like, that is, early medicine in both civilizations. Before the mid-seventeenth century, few diseases entered the discourse of European physicians.[25] They were concerned rather with the overall condition of the vital processes, analyzed by reference to the balance of the Four Humours, or in other ways. Even as the role of disease species grew and spawned elaborate taxonomies, the authority of Galen maintained an important place for humoural reasoning in the medical schools until well into the nineteenth century. The difference between analysis of whole-body states and diagnosis of individual diseases is not a basic cultural difference, in other words, but a matter of strategies that competed within each culture.

It is not surprising that we should find humouralism in Europe and manifestation type theories in China at the elite end of the spectrum of health care. To consider the Chinese case, skilled determination of manifestation type, regardless of the system used for analysis, requires elaborate training in both clinical and philosophical aspects of medicine. Before modern times such training was available to only a small minority of those who provided therapy. The rest could not hope to go far beyond memorizing lists of symptoms structured into particular disorders for which the techniques at their command were useful.

Recent Trends

In the course of modernizing Chinese medicine for teaching in medical schools to students with little exposure to pre-Marxian

---

[24] *Ko chih yü lun* 格 致 餘 論 , page 3. On attack therapy see below, page 177.
[25] See Cohen 1981: 212.

philosophy—to whom the Five Phases are almost as exotic as to a European—the custodians of the tradition are unavoidably moving toward a conceptually simpler, more symptomatic approach to diagnosis. This can be seen in chapter 8 of this book, which describes visceral system manifestation type determination. This is a recent system of analysis which in effect leads the medical student from a list of symptoms without further exercise of judgment to a specific visceral manifestation type. These would hardly differ from diseases except for their restricted number and their fairly systematic definition in terms of disordered functions. As the examples of therapy translated in chapter 8 show, each of these disease entities is related to a specific technique of treatment; for instance, for cardiac system *ch'i* depletion, one "replenishes the cardiac *ch'i* and calms the mind" (8.1.1). This looks like a broad therapeutic strategy; but in chapter 8 most such strategies are identified with a single prescription. The visceral system of analysis has obvious affinities to classical manifestation type determination, but is largely taxonomic.[26]

Its prominence signals a period of accelerated transition in manifestation type determination.[27] A system that can be mastered by memorizing lists of symptoms rather than learning to subt-

---

[26] Compare Shryock 1936: 14–15, 188.

[27] Although visceral system manifestation type determination became a highly ramified and widely used system in the last generation, it developed over a millennium. Its origins go back to the *Chung tsang ching* 中藏經 [Canon kept in the palace repository], attributed to the Six Dynasties physician Hua T'o 華佗 but probably Northern Sung. The system set out in the *Chung tsang ching* depends more heavily than the modern version on pulse diagnosis. Its information seems to come more from earlier classic works than from the author's clinical experience (see Okanishi 1958: 710–24 and Jen Ying-ch'iu 1980: 23–24). A less doubtful early source is Ch'ien I's 錢乙 important pediatric work *Hsiao-erh yao cheng chih chueh* 小兒藥證直訣 (1119), ch. 1.

The visceral system of manifestation type determination is prominent in recent medical-school textbooks such as Pei-ching Chung-i hsueh-yuan ed. 1978: 112–27, Hu-pei Chung-i hsueh-yuan ed. 1978: 75–88, Chang Hsueh-yung et al. ed. 1979: 55–63, and Nan-ching Chung-i hsueh-yuan 1983: 66–86.

ly weigh a few related factors is desirable when physicians are being trained as quickly as possible on an unprecedented scale. Modern medicine, with its emphasis on differential diagnosis, is obviously an influence in the same direction.

The same transition is perceptible when we look closely at current etiology. There is, for instance, an odd inconsistency in the discussions of jaundice in the *Revised Outline of Chinese Medicine*. In the section on causes of medical disorders, jaundice is described in the usual (but not only) classical way as due to moist-hot heteropathy pent up in the splenetic or stomach system (5.1.4.1.3).[28] In the chapters on the visceral systems and on diagnosis, however, jaundice is unconventionally explained by reference to the gall bladder functions (2.1.2.2, 6.2.1.2, 8.3.4). This is clearly a matter of Western influence; in modern medicine jaundice results from deposition in the skin and sclera of bile pigment, due to excess of bilirubin in the blood.

A look at the many textbooks on traditional medicine published in the last quarter-century demonstrates that this change is not an anomaly. We find instead an interesting progression of changing explanations, which I will summarize using only a few representative titles.

The *Outline of Chinese Medicine* (1958) and other publications of the next decade or so give a straightforward classical explanation of jaundice. In *Simplified Teaching Materials on Chinese Medicine* (1971), this is no longer true. Jaundice is listed as a symptom of moist-hot heteropathy in the hepatic and gall bladder systems, associated with gallstones, but elsewhere is said to be a symptom of splenetic and stomach system depletion. This and other books written as late as 1974 were responses to a national campaign to expand public hygiene and primary medical care, and to integrate traditional and modern medicine. Sections on particular diseases in these publications are organized according to Western nosology. Although they are clear about the differences between the Western diseases they describe and traditional disorders, they apply classical manifestation type determination and therapeutic reasoning to the former (for instance, in part 4 of *Simplified Teaching Materials*). We

---

[28] On the early understanding of jaundice see Miyasita 1976.

find similar but not identical inconsistencies in the *Revised Outline* of 1972 and in *Simplified Chinese Medicine* of 1974.[29]

A second major transition also came in 1974, in *Foundations of Chinese Medicine*, a textbook for traditional medical schools, with therapeutic discussions based on classical Chinese nosology. Rather than choosing between classical and modern explanations, this book combines them by arguing that when the splenetic system becomes responsible for circulatory dysfunction, an internal circulation stasis due to moist heteropathy may force the bile to "overflow" into the blood. This did not become the definitive explanation, but in writings up to 1978 the point remained established that jaundice must be explained with reference to all four visceral systems of function, and the old and new explanations must not only coexist but somehow be reconciled.

Since the end of the Great Proletarian Cultural Revolution this demand for synthesis, although not always given priority, is still very much in view. The revised *Foundations of Traditional Chinese Medicine* of 1978, written, like its predecessor, for traditional physicians in training, gives both the old and new explanations, but separately, without reference to each other. The *Unabridged Dictionary of Chinese Medicine* (1982) explains jaundice as a result of bile overflow without mentioning the splenetic or stomach systems. Only the chronic *yin huang* 阴黄 type (6.2.1.2) is related to the splenetic system, but without reference to the gall bladder or bile. Other recent publications, such as the *Internal Medicine* of 1979–80 and *Basic Theories of Chinese Medicine* of 1984, provide substantial discussions of jaundice with full involvement of the splenetic and stomach as well as hepatic and gall bladder functions. At one point in the latter book, the hepatic system's inability to facilitate the assimilative splenetic and stomach functions affects gall bile secretion. At another point, splenetic yang *ch'i* deficiency may indirectly affect the hepatic and gall bladder systems. These etiologies of jaundice are not contradictory. In the classic understanding there are many possibilities for interaction.[30]

---

[29] Nan-ching Chung-i hsueh-yuan ed. 1958: 167; T'ien-chin i-hsueh-yuan 天 津 医 学 院 et al. ed. 1971: 44, 10; below, 5.1.4.1.3, 8.3.4; Ho-pei hsin i ta-hsueh 河 北 新 医 大 学 ed. 1974: 5, 259, 261 (in order of citation).

[30] Pei-ching Chung-i hsueh-yuan ed. 1974: 32; 1978: 16, 68; Chung-i yen-chiu-yuan et al. ed. 1982: 271a, 134b s.v. *yang*

To sum up, since 1971 authors of textbooks have been fluctuating between the old and new explanations. Despite great national stress on integrating traditional and modern medical knowledge, no syncretic explanation has been adopted consistently. This is only one indication that, although the combined practice of traditional and modern medicine is well launched, an integrated etiology is hardly under way. As for the nomenclature of diseases, there is no sign of synthesis. Writers simply choose to organize their therapeutic chapters around either traditional or modern diseases, depending on whether their books are meant for traditional physicians and pharmacists or for less specialized readers.

---

huang 阳黄 , 139b s.v. *yin huang*. Shang-hai Chung-i hsueh-yuan ed. 1979–80: I, 111–17; Yin Hui-ho 印会河 and Chang Po-no 张伯讷 ed. 1984: 37, 123–24. Gall bile was implicated in jaundice before the influence of European medicine was felt, but chiefly with reference to special forms of jaundice. See, for instance, *Ching-yueh ch'üan shu* (1624), *31*: 546b. Che-chiang Chung-i hsueh-yuan ed. 1983: 64 mentions only the hepatic and gall bladder systems in connection with jaundice.

Chapter IV

CONTENTS OF THE BODY

Modern physicians writing about the history of Chinese medicine used to say that the anatomy of traditional physicians "was mostly a product of the imagination."[1] Although it is still not quite usual to study what traditional physicians actually have said before setting down judgments on such topics, a considerable bulk of concrete knowledge about the body's internal structure has emerged. We find in the earliest classics tolerably correct accounts of the peripheral parts of the body through which the circulation tracts pass. There are brief descriptions of the internal organs associated with the visceral systems of function, colored by theoretical correspondences but roughly accurate. These classics include moderately detailed measurements of a good many external dimensions of the body, measured lengths and computed volumes of the alimentary tract's parts, and lengths of the most important circula-

---

[1] Wong and Wu 1936: 34, with particular reference to the anatomy and physiology of the *Inner Canon*. E. T. Hsieh 1921 is more charitable and more detailed with respect to anatomy, but equally based on random reading and even less reliable. There has been remarkably little publication on Chinese anatomical knowledge in Western languages, and no monograph that can be recommended with a clear conscience, but there are useful incidental remarks in the writings of Lu Gwei-djen and Joseph Needham, especially CL99 *et passim*. Watanabe Kōzō 1956 is an excellent study of anatomical ideas embodied in early diagrams and illustrations. For a detailed study of anatomical information in the *Inner Canon* see Wu Kuo-ting 1967.

tion tracts.[2] Later writings accumulated information about the body's bony framework, especially books on forensic medicine and the treatment of fractures.[3]

As we have formed a more comprehensive idea of what anatomical structures Chinese medicine recognized, curious gaps in this knowledge have become obvious. It is plain that traditional anatomy from first to last lacked the detailed and systematic character that we find even in Galen of Pergamon (second century A.D.), and many aspects of the body's contents were not studied at all. The early descriptions and measurements of viscera were repeated verbatim in one book after another for two millennia, with only a very few additional dissections to motivate minor changes.

The circulation tract system undoubtedly reflects early acquaintance with the network of blood vessels (including the capillaries), on which the tracts are modelled in many respects. The course of the tracts follows more closely that of the nervous than of the vascular system; for it is along nerve pathways that signals propagated by acupuncture chiefly travel. But the vascular and nervous systems (and the lymphatic system, also involved in the mechanisms underlying acupuncture) were never distinguished and studied separately.[4]

While the functions of the nervous system were combined with that of the blood vessels in the circulation tract system (*ching-lo* 経絡 or *ching-mai* 経脈), the physical structures of the nervous system were combined in a vague way with those of muscles,

---

[2] TS, *13*; LS, *4* (14, 17), *6* (31–32); more schematic in *Nan ching*, 2 (23, 42–43); see also CL30.

[3] The oldest extant manual of forensic medicine, *Hsi yuan chi lu* 洗冤集錄 (ca. 1247) has been reliably translated into English. For its discussion of bones (chapter 3) see McKnight tr. 1981: 95–106, which reproduces diagrams of skeletons from an edition dated 1854.

[4] The most comprehensive review of fairly recent Chinese and Occidental research on the scientific basis of therapeutic acupuncture as well as acupuncture analgesia is that of Lu and Needham in CL184–262. Chinese works such as Shang-hai shih wei-sheng-chü 上海市衛生局 1958 are also worth consulting. For a brief indication of the range of Chinese research issues see Shang-hai Chung-i hsueh-yuan 1974: 92–102 and Chang Sheng-hsing 张晟星 ed. 1983: 180–201.

sinews, and tendons in the *ching chin* 経 筋 (crudely translatable as "circulation sinews"). The course of this system of twelve branches resembles to a limited extent the peripheral parts of the cardinal tract system (4.2, P216–73), but it does not pass through the visceral systems and has no designated acupuncture loci. Its main functions are *ch'i* circulation and control of the joints. As is true of the circulation tracts, much attention is given to the courses of the *ching chin*, but what the latter are made of and what they look like are never described.[5]

Perhaps most remarkable of all, the idea of separate distribution processes for *ch'i* and *hsueh* (whether we think of the latter as blood or yin vitalities) was never developed. It is not that the two were firmly believed to flow together. How their flows are related and how they can remain distinct while flowing through the same channels—for there was only one system—were not examined in the canons of medicine.[6] The commentators sometimes took up such matters when explaining ambiguous wording, but discussion was not sustained and no conclusion was reached. The point is not that traditional authors were incapable of reaching a conclusion, but rather that this was not an issue of any importance.

The contents of the abdomen were not studied in detail. We can find over the centuries hints of internal organs beyond those for which the visceral systems of function were named by the second century A.D., but these hints had little outcome. Butchers knew of sweetbreads, but the human pancreas, although eventually recognized, did not become a regular part of medical discourse (Miyashita 1969).

---

[5] The classic discussion is TS, *13* (1) = LS, *4* (13). Ho Tsung-yü 何 宗 禹 1981, 1984, and Yao Ch'un-fa 姚 純 发 1982 disagree about whether the recently excavated precursor of the *Inner Canon, Tsu pi shih-i mai chiu ching* 足 臂 十 一 脉 灸 経 , is concerned with an early form of the *ching chin* (for which it uses the archaic graph 溫) rather than with the cardinal tracts. Ho 1984 marshals strong evidence against this proposition. Porkert describes the courses of the *ching chin* in detail (P317–33).

[6] On the claim of Maruyama Masao and Lu and Needham that the circulation tracts were distinct from the blood vessels in classical medicine, see appendix C.

One can easily be led astray, of course, by imposing the expectations of modern medicine on a traditional system with very different views of the body. But even if we consider only the organs that traditional physicians did know, there are still odd blanks in what they knew about them. Scholarly doctors took a variety of positions on several questions that would seem fundamental to anatomy, for instance: Is the triple *chiao* (*san chiao* 三 焦 , substratum of one of the six yang visceral systems, 2.1.6) immaterial, a single organ, three organs, a membrane lining the body cavity, or an abstract division of the yin visceral systems into three areas of function? Is the Gate of Life (*ming men* 命 門 , 2.1.5.1.4) the right kidney, a body between the kidneys, the same as the Cardiac Envelope Junction (*hsin pao* 心 包 , 2.1.1.1.5), or an immaterial locus of vital *ch'i*? These positions were never thoroughly argued out and never settled; at best, a couple of individual propositions were tested and found wanting.[7]

In the *Revised Outline* and other contemporary textbooks, questions like these have been settled—at least for the nonce—but what has settled them is the incompatibility of the Gate of Life and the triple *chiao* with modern anatomy. The former has dropped out of use except to designate certain functions such as the "Fire of the Gate of Life," now understood as the yang *ch'i* concentrated in the renal system (2.1.5.1.4). The triple *chiao* system has become "a generalization for the physical functions of several of the visceral systems within the body cavity," divided laterally into three types (2.1.6). A more recent manual hastens to add "it should also be pointed out that the concepts of superior, medial, and inferior *chiao* now commonly used differ in meaning from the triple *chiao* that originally was one of the six yang systems of function."[8]

Even more significant in recent writings than this pruning of ambiguous classical entities is the continuity of the old gaps. Despite the mass of detail in the *Revised Outline* (of which only one fifth is translated here), like all other books of its sort it gives no anatomical or physical description of the viscera. The authors emphasize that they "cannot simply impose Western medicine's conception of the internal organs" (2.0). Indeed what we learn about the Chinese conception is not anatomical but physiological and

---

[7] For a review of these and other points of contention see below, pages 125ff, and Jen Ying-ch'iu ed. 1980: 181–93.

[8] Pei-ching Chung-i hsueh-yuan 1978: 18.

pathological—as usual, not what the viscera are but what they do in health and sickness. In order to keep constantly before the reader the emphatic differences between these functions and those of the organs that bear the same names in modern medicine, I translate *tsang-fu* 臟 腑 in chapter 2 and elsewhere not as "viscera" but as "visceral systems of function" (abbreviated as "visceral systems"), and similarly for the individual *tsang* and *fu*.[9]

The *Revised Outline* also does not describe the circulation tracts. Even their courses are traced only perfunctorily, so much so that the reader who wishes to understand the underlying doctrines of acupuncture must refer to specialized works. The tracts are "the pathways along which the *ch'i* and blood are transported within the human body" (4.0), but nothing is said about whether the pathways of *ch'i* and blood coincide, either completely or in part. We are told that "the motion of the blood depends upon propulsion by the *ch'i*" (3.2). Is this direct physical propulsion in the same channels? The further statement that "if the *ch'i* moves the blood moves, and if the *ch'i* is static the blood coagulates" does not clear up the vagueness, for in classical Chinese science assertions such as these can apply equally to relations of resonance in which one entity affects another at a distance.

There is an obvious modern objection to the idea of a single circulation for *ch'i* and blood. The courses of the traditional circulation tracts do not coincide with that of the modern vascular system, as the authors of the *Revised Outline* are aware (4.4.1). To say that blood flows in the circulation tracts is to imply that the tracts, as

---

[9] Since the *tsang-fu* are simultaneously structural and functional entities, the choice of translation is a heuristic matter. I prefer a terminology that reminds the reader of both their visceral and physiological aspects, but I see nothing wrong with the decision of some translators, who emphasize similarities with modern medicine, to translate their names simply as "heart," "liver," etc.—so long as they do not obscure the differences between the *tsang-fu* and the viscera of modern medicine.

The forms of the two words that we find in the classics, *tsang* 藏 and *fu* 府, originally both meant "storehouse, treasury" (the sense of *fu* as "headquarters, official residence" is post-Han). Since there is no etymological basis for different translations, I simply translate *tsang* and *fu* when they occur separately as "yin (or yang) visceral systems of functions."

carriers of blood, are a crude and inaccurate approximation to the vascular system. This is not an admission without political consequences. Once made, it is hard to dismiss the pressure from modern M.D.'s to replace the latter, as obsolete, by the blood vessels.[10]

Yet acupuncture and moxibustion demonstrably act on the *ch'i* loci not along the blood vessels but along the tracts. The simplest reply to the modern physician's objection is that *ch'i* flows in immaterial tracts, as traced in the classics but hidden to modern anatomists, and blood in its own network of vessels, which the classics do not trace but modern medicine has charted in the utmost detail. This defense has not become fashionable, for it has its own all too obvious shortcomings. One would expect an introductory textbook to offer some solution to a question that might occur to any bright student. What we find instead in the latest publications is the same vagueness and inconsistency with respect to anatomy and physical form that runs through discussions of the tracts in writings centuries old. The tracts are pathways of blood as well as *ch'i*, we are assured, even though they do not coincide with the modern blood vessels. Still, "it is likely that the tract system includes the nervous, endocrine, and vascular systems" (4.4.3.3). And that is that.[11]

---

[10] One result of this pressure was a tendency in publications of the Cultural Revolution period on acupuncture either to concentrate on the acupuncture loci and discuss the circulation tract system separately in an appendix, or to emphasize the uncertain status of the system with respect to anatomical entities. An example of the former approach is Shang-hai shih chen-chiu yen-chiu-so ed. 1970, especially pages 182–92; the same approach is maintained in the revised version, Chang Sheng-hsing ed. 1983, especially pages 180–201. For the second approach see the Academy of Traditional Chinese Medicine ed. 1975, especially page 34.

[11] I follow Lu and Needham in translating *ching-lo* 経 絡 and *lo mai* 絡 脉, etc., as "tracts." Unlike other prevalent translations—"meridians," "conduits"—this one leaves open the question of whether a particular writer considers them material tubes. Below I will discuss the term *ching-sui* 経 隧, which authors used when they wanted to picture the cardinal tracts as conduits (page 135). Note that "meridian" cannot be considered a literal translation of *ching* in medicine, where it occurs in apposition to

It would miss the point to account for these gaps in recent writing by ignorance of elementary anatomy, inferior critical capacity, stunted curiosity, or the like. Anatomy has been taught for some time to every student in schools of traditional medicine, and the authors of the *Revised Outline* and similar books are demonstrably curious and critical when they want to be.

The best working hypothesis when studying science in another culture is that when writers consistently do not give a topic the emphasis you think it ought to have, they and people like them do not consider it as important as do you and people like you. That means, not that there is something wrong with them, but that you have not yet understood them.

In traditional medicine the tissues and internal structures of the body are unimportant by comparison with metabolic processes. That is why they receive so little attention. The simple and symmetric metabolic system was based on early, sketchy anatomical knowledge, which was adequate for constructing and refining that system. The goal of this effort was not a perfected description of the body, but an understanding of function and dysfunction that could guide therapy. The symmetry is ultimately that of functions, not of structure.

In Europe, in the Renaissance and later, anatomical knowledge far outstripped its medical applications. By 1700 physicians could still only guess about how lesions in dissected corpses corresponded to symptoms in live patients. Anatomy was valued because medicine in its upper reaches was a scholastic profession. Members of the Royal College of Physicians in England and their counterparts in Western Europe were honored by their peers for their erudition, regardless of whether they chose to serve the afflicted. Thus anatomy, although not a practical art, had its social uses; it could be mastered *without* long therapeutic experience. The learned and clinical aspects of medicine coalesced in the eighteenth and nineteenth centuries; the correlation of disease with morbid anatomy and the development of relatively safe surgery made anatomy finally pertinent to therapy.

In China, all along, the reputation of the doctor, enhanced though it might be by erudition, was settled at the sickbed. The closer we come to therapy, the greater the curiosity we find, the

---

lo, not to *wei* 緯 (meridian of latitude). The latter is implied when *ching* is understood as "meridian of longitude."

more critical the approach. Since traditional medicine still does not require cutting into the body, there is no urgency about resolving the discrepancies between traditional and modern anatomy. Since it is evident to all concerned that when they are reconciled it is the traditional understanding that will have to yield, it is simpler to let the matter lie.

So much for what is not said in the *Revised Outline* about the contents of the body. What is said deals with three types of substratum for distinct functions. First there are the eleven visceral systems, along with the Cardiac Envelope Junction system and various auxiliary systems, mentioned in passing (chapter 2, especially table 2.1).[12] The visceral systems ferment food, extract and store the vital essence from it and from air, maintain and regulate the distribution of the essence, and expel the residues. Secondly there is the circulation tract system, which provides a network through which the nutritive essences are distributed throughout the body, and through which heteropathy may be transmitted inward from the body's periphery to invade the visceral systems (chapter 4). Finally there are the various fluid and pneumatic sources of vitality, some extracted by the visceral systems and some inborn, stored and moved both through and outside the circulation system (chapter 3; see especially 3.1.3). All three categories have been simplified and systematized over the past two millennia. The change has been most decisive over the past generation, with unmistakable influence from modern medicine.

Visceral Systems of Function

The eleven basic visceral systems comprise five pairs, each pair including one each from the five yin (*tsang*) and six yang (*fu*) systems (2.0). It is likely that this conception of five pairs originated to structure rudimentary knowledge of the viscera according to the yin-yang and Five Phases theories. By the time of the earliest surviving writings a sixth yang system, the enigmatic "triple *chiao*"

---

[12] The auxiliary systems receive little attention in recent textbooks, but are more adequately described in Nan-ching Chung-i hsueh-yuan ed. 1958: 60–62.

(*san chiao* 三 焦.) system, had been added.[13] The motive was evidently to associate the yang systems with the Six Warps.

The ensuing development is worth following. It is typical of how conceptions of the visceral systems evolved. This example will show how important in that evolution reasoning about functional correspondences was, seldom posing problems that dissection could have solved. It will also show how the agenda for discussions of body contents and processes was set by the *Inner Canon*, vague and internally contradictory as it was, and systematized by the *Canon of Problems*. Afterward, as the emphasis moved to therapy, we find new views on anatomical and physiological topics consistently stated in the old language (which was thus often tacitly modified in meaning) and engaged in dialogue with the old ideas.

---

[13] *San chiao* is usually translated "triple heater," "triple burner," "triple warmer," "three coctive regions," etc., but these are fanciful extrapolations from the common but obviously irrelevant sense "to scorch" for *chiao* (Morohashi 19119, sense 1; the word may also refer to a scorched smell or color, senses 2, 5, but the only other related sense, "to toast," sense 3, occurs only as an old dictionary definition, with no *locus classicus*). *Chiao* does not mean "to heat," "to burn," "to warm," or "sodden, easily boiled" (the *OED* definition of "coctive"). I prefer to keep the issue open by making it clear that I do not understand the term.

The oldest occurrence of the term *san chiao* is in *Shih chi* 史 記 , *105*: 13–14. This work was completed between 100 and 90 B.C. The pertinent passage occurs in a biography of the physician Pien Ch'ueh 扁 鵲 (tr. Bridgman 1955). His legendary *floruit* is 501 B.C. No one has yet proven when in the interim the biography copied into the *Shih chi* was written; 400 and 200 are equally plausible guesses. In any case the document is almost certainly as old as the recently discovered medical MSS published in Ma-wang-tui 1979.

As for the anatomical substratum of the *san chiao*, early sources disagree about whether it has one, three, or none, giving rise to many divergent later guesses, some of which have already been noted (page 120). As the *Revised Outline* points out (2.1.6), there is still no agreement about the configuration and functioning of the triple *chiao* system.

The triple *chiao* system had no yin counterpart in the *Inner Canon*.[14] The author of the *Canon of Problems* perhaps considered this a violation of symmetry. In order to create twelve visceral systems he paired it with the "Gate of Life" (*ming men* 命 門), mentioned separately in the *Inner Canon*, which he identified with the right kidney. This had a theoretical advantage that the author stressed: the ensemble could be considered either five pairs (of viscera) or six pairs (of functions), and thus could correspond to both the Five Phases and the Six Warps:

> The Gate of Life is the abode of the essence that brings about new configurations (*ching-shen* 精 神 , pages 193–96). In men the reproductive essence is stored there, and in women the womb is fastened there. Its *ch'i* flows through [*or* with that of] the [left] kidney. Thus we may say that there are six yin visceral systems. . . . For each of the five yin systems (*tsang*) there is a yang system (*fu*). The triple *chiao* is also a yang system, but it is not associated with the five yin systems. Thus we may say that there are five yin visceral systems.

This sixth pairing created much confusion for later scholars, because the *Inner Canon* had already used a different correspondence to make up the twelve branches of the circulation system. It paired with the triple *chiao* tract the Cardiac Envelope Junction tract (*hsin pao lo* 心 包 絡), also called "Master of the Heart" (*hsin chu* 心 主). As the *Canon of Problems* puts it, "The Hand Minor Yin [car-

---

[14] There is a puzzling passage that mentions "twelve visceral systems" in SW, *3* (8). It outlines what it calls twelve visceral "offices" (*kuan* 官 ; see further discussion below). Actually only eleven offices are named, but there are indeed twelve components, since the splenetic and stomach systems are combined in one "office." The twelfth is named after the acupuncture locus *shan chung* 膻 中 (JM17), and is not otherwise identified or correlated by yin-yang pairing with the others. This would seem to be a variant tradition not otherwise represented in the *Inner Canon* (and altogether missing from TS). Some commentators arbitrarily identify *shan-chung* with the Cardiac Envelope Junction to explain away the anomaly (see below, page 131, note 19).

diac] tract and the Heart Master are separate tracts, so the Heart Master and the triple *chiao* are related as outer and inner [i.e., as a yin-yang pair]. Both have names but no shapes [that is, anatomical substrata]."[15] Scholars of this classic over the centuries, assuming that the doctrines of the early literature were unitary, have found several ingenious ways to prove that the Gate of Life and the Cardiac Envelope Junction are the same thing, simultaneously a visceral system of functions and a circulation tract that passes through it, or at least is connected with it. Once that assumption, ultimately untenable, is set aside, there is no confusion to explain away. In the texts translated above the author says plainly that the first association is of visceral systems, and the second of circulation tracts.[16]

---

[15]*Nan ching*, Problems 39 (cf. 36) and 25. The Heart Master is the hand attenuated yin tract. The idea of a Cardiac Envelope Junction was probably suggested by observation of the parietal pericardium, but the Cardiac Envelope tract as classically described does not represent the pericardium structurally or functionally, and cannot be equated with it (the *Revised Outline* does not equate them, 2.1.1.1.5). The Cardiac Envelope Junction tract not only has no associated organ, as *Nan ching* Problem 25 emphasizes, but its circulatory functions do not differ essentially from those of the cardiac tract. The canonical enumeration of the twelve tracts occurs in TS, *8:* 95-113 and LS, *3* (10): 25-30. Hans Ågren (forthcoming) argues plausibly that the point is not the vague recognition of the pericardium but the splitting of cardiac functions. The more clinically oriented annotators justify the division of cardiac functions between two tracts on the ground that the two are read separately on the radial pulses. See the commentaries collected in *Nan ching pen i* 難經本義 , *1:* 31-32, and *Nan ching chi chu* 難經集註, *3:* 48a-49a.

[16] For some of the more interesting attempts to identify the Gate of Life with the Cardiac Envelope Junction see Jen Ying-ch'iu 1980: 181-86, 207. The picture was further complicated by the disagreements already mentioned about the substratum of the triple *chiao* system, and by the fact that in the *Inner Canon* the Gate of Life is associated not with the kidneys but with the eyes (LS, *2* [5]: 14); the association with the eyes does not appear in the corresponding passage of the TS version (*10* [8]: 161), but is quoted in *Chia i ching*, *2* (5): 25a.

While the scholiasts were trying to resolve the contradictions
generated by their own assumptions, those intent on the medical issues had to find a rough working consensus. This they did gradually by making the Cardiac Envelope Junction a visceral system as
well as a circulation tract, either associating it with the Gate of Life
or ignoring the latter in this connection. The massive *Imperial
Grace Formulary* (*T'ai-p'ing sheng hui fang* 太 平 聖 惠 方 ,
992), discussing the mutual relations of the tracts, interjects the
Gate of Life without saying why it does so: "The hand Heart
Master tract is associated with the triple Chiao tract, which is called
'hand minor yang,' as well as with the Gate of Life. The hand
Heart Master has a name but no visceral system, and the triple
chiao has a location but no shape. Thus the circulation tracts make
up an outer-inner pair." Li Kao's 李 杲 (1180–1251) *This Is No
Simple Matter* (*Tz'u shih nan chih* 此 事 難 知), compiled by his
disciple Wang Hao-ku 王 好 古 in 1308, goes a great deal further. Li lists thirteen visceral systems (*tsang-fu*). Among the six
yin systems is "the Cardiac Envelope, another name for which is
Gate of Life"; the womb becomes a seventh yang system of functions.

Li Ch'an 李 梴 in his *Introduction to Medical Studies* (*I hsueh
ju men* 醫 學 入 門 , 1575), an unprecedentedly systematic
textbook, went further and tried to find an anatomical structure to
underlie a Cardiac Envelope Junction visceral system, producing the
first recognizable Chinese description of the outer fibrous layer of
the pericardium, assigning the inner serous layer to the cardiac system. Li had obviously observed a dissection, in which he had difficulty delimiting the location of what he considered the Cardiac Envelope, since he describes it as penetrating or passing obliquely
alongside the diaphragm, and connected to the lungs as well as the
heart. But the two layers of the pericardium ring true: "The yellow [or brown] fatty substance (*huang chih* 黃 脂) that spreads
and envelopes [the heart] belongs to the cardiac system. Outside
this spreading fatty substance there is a fine sinewy silk-fiber-like
membrane, connected to the cardiac and pulmonary systems; this is
the Envelope Junction."[17]

---

[17] *T'ai-p'ing sheng hui fang*, 1: 4; *Tz'u shih nan chih*, 1: 6a (XI,
7617); *I hsueh ju men*, 1: 105–19. The passage translated is
found in a footnote on page 117 of *I hsueh ju men*. Note that Li
writes *hsin pao* for "Cardiac Envelope" with *pao* 胞 , which nor-

These examples do not exhaust the ambiguities and contradictions that arose from what were originally separate correspondences of the three *chiao* functions in the visceral systems and circulation tracts. It would not be accurate to claim that the matter had been investigated and settled by the middle of the twentieth century; but it had become usual to consider the Cardiac Envelope Junction as the twelfth visceral system as well as the twelfth circulation tract, and at most to mention the Gate of Life in passing as terminologically, structurally, or functionally equivalent. Although the physiological functions associated with the two are traditionally distinct—for instance, the Cardiac Envelope Junction protects the cardiac system and the Gate of Life stores the essences secreted by all the visceral systems—this was not a pertinent objection. It was not made.

In summaries of traditional medicine published since 1949 the Gate of Life is not even mentioned in connection with the visceral systems. We find new ambiguities and contradictions due to awareness of modern anatomy. The *Lectures on Traditional Chinese Medicine* of 1972 reminds its readers that the visceral systems of function differ from the viscera of modern medicine, as do all textbooks of the last generation save for a few published in the last stages of the Cultural Revolution. It notes that the description of visceral system functions and pathology is much cruder than that of the modern viscera due to "historical limitations." After this warning against clear-cut equations it proceeds to make one. "The Cardiac Envelope is the cardiac system's (*hsin* 心) enveloping membrane, the peripheral tissues associated with the heart (*hsin-tsang* 心 脏)."[18]

The definition of *hsin pao lo* in the *Glossary of Selected Chinese Medical Terms* of 1973 (a precursor of the *Unabridged Dictionary of Chinese Medicine*) modernizes the notion that the Cardiac Envelope Junction is both a visceral system and a circulation tract. In explaining why the Cardiac Envelope is called a "junction" (*lo* 络), a word that usually designates points where cardinal and reticular

---

mally means "womb." Chinese authors before 1900 were equating the Heart Master with the Western pericardium, e.g., Yeh Lin 葉 霖 in his *Nan ching cheng i* 難 経 正 義 (1895), comment on Problem 25, 2: 47.

[18] Liao-ning Chung-i hsueh-yuan 辽 宁 中 医 学 院 ed. 1972: I, 3–4.

tracts meet, and that by extension names reticular tracts (*lo mai* 絡 脉, 4.0, CL 16–17), it begins: "Cardiac Envelope Junction (short form 'Cardiac Envelope') is the outer membrane of the heart (*hsin-tsang*). Attached to it is a reticular tract, the pathway for the flow of *ch'i* and blood. The Cardiac Envelope and cardiac systems of functions are both related to the activities of the central nervous system. If an external heteropathy invades the cardiac system, it is the Cardiac Envelope that is first affected." This last idea goes back to the classical description in the *Inner Canon*: "The cardiac system is the great master among the five yin and six yang visceral systems. It is where the body's governing vitalities (*ching-shen*) abide. Its yang viscus (*tsang*) is hard and impenetrable, so heteropathy cannot [ordinarily] settle there. If it does so, the cardiac system is damaged, its vitalities leave it, and the person dies. Therefore heteropathy resident in the cardiac systems resides in its Envelope Junction. This Envelope Junction is the tract of the Master of the Heart." In other words, the relation between the cardiac system and the Cardiac Envelope tract (not, in the *Inner Canon*, a visceral system) is based on an analogy with the relation between a monarch and a vassal who protects him from evil. This analogy is explicit in the *Basic Questions*.

The *Lectures* of 1972 (the high Gang of Four era) derided this metaphor: "The ancients also had a saying that 'the cardiac system is the office of the monarch' and can receive no heteropathy, so that the Cardiac Envelope receives heteropathy in its stead. This is trash meant to protect the feudal ruling class, and should be criticized." One can see a new issue on the horizon. If ideas derived from discredited political metaphors are to be "criticized," how many concepts of traditional medicine will survive such scrutiny?

As the tide of the Cultural Revolution ebbed, this question receded, and along with it, to a considerable extent, the tendency to mix freely traditional and modern notions. In the *Simplified Dictionary of Chinese Medicine* (1979), the second precursor of the *Unabridged Dictionary*, and in the 1982 version of the latter, note how the definition has been reworded to avoid equating cardiac system and heart. "Cardiac Envelope Junction: an organ (*tsu-chih ch'i-kuan* 组 织 器 官) peripheral to the cardiac system (*hsin*). The Cardiac Envelope is the outer membrane of the cardiac system. Attached to it is a reticular tract, the pathway for the flow of *ch'i* and blood. Together they are called the Cardiac Envelope Junction, conventionally shortened to Cardiac Envelope." The definition goes on to repeat the idea that the Cardiac Envelope receives heteropathy in the cardiac system's stead, citing the passage from the *Inner Canon* as authority. The new confusions of a few years before have been brought under control, but the old confusion survives in Westernized form in the description of the Cardiac Envelope Junction as "an organ."

To call them confusions, however, is purely a historical statement. The authorities of any medical tradition, if we read those of different times side by side, contradict each other in many ways. The synthesis that makes a classical system of medicine possible reconciles these differences.

It is only reasonable to expect that a synthesis will emerge from the many efforts reflected in recent writings to reconcile these several views of the Cardiac Envelope Junction. The eventual shape of such a synthesis is not predictable. An important new textbook, *Basic Theories of Chinese Medicine* (1984), is even more ambiguous than its immediate predecessors. It writes of the Cardiac Envelope Junction as "the integument wrapped round the heart" and quotes without comment a seventeenth-century essay that describes it as "resembling an upright bowl, with the cardiac system located in it."[19] These two claims are not at all equivalent.

Before passing on to the circulation tracts, another general question about the visceral systems calls for attention. What is their role in the economy of the body? The *Revised Outline* asserts that the five yin systems store vitalities (*ching ch'i*) and the six yin systems ferment food, separate the pure product, and transport residues to be eliminated (2.1). Its discussions of the individual visceral systems indicate that on the whole the yin systems control and regulate vital functions, while the yang systems receive, digest, store, transmit, and excrete vital substances and residues. These two characterizations are inconsistent. When the yin systems are described, only the renal and hepatic are said to store anything (and at the same time to control storage, 2.1.2.1.2 and 2.1.5.1.1).

---

[19] Chung-i yen-chiu-yuan et al. ed. 1973: 16; TS *9* (2): 127, LS *10* (71): 105; SW *3* (8): 49, which speaks not of *hsin pao lo* but *shan chung*, considered by commentators on doubtful grounds to be its location; Liao-ning Chung-i hsueh-yuan ed. 1972: I, 4; Chung-i yen-chiu-yuan et al. ed. 1979: 193–94; *idem* 1982: 77a; Yin Hui-ho 印 会 河 and Chang Po-no 张 伯 讷 ed. 1984: 31, citing *I kuan* 醫 貫 (1617?), *1*: 3.

The distinction between storing and processing is not a generalization based on individual characterizations, but goes back to a famous passage in the *Inner Canon*: "What we call the five yin visceral systems store *ching-ch'i*, without discharging anything they can be full but not replete. The six yang visceral systems transport and transform substances (*wu* 物) without storing them; they can be replete but not full."[20]

Leaving aside the complicated question of fullness versus repletion, this gloriously straightforward dictum, no doubt true for one of the bodies of doctrine that came together in the *Inner Canon*, is violated in chapter after chapter. Nor is storage the simple matter one expects it to be. Among the "substances" the yin visceral systems are said to store are five aspects of spiritual force (*shen* 神). *Shen* may indeed be playing its frequent role as the body's governing vitalities, but the fact remains that a force is not a substance.[21] Still this passage with its neat antithesis has been quoted for two thousand years, despite the inconsistency, because of its epigrammatic quality and the authority of its source. It is nevertheless the sense of the *Inner Canon* as a whole, as well as that of later writings to the present day, that the yin systems regulate and the yang systems are responsible for processing.

If this resembles a modern factory, can we find machines in it? The sources do not mention them. They do not say that the visceral systems do the processing. I have yet to find in medical writings evidence for mechanical interpretations of body processes (as distinguished from occasional figures of speech) before the advent of

---

[20] SW, *3* (11): 67 = TS, *6* (4): 90. TS implausibly reads *ching shen* for *ching-ch'i*; see P110. "Discharging" is *hsieh* 泄 , equivalent to *hsieh* 瀉 .

[21] TS, *6* (4): 89 = SW, *7* (23): 133–34. I do not understand the distinction between fullness and repletion in the quotation, and all of the commentaries I have examined are forced in their interpretations. "Replete" (*shih* 實) has a number of meanings in the *Inner Canon*. Porkert in his discussion of this passage connects repletion with a pathological nutritional condition—a normal sense—but that is not what the text seems to be about (P110–11).

European influence.[22] This is unexpected, considering the prevalence of food-processing machinery as early as the Han period.[23] Then again, the *Inner Canon* and its successors do not say that their storehouses are empty of machinery. Their imagery does not include workers either. Perhaps each visceral system's underlying organ or organs, so perfunctorily described, fill that role—but the point is not made. The documents are not concerned with who performs the labor, and with what tools. What they dwell on is how the operations are ordered. The visceral systems may be storehouses by etymology, but the prevalent metaphor for them is *kuan* 官 , an executive and the office he sits in: an office in a bureaucracy.[24]

It is well when pondering such questions to keep in mind that the visceral systems of function, like the political world and the natural world as every medical author thought of them, made up a bureaucracy. The circulation system was its transportation and communication network, and the various vital substances were their material and energetic resources. Processing machinery, however essential to getting the work done, would be no more germane to discussion on this plane than to the annual reports of present-day manufacturing companies, preoccupied with the responsibilities and achievements of their officials, and above all with the challenges faced by the corporate entity.

Circulation Tracts

Now let us briefly consider the circulation tracts. For reasons that are not stated, the *Revised Outline* is primarily concerned with drug therapy, which occupies roughly four fifths of the book. Acupuncture and moxibustion are discussed only in passing (4.3.3, 10.2.2). Lack of concern for these techniques is by no means ir-

---

[22] On the claim of Lu and Needham that the heart and lungs were considered pumps in classical medicine, see appendix C.

[23] See, among other sources, Needham et al. 1954- : IV.2, 174–211, and a discussion of fermentation and related processes promised in VI.1, section 40.

[24] For an extended metaphor in which all the visceral systems are described as officials, see SW, *3* (8), discussed in note 14 above. Discussion in P, chapter 3, *passim*.

regular, even before modern times, as we will see (page 179). The circulation system takes on special importance for the physician who performs acupuncture and moxibustion, or who does drug therapy in the tradition of the *Treatise on Cold Disorders*. Since neither of these emphases is reflected in this book, its discussion of the tracts is generally superficial. What it has to say about the courses and therapeutic functions of the tracts (4.2.1, 4.2.2) is inferior in clarity and cogency to the descriptions in other Chinese publications available in Western languages. That part of the discussion is therefore omitted from this translation, and the reader is referred to more useful sources.

As in the case of the visceral systems, once we have set aside the assumption that the earliest medical writings convey one consistent and unitary doctrine, an attentive rereading reveals how gradually the beginnings of synthesis appeared. The system of twelve circulation tracts known from the *Inner Canon* was, we now realize, a recent creation when the components of that book were written (probably in the first century B.C.). Some chapters, I have already mentioned, are earlier than others, and contain less elaborated ideas.

Some writings included in the *Inner Canon*, for instance, discuss additional major circulation tracts with uncertain relations to the twelve that are associated with the Six Warps. We find alongside the cardinal twelve, for instance, a group of eight that later, in the authoritative schema of the *Canon of Problems* (probably second century A.D.), were given more peripheral status as auxiliary tracts (4.0). In the *Inner Canon* there is also a group of eleven, ten of which were ignored in the synthesis of the *Canon of Problems* (the eleventh overlapped the group of eight). Whether the chapters that include these two groups of additional tracts are among the earliest has yet to be determined, but they clearly represent variant traditions.[25]

Excavations in Hunan in 1973 have given us sophisticated precursors of the *Inner Canon*, perhaps of ca. 200 B.C., which in some instances agree with it word for word. Their circulation sys-

---

[25] On the evolution of the *Inner Canon* see pages 89–90 above. For the first group of tracts, see TS, *10* (1–6): 143–55, SW *16* (60): 290–91, and the completed schema in *Nan ching*, Problem 28. The second group of tracts is discussed in TS, *30* (26): 582–84 and SW *11* (41): 205. See also Epler 1980: 337–38.

tem contains eleven tracts, not twelve. These are not, in fact, spoken of as tracts (*ching lo*, etc), but as vessels (*mai*, a word that also implies pulsation). R. F. Bridgman notes that these early texts do not specify what circulates in this general network, or indeed that there is a circular flow. He suggests that the system is not based on a rudimentary knowledge of the vascular system, but was instead assembled from knowledge of pathways by which pain is transmitted. This is a suggestive observation, even though it cannot be correct, for earlier non-medical works speak of free flow in "blood vessels" (*hsueh-mai*). The associations of vessels with body parts in the recently excavated manuscripts do not correspond to those in the *Inner Canon*.[26]

Medical writings from the *Inner Canon* on give detailed information about the circulation tracts, but do not describe, trace, or picture a separate network for "blood" (*hsueh*), which in the more systematized chapters of the *Inner Canon* means not just blood but the relatively *yin ch'i* vitalities (see page 51). We are told in the primary sources that both *hsueh* and *ch'i* are distributed by the tracts. Conversely, the network that carries *hsueh* along with *ch'i* may be referred to as tracts, vessels, or conduits (*sui* 隧 , literally, "tunnel," a word applied to the cardinal tracts only). Sometimes all three words are used in successive sentences, as in a passage in the *Inner Canon* on treating abnormal levels of *ch'i, hsueh,* and other vitalities by acupuncture:

> When the *ch'i* is excessive, drain the cardinal conduit (*ching sui* 経 隧), avoiding injury to the tract (*ching*) and without letting the *hsueh* or *ch'i* leak out.

---

[26] The two MSS that describe the precursors of the *ching-lo* system set out in LS, *3* (10) and elsewhere, both of them versions of a book named by their discoverers *Yin-yang shih-i mai chiu ching*, are published in Ma-wang-tui 1979. They have been edited and translated into Japanese in Akahori 1981. The most useful studies of the physiological texts are Akahori 1978 (English summary in 1979b), 1979a, and 1981, and Bridgman 1981, especially page 10. Both Akahori and Bridgman assume, as did the Chinese editors of the silk MSS, that all three texts are concerned with the circulation system. For controversy about this assumption see Yao Ch'un-fa 1982 and Ho Tsung-yü 1984. A brief summary of the medical finds is Harper 1976.

> If inadequate, replenish the cardinal conduit without
> letting the *hsueh* come out. . . . When the hsueh is
> excessive, drain the cardinal tract (*ching*) in which
> the level is abnormally high, making the *hsueh* come
> out. If the *hsueh* is inadequate, replenish the
> depleted tract. Insert the needle squarely in the ves-
> sel (*mai*) and leave it there for some time. When the
> *hsueh* has flowed in and the vessel has enlarged,
> quickly remove the needle without letting *hsueh* leak
> out.

This passage has to do with bloodletting. In using needles to restore the balance of vitalities classified by yin-yang and the Five
Phases it is possibly later than those in which excess blood is simply
drained from the body, and earlier than those in which needling
regulated the energetic levels without releasing blood. In any case,
hsueh here means both the yin aspect of the *ch'i*, responsible "when
it is excessive for anger, and when it is deficient for melancholy,"
and the physical blood that seeps from the site of the puncture. The
easy movement from a word meaning "tunnel" (a term that appears in several chapters, appropriate for the deeper parts of the
cardinal tracts) to the ordinary words for cardinal tract and vessel
shifts the emphasis, not between different parts of the circulation,
but between different ways of thinking about one part of it. In the
last four sentences "tract" (*ching*) and "vessel" (*mai*) are plainly
interchangeable. There are many such unambiguous examples.
There is no warrant for considering the flows of *ch'i* and *hsueh*
separate.[27]

---

[27] TS, *24* (4): 412–13. In characterizing the passage at the beginning of this paragraph, I follow Epler 1980: 357–58. His translation is based on the inferior text in SW, *17* (62): 308. Referring
to a modern dictionary, he remarks that "it is not clear what vessel is meant" by *ching sui*, but among other occurrences this term
is used in TS, *13* (4): 237 = LS, *4* (17): 42, to designate as the
"great cardinal conduit" (*ta ching sui* 大 経 隧) the combined
length of the twelve cardinal tracts plus four of what ultimately
became the eight auxiliary tracts. This, it seems to me, carries
greater weight than the opinion of Yang Shang-shan, the annotator of TS (666/683?), that in the passage translated the *ching*

The circulation system was not invented in the *Inner Canon*. It had been evolving for centuries beforehand, and continued to evolve after the discussions ultimately collected in the *Inner Canon* were written.

In early philosophic writings *hsueh-mai* means simply individual blood vessels or their ensemble. Deane Epler, in a valuable first attempt to reconstruct the evolution of ideas about circulation, has called this earliest understanding organic and mechanistic. I detect no machine analogies in it, and prefer to think of it as the intelligent butcher's view.

In a process already under way in the earliest known medical writings, continued in stages traceable within the *Inner Canon*, this older view was fundamentally transformed into an abstract new conception which Epler and Ågren have called functional and synchronistic. Epler has tentatively reconstructed the stages of mutation. In the Ma-wang-tui manuscripts (buried 168 B.C., written over the half-century or so preceding) the eleven branches of the circulation are called vessels, not tracts. In the biography of the well-born physician Ch'un-yü I 淳于意 (154 B.C.), cardinal and reticular vessels or parts of vessels (*ching mai* 経脉, *lo mai* 絡脉) appear, and orthopathic *ch'i* and blood move in them. The heteropathic *ch'i* responsible for a medical disorder advances in stages identified by the Six Warps, and the character of the disorder is analyzed using yin-yang theory. There is no hint of *ch'i* and blood moving separately.

Epler then traces through various chapters of the *Inner Canon* the crucial transition from an ensemble of twelve vessels each divided into a cardinal, reticular, and third-order part (*sun mai* 孫脉 or *sun lo* 孫絡), to a network of twelve cardinal tracts (*ching mai*), joined in a symmetrical network by the reticular tracts (*lo mai*), subdivided by the finer structure of the third-order tracts. By the time the *Inner Canon* was compiled from these diverse writings, the tracts are no longer tubes carrying aerial essence and plain physical blood. *Hsueh* never entirely loses its material meaning of blood, but it has become an abstract term to denote as well the relatively yin vital energies, just as *ch'i* long before had been abstracted from the air we breathe. In the conceptually more elaborate and presumably later parts of the *Inner Canon*, "vessel" has become just

---

sui is a reticular tract that joins the two hand cardinal tracts (page 412). See also pages 168–69 below.

another word for "tract."[28] Their difference is, like many differences we have already considered, that between aspects of the same thing (as yin-yang, the Five Phases, and the Six Warps are ways of emphasizing in analysis different aspects of *ch'i*). "Vessel" is used mainly when the point is the ability of the tracts to hold and convey substances such as *ch'i* and *hsueh*.

The term "pulsating vessel" (*tung mai* 動 脉) means "artery" in modern medicine. In traditional medicine it does not imply arteries as distinct from veins, but can be used instead of "tract" whenever attention is to be drawn to the phenomenon of pulsation. This can be seen in the first question of the *Canon of Problems*: "The twelve cardinal tracts all have their pulsating vessels, but we palpate solely the inch-mouth pulse [i.e., the radial pulse, 6.4.1.1] as a technique for deciding between life and death, good and bad fortune, as they involve the visceral systems of function. What can be said about this?" The reply does not identify the locations on each tract where the pulse could be taken—the inch-mouth pulse was not in fact the only one used—but the most astute commentator on this classic, Hua Shou 滑 壽 (1361), lists the acupuncture loci on each tract where pulsation may be felt. He goes on "When we call them cardinal tracts [*ching*, which also means 'regular'] we are referring to the fact that the flow of the constructive and defensive *ch'i* is regular and unceasing. When we call them vessels we are referring to the longitudinal allocation of the *hsueh* and *ch'i* and their movement throughout the body."[29] The distinction is between aspects, not things.

Mai alone in many contexts means "pulse," and thus always implies pulsation. The pulse makes it possible to determine by palpation the state of the circulation system. This implication is frequently so strong that in many passages of the ancient books it is impossible to make a clear choice between translating "vessel" or

---

[28] Epler 1980; note that this is not an attempt at a definitive analysis; see also Ågren, forthcoming. The biography of Ch'un-yü I in *Shih chi* 史 記, *105*: 19–62, contains a number of medical case records in which theoretical arguments are used for prognosis as well as therapeutic reasoning. They have been studied in Bridgman 1955. In 1981 Bridgman considered them alongside the Ma-wang-tui MSS in order to summarize the state of Chinese physiology ca. 200 B.C.

[29] *Nan ching pen i* 難 經 本 義, *1.* 1 (item 1).

"pulse." For instance, one chapter of the *Inner Canon* on depletion and repletion reads "when the *mai* is replete the *hsueh* is replete, and when the *mai* is depleted the *hsueh* is depleted; that is the normal situation. When this [relation] is violated medical disorder occurs." Yang Shang-shan, the earliest commentator on the *Grand Basis* (ca. 600), comments: "*Mai* refers to the inch-mouth and *jen-ying* pulses (*ts'un-k'ou jen-ying* 寸 口 人 迎 , the radial and carotid pulses). *Hsueh* refers to the *hsueh* in the cardinal vessels (*ching-mai*)." Wang Ping, the editor and annotator of the *Basic Questions* (672), comments: "The *mai* is the depository of the *hsueh* [P187–88]; therefore their repletion and depletion must be identical. When [the identity of their vital state] is violated and they do not correspond, medical disorder occurs." Yang is emphasizing the pulse and Wang the circulation system—not merely the blood circulation, for in the same chapter Wang speaks of alimentary *ch'i* being "distributed through the cardinal vessels." Thus he asserts that both *ch'i* and *hsueh* travel through the *ching-mai* as a whole, not through separate parts. One cannot say that Yang's reading of *mai* is correct and Wang's wrong, or vice versa. Their interpretations are convergent.[30]

In the case of the circulation tracts as in that of the visceral systems, we can see that the *Inner Canon* is only one step in the formative stages of medical theory, neither the beginning nor a full-blown, coherent system. We do not find a systematically organized treatise on the tracts that draws on all previous literature until the *Canon of the Pulse* (*Mai ching* 脉 経, ca. A.D. 280).

The discussion of the cardiac envelope junction a few pages earlier has already made the point that the understanding of the tract system once again is changing rapidly as interaction with Western medicine accelerates. But concentration on such details cannot give a true picture of the changing situation, since the fundamental issue in this encounter of two medicines is the very existence of the circulation tracts. I have already discussed the doubts that modern anatomy inspires (pages 120–22). It is not that such doubts could be inspired only by Western anatomy.

---

[30] SW, *14* (53): 251–52 = TS, *16* (1): 3–6, in TIZ only. The chapter as a whole asserts that the state of the body, of food intake, and of the pulse must correspond to that of *ch'i* and *hsueh* as signalled by certain symptoms, or serious illness will ensue.

Wang Ch'ing-jen 王清任 , who in 1830 challenged many received ideas about the *tsang-fu*, had received from seventeenth-century Chinese books one or two vague notions that, apparently unbeknownst to him, originated in the West, such as the idea that the brain, not the heart, was the seat of memory. Many have suspected, but no one has succeeded in demonstrating, that his intense motivation to understand the anatomical substrata of the visceral systems of function was due to European sources, direct or indirect.

Wang revised and bettered in many but not all respects the stereotyped descriptions and crude illustrations of the organs that had been copied from one book to another for centuries. But his greatest achievement was to ask genuinely anatomical questions of the ancient authors. His *tsang-fu* were not merely material substrata. He is the first author since those who composed certain parts of the *Inner Canon* of whom it could be said practically without qualification that he saw the *tsang-fu* as organs pure and simple. Undoubtedly the major reason was his examination of hundreds of disinterred corpses and attendance at public executions when the sentence was disembowelment. In this curiosity he had no predecessors (it led him to trust hearsay as well).

One of Wang's remarks on the circulation system indicates that he was prepared to see the tracts as anatomical structures or not at all: "The ancients said that the *ching-lo* were blood-pipes (*hsueh kuan* 血管), with two of them growing outward from each viscus, with the exception of four from the urinary bladder. I have personally seen more than a hundred sets of viscera; in none of them were outward-growing blood-pipes perceptible." Wang concluded, as a result of this radical reinterpretation, that the traditional tract system was a misunderstanding. He argued that there were two entirely distinct circulation systems, one for blood (*hsueh*) and one for air (*ch'i*). The blood circulation did not pass through viscera, and only the *ch'i* tubes pulsated. He was consciously rejecting the traditional view, and certainly not adopting an Occidental one.

Why did Wang's empirical investigations not lead him to rediscover what every medical student in sixteenth-century Padua saw? It is true that the prohibition against dissection of human cadavers had forced him to observe passively corpses either partly decayed or freshly killed, but that did not prevent him from making other observations that were both original and accurate. His orientation remained clinical. He insisted on anatomical hypotheses compatible with established methods of diagnosis, and with a holistic approach to treatment: "It is easy to determine prognosis from the pulse, but hard to know what the disorder is. The essential secret of successful therapy is a clear understanding of *hsueh* and *ch'i*." If Wang was not prepared to see the body in a wholly new way oriented toward the identification of localized lesions, we can recognize that he was examining the abdominal contents of cadavers with transformed eyes. What he saw was neither Galenic nor modern anatomy, but it was anatomy.[31]

In 1901 Pao Hui 寶 輝, one of the first physicians to compare classical and modern medicine, discussed more concretely the relation between the tracts of the former and the blood vessels of the latter. He equated the cardinal tracts (4.2) with the arteries, and the reticular tracts (4.0) with the veins—an identification that is not anatomically or physiologically plausible.[32] Attempts to find a more satisfactory explanation of the tract system continued, but in the first half of the twentieth century, traditional physicians on the whole were too little informed about Western medicine to consider the problem urgent. Modern physicians who had informed themselves about the traditional art tended to be highly skeptical about the existence of *ching-lo* distinct from the vascular system.[33]

It was the Cultural Revolution policy of actively combining the two traditions, and encouraging modern research on Chinese medicine, that made the anatomical status of the circulation tracts a matter of frequent concern. This policy did not become an official

---

[31] *I lin kai ts'o* 醫 林 改 錯, *1*: 10–14, 25–27; the quotations are from pages 10 and 27. There is a good discussion of Wang's life and discoveries in Ma K'an-wen 馬 堪 溫 1963. On evidence for Western influence see Fan Hsing-chun 1944: 682–83 and Jen Ying-ch'iu ed. 1980: 155, 157. Information on Western knowledge of the body available in early Chinese translations is summarized in Peterson 1973: 307–11.

[32] *I i hsiao ts'ao* 醫 醫 小 草 , page 13. Oddly enough, this equation was still being made by Ch'en Pang-hsien 陳 邦 賢 in his old standard history of Chinese medicine (1937: 16). For other comparisons see Ch'üan Han-sheng 1936.

[33] For instance, Liu Yao-hsi 劉 曜 曦 1929. For a general discussion of conflicts in the Republican period see Croizier 1968: part 2.

priority until 1958, and did not have wide repercussions until the mid-1960s.[34]

Recent discussion of the circulation system is interesting. The *Outline of Traditional Chinese Medicine* of 1958, an authoritative textbook, does not provide any modern rationale of the circulation tracts, calling them simply a "naturally occurring function of the human body." From the 1960s on, the general pattern is that handbooks of traditional medicine meant for popular education and lower-level training state briefly that the tracts are pathways for the effects of acupuncture and other phenomena, and move on to enumerate the loci. The anatomical status of the tracts is not discussed. As the Cultural Revolution intensified, emphasizing new therapies and lowering qualifications for practice, even this limited attention was further attenuated. The *Simplified Materials on Traditional Chinese Medicine* of 1971, for instance, in its extensive discussion of "new acupuncture therapy," does not mention the circulation system or relate loci to it.[35]

The medical-school textbooks published between 1960 and 1978, although they describe at length the courses and functions of the parts of the circulation system, also characterize the *ching-lo* only as lines of connection between phenomena. They do not take up

---

[34] Croizier 1976, especially page 349. This source is informative about modern physicians' and administrators' attitudes, but not about those of traditional physicians in recent decades. See also Shang-hai shih chen-chiu yen-chiu-so 上 海 市 針 灸 研 究 所 ed. 1970: 183.

[35] Nan-ching Chung-i hsueh-yuan ed. 1958: 73; T'ien-chin i-hsueh-yuan et al. ed. 1971: 217–301. Strictly speaking, such methods as auricular acupuncture and acupuncture analgesia were not considered part of the "new therapies."

"New acupuncture therapy" was a response to calls for greatly simplified training as well as methods that combine needling and injection of drugs and other materials into the loci. In books like the one mentioned, traditional acupuncture is subsumed under this new rubric, but in the process is reduced to a small number of loci and their uses, to be memorized quickly. The "new acupuncture therapy" is not mentioned in the *Revised Outline*, except for a paragraph on new loci (4.3.3.4). It is broadly surveyed in English in Academy of Traditional Chinese Medicine ed. 1975: 269–90.

their anatomical status, but at least they ask what they are. *Lectures on Acupuncture*, a text of 1960, is more detailed in this regard than the *Revised Outline* (cf. 4.4.3):

> While acupuncture is being applied, the patient may feel a sensation of soreness, distention, heaviness, or numbness spreading in a certain direction. While therapeutic massage is being applied, the patient may feel a sensation of soreness, distention, warmth, or heat spreading toward a certain location. When someone has reached a certain level in the practice of breath control (*ch'i kung* 气 功), he may feel hot *ch'i* circulating in a certain location. These connections of physiological function provide a basis for determining the courses of the circulation tracts. When disease occurs in the human body, internal pain may be reflected in certain locations on the surface of the body, or may be related between various parts of the body, or this symptom and that may occur in combination. These connections of disease symptoms provide another basis for determining the course of the circulation tracts. During acupuncture or massage therapy, experience proves that cardinal tract loci in the extremities can be used to remedy pain in distant locations, and superficial loci can be used to treat afflictions within the viscera. These connections of therapeutic capabilities of loci between far and near or interior and exterior provide another basis for determining the course of the circulation tracts. . . . The courses of the tracts, then, are generalizations of these numerous phenomena of connection, and are based on clinical practice.[36]

---

[36] Shang-hai Chung-i hsueh-yuan ed. 1960: 28. Shang-hai shih Chung-i hsueh-hui 上 海 市 中 医 学 会 ed. 1960, a monograph on the circulation tracts, appears to be an expansion of parts of this book. The passage translated and other discussions of the status of the circulation system do not appear in it.

The 1978 edition of *Foundations of Chinese Medicine* is the first basic medical-school textbook to summarize research on anatomical correlates of the tracts, but what we find is merely a rewritten version of section 4.4.3 of the *Revised Outline*, without the detailed information on the anatomy and functions of the loci given in 4.4.1 and 4.4.2. The *Revised Outline*, then, although it is not a medical-school textbook but meant for study by modern physicians, gives the most comprehensive outline of anatomical and other correlates in any general treatise I have read. Among handbooks entirely devoted to acupuncture and moxibustion accessible to me, only *Acupuncture and Moxibustion* (1974) exceeds it in scope and thoroughness.

The 1984 revision of the *Foundations* textbook eliminates the latter's discussion of anatomical correlates. Given the wide use of this introductory work on medical colleges (the first printing of the new version was over 60,000 copies), the reaction against the Cultural Revolution seems in this respect as in others to have lessened motivation in medical education for scientific explanations of traditional concepts. The current state of research has been well summarized in the 1983 *Handbook of Acupuncture and Moxibustion Therapy:* "questions answered by the circulation tract [hypothesis] include some for which preliminary solutions have already been found (for instance, the connections following definite patterns between all parts of the organism), some which have not yet been clarified (for instance, the distribution routes of the tracts inside and at the periphery of the body), and some that so far have been very little studied (for instance, the patterns of circulation and flow of *ch'i* and blood in the tract system)."[37]

This survey of the last quarter-century's publications suggests that the policy of combining the two medicines has not decisively influenced teaching about the circulation tracts. It has finally become usual to ask what they are as well as what they do, but the answer is usually still in terms of what they do. The emphasis is clearly on

---

[37] Pei-ching Chung-i hsueh-yuan ed. 1978: 49–51 and the revision in Yin Hui-ho and Chang Po-no ed. 1984: 64–92; Shang-hai Chung-i hsueh-yuan 1974: 92–102. Oddly enough the latter discussion does not cite the research reports that it summarizes. The 1960 textbook cited in the last note gives 39 citations but is less comprehensive than the Shanghai work.

their role in acupuncture and moxibustion more than on their role in *ch'i* and *hsueh* circulation.

We can see political patterns in the fluctuations about this norm. Writings that deal only or primarily with the loci, ignoring the tracts, are generally products of the mass education campaigns of the Cultural Revolution, which took the synthesis of old and new seriously when training barefoot doctors, red medical workers, and others expected to mix traditional and Western techniques. Ignoring or paying minimal attention to the tract system facilitated this synthesis, and meant that much less to learn in an accelerated curriculum. With the end of the Cultural Revolution campaigns of that sort ceased, but the tracts can still be ignored in texts for low-level medical personnel.[38]

In books for medical students and modern physicians, presentation of the tract system has been relatively traditional. Such topics as anatomical correlates are taken up, when they are taken up, as supplementary digests of research findings—an unusual and uncommitted genre within textbooks, which normally present their doctrine in authoritative form. These accounts of research are always presented tentatively. Traditional and modern workers, we are told, "have come to the conclusion that the channels *are closely related to* the nerves, blood vessels, and body fluids. But as the theory involves some unsolved problems of modern medicine and biology, further investigation remains to be done."[39] Even the *Revised Outline*, exceptional for its detail concerning the issue, makes no claim that the loci or tracts are identical with known anatomical or histological structures.

But the problem of accounting for the tracts will not go away. The presence of Western medicine keeps it on the agenda. If the

---

[38] Although no acupuncture handbook known to me entirely ignores the question of what the tracts are, discussions of this issue are often perfunctory. Some, such as Shang-hai shih chen-chiu yen-chiu-so ed. 1970, meant for part-time and low-level medical personnel, and much occupied with "new acupuncture therapies," ignore the circulation system in the text and take up its reality in an appendix (pages 182–85). The same arrangement is followed in a revision, Chang Sheng-hsing 张 晟 星 ed. 1983: 180–85; the quotation is taken from page 185. See also Lucas 1982: 122.

[39] Academy of Traditional Chinese Medicine ed. 1975: 34, my italics.

functions of the *ching-lo* prove that the *ching-lo* exist, why do they not exist as physical structures? If their functions are merely "closely related to" those of the nervous, vascular, lymphatic, and other systems, what is the point of calling the tracts a distinct system and tracing their separate courses? In fact, since Chinese physicians do not perform any therapeutic procedures on the tracts, but only on the loci, why regard the former as anything more than a set of imaginary lines useful for remembering the latter and tracking complicated therapeutic effects?

In discourse as functionally oriented as that of traditional medicine it is enough that, as Lu and Needham put it, "the acu-tracts have a certain reality . . . as lines of equivalent physiological action."[40] But modern physicians who do not accept this functional orientation are apt to reply that a circulation system that does not exist anatomically can be dispensed with, or frankly represented as a fiction. We have just seen that some handbooks for low-level medical workers do in fact dispense with it.

The tension was made even more uncomfortable in 1963 by the debacle of the Bonghan corpuscle. Professor Kim Bonghan 金鳳 漢 of Pyongyang University in North Korea announced in that year that he had discovered special cell structures that correspond not only to the loci but to the *ching-lo*. His discovery was given much publicity in China and elsewhere, but could not be verified. The so-called Bonghan corpuscles quickly fell into oblivion in China, but the incident remained embarrassing.[41] I have seen no sign that Chinese researchers are chasing a similar chimera.

In order to trace the vicissitudes of the major body systems in traditional medicine, I have considered a small component—the cardinal envelope junction—and a large one—the circulation tracts. In both instances we can see considerable diversity of understanding before modern times, and the first effective moves toward standardization of doctrine in the last generation. This standardization has been greatly impeded by the influence of Western medicine, not because such influence is undesirable but because it has been accepted unsystematically and in a way that makes theory less coherent rather than more so. In any case it raises questions that would not

---

[40] CL191; see also Porkert's discussion of the reality of the *ching-lo* in P197–98 and Kao To 髙鐸 1984.

[41] *Jen-min jih-pao* 人民日報 , 1963.12.14, page 4; Croizier 1968: 203–4; CL186–87, and 4.4.1 below.

have been asked within the Chinese tradition. We can see in the responses to these questions, as in those raised earlier with respect to the etiology of jaundice, signs of an unsettled short term and a questionable long term.

Vital Substances

Finally let us examine the substances that circulate through the viscera and peripheral parts of the body to sustain growth and life. Chapter 3 of the *Revised Outline* divides these into *ch'i*, blood, *ching*, and the dispersed body fluids (*chin-yeh* 津 液). It also discusses mucus, a pathological substance. We are told that the dispersed fluids and mucus are each of two types, and the descriptions indicate that each class is a yin-yang pair (3.4–3.5). *Ching* is paired in a yin-yang relation with *ch'i* (3.6).

We have already seen that in the ancient books *ching* was also paired with *hsueh* (now understood mainly as blood), and *ch'i* and *hsueh* themselves made up a yin-yang pair (see table 2). In this alignment *ch'i* and *hsueh* are the relatively yang and yin aspects of the general body vitalities, collectively called *ch'i* or *ching-ch'i*.[42]

All the body substances are seen by the *Revised Outline* as "substantial liquid matter," distinct but interacting in ways mentioned throughout the book. Five types of *ch'i*—constructive *ch'i*, defensive *ch'i*, and so on—are introduced. These are not different fluids, but characterizations of the body's *ch'i* "according to its various functions" (3.1). Clearly substance and function are not entirely separate.

Before the beginnings of medicine as a discrete science, in early philosophic writings such as those we have already examined (page 45ff), air, blood, semen, sweat, and the like are not neutral materials, but concrete, vital stuff. In such writings they are always discussed in relation to issues of right action and the social good. Rich in meaning though these conceptions of body substance are, they are seldom abstract.

In the classical medical theory that the *Revised Outline* is adapting to contemporary needs, the yin-yang relations remind us that discourse is not about simple substances, but about elaborate concepts that, while they remain rooted in the body fluids of common

---

[42] See pages 51–53 and the more comprehensive table in P195.

Table 2
Relations of Body Substances in Classical Medicine

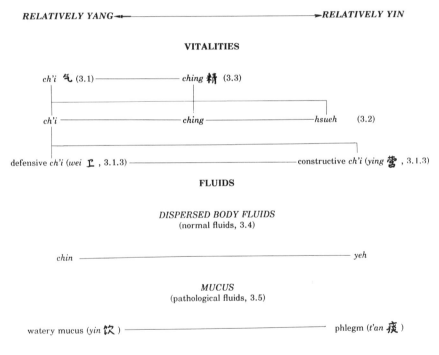

RELATIVELY YANG ◄──────────────────────────► RELATIVELY YIN

VITALITIES

ch'i 气 (3.1) ─────── ching 精 (3.3)

ch'i ──────────── ching ──────────── hsueh   (3.2)

defensive ch'i (wei 工 , 3.1.3) ────────── constructive ch'i (ying 營 , 3.1.3)

FLUIDS

DISPERSED BODY FLUIDS
(normal fluids, 3.4)

chin ───────────────────────── yeh

MUCUS
(pathological fluids, 3.5)

watery mucus (yin 饮) ───────────── phlegm (t'an 痰)

experience, are far abstracted from them. Today they have become once again "substantial liquid matter" involved in dynamic processes. This new picture, based at some remove on biochemical and biophysical views of body substances, is far from a return to the archaic conceptions. The concrete molecules of modern science are themselves an enormous feat of abstraction from the lay view in which blood and other fluids are still imbued with the mysteries of life and death.

In order to provide a brief idea of how recent Chinese medicine is a momentary stage in a long evolution, I will comment on each of the substances introduced in chapter 3 below, with special attention to *hsueh* and then to constructive and defensive *ch'i* (which are easily misunderstood unless the relationship of *ch'i* and *hsueh* is clear).

Ch'i, we have seen in the discussion of its pre-medical meanings, incorporates not only the energies that drive dynamic processes but the functions that they comprise and even the stuff that persists as particular things come into being and pass away. The protean character of *ch'i* is well illustrated in a passage from the *Inner Canon* that includes in the category of *ch'i* all of the life-maintaining substances described in chapter 3 below, including "blood." It adds a sixth stuff which (at least to modern readers) is not at all obviously a *ch'i*—certainly not "substantial liquid matter"—namely the circulation vessels (*mai*):

> Yellow Lord: I have heard that in humans there are *ching, chin, yeh, hsueh,* and *mai*. I had thought of them as one *ch'i*. Now it seems that they are distinguished with six names! I do not know why this should be so.
>
> Ch'i-po: When the two spiritual forces [*shen* 神, the male and female *ching*, P181] conjugate, they unite to shape a physical form [*hsing* 形]. They [thus] always come into being before the body [of the offspring, for they provide its initial endowment of vitality as well as its form]. This is called *ching* (3.3, P176–79, 182).
>
> Yellow Lord: What is called *ch'i* ?
>
> Ch'i-po: When the superior *chiao* 焦 [in which the defensive *ch'i* is produced; 2.1.6] sends it spreading outward, disseminating [the refined matter of] food, it steams into the flesh, filling the body and

moistening the hair as mist and dew soak [the earth]. This is called [defensive] *ch'i* (3.1.3).

Yellow Lord: What is called *chin?*

Ch'i-po: When the interstices between skin and flesh leak, sweat exudes freely from them. This is called *chin* [, the yang aspect of the dispersed body fluids, 3.4].

Yellow Lord: What is called *yeh?*

Ch'i-po: When food enters and the alimentary *ch'i* reaches an adequate level, it irrigates and flows into the bones. As the bones and joints contract and extend, it [is carried upward to] moisten and replenish the brain and the medulla, and to make the skin sleek. This is called *yeh* [, the yin aspect of the dispersed body fluids].

Yellow Lord: What is called *hsueh?*

Ch'i-po: When the medial *chiao* receives the [constructive] *ch'i* [from food] it extracts its juices, transforming and reddening them. This is called *hsueh* (3.2).

Yellow Lord: What is called *mai?*

Ch'i-po: When it banks in the constructive *ch'i*, it leaves the *ch'i* nowhere to escape. This is called *mai*.[43]

This is not a definition of *ch'i*. One was hardly needed. By the time of the Inner Canon the broad significance of the word had already been fixed in everyday speech and learned writing. Here we have simply an enumeration of six diverse aspects, defined purely by their roles in metabolism and circulation. This is one of the few passages in early medical literature that specifies *hsueh* is a red liquid. It does so only indirectly, by reference to the extraction and reddening of juices—functions again. If the reader compares this dialogue with chapter 3 below, the differences in how the various *ch'i* are described will speak for themselves.

---

[43] TS, *2* (2): 10–11 = LS *6* (30): 58–59, also quoted extensively in Wang Ping's annotation to SW, *17* (62): 305. On the whole I follow the LS text of this passage, which differs slightly from TS. The relation of the medial *chiao*, constructive *ch'i*, and *hsueh* is further discussed below, pages 152–53.

The *ch'i* of the body can be separated into any number of aspects that differ in function. Most of these are named by adding a qualifier to *ch'i*, as in "constructive *ch'i*" and "defensive *ch'i*." Section 3.1 of the *Revised Introduction* lists only a sample of the aspects used to describe vital and pathological processes. Most of the large array found in premodern writings have recently dropped out of use.[44] Their main use in the classics was in refining understanding of physiological and pathological processes.

Perhaps the last major innovation of this kind came at a time when most medical authors were preoccupied with therapy or elementary instruction, in Wu Yu-hsing's 吳有性 *Treatise on Warm-factor Epidemic Disorders* (1642). Wu proposed that, in addition to the Six Excesses responsible for disease of external origin (5.1), there exist varied "heterogeneous *ch'i*" (*tsa ch'i* 雜氣) that enter through the nose and mouth rather than, as the former do, predominantly through the pores. A subgroup, the especially virulent "deviant *ch'i*" (*li ch'i* 戾氣), are responsible for serious epidemics. Wu's key point was that "because illnesses are diverse, we know that the [heteropathic] *ch'i* cannot be the same. It appears that at a certain time a certain *ch'i* enters only certain visceral systems and circulation tracts, causing the onset of only a certain illness. That is why [in an epidemic] everyone's disorder is the same. This perhaps proves that [the incidence of the epidemic] has nothing to do with [similar predisposing conditions in] the visceral systems and circulation tracts [of every patient]. Since [epidemics] cannot be explained solely by reference to year or season, it appears that they cannot be determined by phase energetics," the prevalent theory that explained disease of external origin by Five-phases and Six-warps cycles of environmental influence (P55–106). The heterogeneous *ch'i* were, in other words, specific etiological agents. This was a radical departure from the traditional heteropathy, which differed only according to origin in the environment or the

---

[44] P168–73 lists 32 epithets of *ch'i* that occur in early medical writings. Many of these have dropped out of use in the last generation. Chung-i yen-chiu-yuan et al. ed. 1973: 66–74, a rather comprehensive glossary of traditional medicine, gives only fourteen such two-character compounds. The three types of *ch'i* treated as synonymous in 3.1.1 below are not clearly distinguished in the 1973 reference work, but are quite distinct in Porkert and his classical sources.

body. The contrast with the Yellow Lord's affirmation that *ch'i* are fundamentally one is obvious.[45]

Such exceptions aside, curiosity about metabolic and disease processes, even in the twentieth century, has been largely satisfied by looking back to the *Inner Canon* and its towering accretion of commentaries, systematic rearrangements, digests, and textbook recapitulations, along with a few important handbooks of etiology along the lines of *Origins and Symptoms of Medical Disorders*. The authority of these sources is now being replaced by germ theory and other doctrines of modern medicine that have become familiar to every Chinese.[46]

Since in defining the body fluids metabolism is central, let us see how it is classically described. The clearest early description occurs in one of the *Inner Canon's* chapters on the constructive and defensive *ch'i*. Since it is discursive, let me summarize what is pertinent, translating only key parts.

Food enters the stomach, and its essential *ch'i* is forwarded upward to the pulmonary tract for distribution to the visceral systems. The purer fraction is the constructive *ch'i* (*ying*); the more turbid, the defensive *ch'i* (*wei*). The former circulates in the pulsating vessels (*mai*), the latter outside them, without ceasing. The defensive *ch'i* exits from the superior *chiao* at the cardiac orifice of the stomach and circulates, "normally travelling alongside [*or* with] the constructive *ch'i*," and being reunited momentarily with it (the language is that of astronomical conjunction) once a day, after fifty revolutions. As for the constructive *ch'i* that ultimately exits from the medial *chiao* (dorsal to the superior *chiao* at the cardiac orifice), first "the residue is separated out, the liquid part (*chin-yeh*) distilled off, the subtle essence transformed"—that is, digestion must be

---

[45] *Wen i lun* 溫疫論, first three sections of chapter 2, especially page 42b. There is an unreliable translation of some relevant portions, accompanied by an interesting discussion, in Dunstan 1975: 35–43.

[46] Liu Ts'un-yan 1971 is a singularly uncomprehending attempt to prove that in the twelfth century Taoist priests were observing the microorganisms of pulmonary tuberculosis through compound microscopes. His primary source, *Wu-shang hsuan-yuan san t'ien yü t'ang ta fa* 無上玄元三天玉堂大法, clearly states that its demonic heteropathies are of normal demonic size and are seen through visionary meditation.

completed—"and sent flowing upward into the pulmonary vessel; only there [in the pulmonary system] will it be metamorphosed into *hsueh*, which is supplied to vivify the whole body. None [of the body substances] is as noble; that is why only it [i.e., constructive *ch'i*, and not defensive *ch'i*] can travel in the cardinal conduits. . . . Constructive and defensive *ch'i* are *ching ch'i* 精 氣 , and *hsueh* is *shen ch'i* 神 氣 . Thus *hsueh* and *ch'i* differ in name but are of the same category." The difference, like that of other vital substances, is aspectual, not material. Constructive and defensive *ch'i* are vitality seen as emergent from food and drink, available to maintain or change the body's configurations (Porkert's *ch'i* as structive potential); *hsueh* is vitality seen as formative, acting within the body (*ch'i* as configurative force). The *ch'i* and *hsueh* are yin and yang in relation to each other, not at all the same but "of the same category." The excretory functions, finally, are located in the inferior *chiao*.[47]

This is an interesting account, but not at all a comprehensive one. It says nothing, for instance, about the role of *ch'i* derived from breathing. At a minimum, it needs to be supplemented with another passage from the *Inner Canon:*

> When food enters the stomach system, its residues, essential fluids, and genetic *ch'i* (*tsung ch'i* 宗 氣 , 3.1.2, P171) separate among three conduits. As a result the genetic *ch'i* accumulates in the chest. It exits into the windpipe, passing through the cardiac and pulmonary systems and actuating the respiration.

---

[47] TS, *12* (1): 201–5, part only in the TIZ ed.; LS, *4* (18): 43–44. The two versions differ in several small but significant respects; I follow the generally superior LS text except where a copyist's error has the *wei ch'i* coming from the inferior *chiao*. See Kuo Ai-ch'un ed. 1982: I, 359–61, for a comprehensive discussion of variants. Part of the text summarized here is translated in CL30, but cited from *Nan ching* rather than *Huang ti nei ching*. For a rigorous discussion of the last quotations see P179–82, 186. Porkert points out that in LS, *1* (4): 9, the yin and yang parts of the body's interior are also said to differ in name but to belong to the same category.

> As for the constructive *ch'i*, the liquid [part of the food] is separated and is sent flowing into the pulsating vessels. It is then transformed into *hsueh* and circulated to the extremities. In the inward direction it is sent flowing into the yin and yang visceral systems. This happens in a way that corresponds with the divisions of the day [, that is, maintaining a regular daily fifty circuits].
>
> As for the defensive *ch'i*, the most impetuous part of the rough *ch'i* is sent forth and circulates first in the extremities, the interstices in the flesh *(fen jou)* 分 肉 , and between the flesh and skin, never ceasing.[48]

The food and drink is separated into three fractions and forwarded to the triple *chiao* (here clearly three distinct ensembles of functions). As we have seen, the useless part in the inferior *chiao* is excreted. The liquid fraction in the medial *chiao* is further fractionated. Its finest part becomes the constructive *ch'i*. This quotation is as unclear as the first about whether it is the constructive *ch'i* or the liquid from which it is separated that flows into the tract system for further processing. That activity somehow yields *hsueh* without destroying the constructive *ch'i*; the latter plays a principal part in the circulation. The remainder from the separation of constructive *ch'i* and liquid is the dispersed body fluids.

The original light fraction in the superior *chiao* not only yields the defensive *ch'i* that because of its "impetuosity"—equated by some commentators with slipperiness—moves outside the tract network, but also the genetic *ch'i* responsible for respiration. Again this is not a separate kind of stuff, but a designation for the combination of vital *ch'i* from inspired air and that from food. At least that is the later view, assembled from brief discussions on different topics in various of the *Inner Canon's* writings.

The missing piece is found in a chapter on the Five-Phases affinities between the visceral systems and foods of different flavor:

---

[48] TS, *12* (2): 206 = LS, *10* (71): 104. LS reads *hsin mai* 心 脈 , "cardiac vessel" for *hsin fei* 心 肺 , "cardiac and pulmonary systems." Both readings are consistent with theory, but *Chia i ching*, *12* (3): 6a, agrees with TS. Kuo Ai-ch'un ed. 1982: I, 266–67 emends LS accordingly.

When food first enters the stomach system, the essential part first emerges from it and arrives in (*chih* 之) the two *chiao* [i.e., the superior and medial], so that they irrigate the yin visceral systems, separately moving along the pathways of the constructive and defensive *ch'i*. The part of the great *ch'i* (*ta ch'i* 大 氣) that has become static and does not circulate accumulates in the chest, in what is called the "reservoir of *ch'i*" (*ch'i hai* 氣 海). It exits into the pulmonary system, following the course of the windpipe so that [the *ch'i*] moves outward on exhalation and inward on inspiration.[49]

In the commentaries we can see much patchwork reconciling the discrepant terminologies of the different traditions recorded side by side in the *Inner Canon*. The great *ch'i* plays the same role here with respect to the respiration as the genetic *ch'i* played in the passage quoted earlier. That is a matter of historical interest, but more to the point is the understanding that later students of classical medicine shared.

There are, as I have noted, several texts in the *Inner Canon* itself that attempt to clarify other texts in the same book. The first attempt to impose straightforward statement on the heterogeneity, vagueness, and frequent internal contradiction of the *Inner Canon* as a whole is the *Canon of Problems* (probably second century A.D.)—a book that played a large role in shaping subsequent understanding of the *Huang ti nei ching*. It cuts through all the ambiguity of the passages just discussed to set out several influential equations:

"Why, since the five yin systems are [hierarchically] on the same level, are only the cardiac and pulmonary systems located above the diaphragm?" "The cardiac system = *hsueh*, and the pulmonary system = *ch'i*. *Hsueh* is constructive (*ying*), and *ch'i* is defensive (*wei*). Following each other as they ascend and descend, they are called constructive and

---

[49] TS, *2* (4): 15 = LS, *8* (56): 86. Here the LS text is superior. "Great *ch'i*" is ordinarily understood as a term for environmental air, *t'ien ch'i* 天 氣 , after it has been inhaled (P169.7).

defensive. They travel throughout the circulation
tracts (*ching-lo*) and make a circuit outside them.
That is why the cardiac and pulmonary systems are
made to be above the diaphragm."[50]

The reasoning of this answer as a whole is not obvious, as the
forced explanations of the commentators make clear, but the point
is evidently the importance of the cardiac and pulmonary functions
with respect to this circulation. An office with more important
responsibilities deserves a better location.

This statement is not as audacious as it looks. Calling *hsueh*
constructive does not equate it with constructive *ch'i*. What corresponds is functions, not physical or chemical identities. The
Canon of Problems is saying that the cardiac and pulmonary systems, paired by their location, exercise a regulatory influence over
hsueh and *ch'i*. *Hsueh* and *ch'i* together carry out the basic functions for which constructive and defensive *ch'i* are named. Constructive *ch'i* and *hsueh* carry out the same ensemble of functions,
we know from other sources, but with a different division of responsibility.

The danger of reading such statements as though they were
written by modern physicians becomes even clearer when we examine *Stepping-stone to Medicine*, a textbook of 1751 that was long
popular in south China:

Ch'i has no physical form, but *hsueh* is substantial. *Ch'i* is yang, and is responsible for protecting
the outer aspect; thus it is called "defensive" (*wei*).

---

[50] *Nan ching*, Problem 32. The first sentence of the reply is a verb-
less equation with *che* 者 ; the second uses the equational verb
wei 為 . The commentators do not make much of this assertion.
Hua Shou in *Nan ching pen i* (1361), 2 (32): 38, the leading
premodern commentary, ignores it. Those who do not ignore the
equations understand them as correspondences mediated by the
cardiac and pulmonary systems, which govern *hsueh* and *ch'i*
respectively. The connection is, as usual, through function rather
than substance. A good example is *Nan ching ching shih* 難 經
經 釋 , *1* (32): 24. This commentary (1727) is excellent for its
analysis of divergences between the *Inner Canon* and the *Canon
of Problems*.

Hsueh is yin, and is responsible for circulation within; thus it is called "circulatory" (*ying*). Because *hsueh* is yin and substantial, its motion must be sequentially along the circulation tracts. Thus it enters the pathways of the pulsating vessels, through which, after filling the inner aspect, it reaches the outer. Because *ch'i* is yang and formless, its motion is so impetuous that it passes outside the pathways of the vessels without moving along the circulation tracts, first filling the outer aspect before turning back inward. . . .

Ch'i is unitary. When it is moving outside the vessels it is called defensive *ch'i*; when it is moving within the vessels it is called circulatory (= constructive) *ch'i*. When it collects in the chest [i.e., the cardiac and pulmonary systems] it is called genetic *ch'i*. Three names there may be, but *ch'i* is indivisible.

To the impatient reader this passage appears to be equating *ying* with both *ch'i* and *hsueh*. That impression does not survive careful rereading. The equation in the first paragraph is the familiar one of the *Canon of Problems*, but note that the author of *Stepping-stone to Medicine* is reading *wei* and *ying* as characteristics of *ch'i* and *hsueh*, not as corresponding substances. *Ying* in such usages means "circulatory." That is why in the first paragraph, as in the *Canon*, *ying* and *wei* are not called *ch'i*. In the second paragraph, *ying*, as clearly labelled *ch'i* that circulates within the pulsating vessels, is not *hsueh* but one aspect—one activity—of unitary *ch'i*.[51]

Classical physicians took assertions such as "*hsueh* is constructive and *ch'i* is defensive" to mean that certain aspects of the body's vitalities correspond in respect to certain functions under consideration, and not necessarily in others. The body's metabolic vitalities break down into yin and yang aspects called *hsueh* and *ch'i* when the subject of discourse is the nutritive circulation in the circulation tract system. The same vitalities break down into yin and yang aspects called *ying* and *wei* when the topic is the complementarity of circulations inside and outside the tract system.

---

[51] *I pien* 醫碥 , *1*: 21-22.

The *Canon of Problems* did not say the final word on the production of *hsueh*. Later classical physicians remained so engrossed in vitalities and the functions they perform that they paid little more attention to physical and chemical substances in the body than the *Inner Canon* had done. But they did add to the clarity and consistency of functional explanation. I will give only one example, which demonstrates that added clarity was not always a desideratum.

The last three quotations from the *Inner Canon* may be read as saying that constructive *ch'i* is first separated from the liquid essence of nutriment in the medial *chiao* and then transformed into *hsueh* but continues to exist after this process is complete. The *ch'i*, since it is separated from liquid, is presumably not liquid; *hsueh*, when considered as material, is liquid blood. Why should *ch'i* be separated from a liquid and then become a different liquid? The cumbersome character of this schema reflects a basic ambiguity in the *Inner Canon's* explanations, which I have maintained in the translations above. Is the constructive *ch'i* the material from which *hsueh* is produced, or the agent that produces it? Both possibilities are open, and are left open by most commentators. They are not asking either/or questions of that kind.

Ma Shih 馬蒔 (1580) resolved the ambiguity, making the constructive *ch'i* the transforming agent, acting upon one liquid to transform it into another. Here he is commenting on the *Inner Canon's* assertion that *hsueh* and *ch'i* as extracted from food and air are "of the same category": "*Hsueh*, then, is the product of constructive *ch'i*; in fact it is *ch'i* made divine (*shen hua* 神化)." In other words, *hsueh* is *ch'i* raised to a second level of essentiality (*shen*) that lets it determine, produce, and maintain the body's configuration of vitalities (P183). Ma continues a few lines on: "Consider the statement above that, 'as for the constructive *ch'i*, the residue is separated out, the liquid part distilled off, the subtle essence transformed, sent flowing upward into the pulmonary vessel, and transformed into *hsueh*.' Thus *hsueh* is transformed by [or due to] constructive *ch'i* and formed from [or due to] yin fluid (*yeh*). Sweat is the yin fluid of the cardiac system, so that sweat and *hsueh*, although they differ in name, are also of the same material substratum (*wu* 物)." This assertion still contains some leeway for interpretation, as the alternative phrases in square brackets indicate, but I do not see how the role it gives constructive *ch'i* can be anything but active.

Just as the ambiguity of constructive *ch'i* as material and agent did not generate anxiety earlier, its resolution did not mandate emulation by later scholars. Chang Chieh-pin, perhaps the best and certainly the most widely studied later commentator on the *Inner Canon* (1624), described *ying* in a way that lets it be seen as both agent and substratum, for instance: "The purer part corresponds to yin. Its tendency is to segregate the most essential part (*ching chuan* 精專). Thus the *hsueh mai* is produced by transformation and circulates in the cardinal vessels. That is the constructive *ch'i.*"[52] In view of Chang's intelligence and erudition, there is only one rational conclusion: he did not wish to be more precise than he was. Constructive *ch'i* could remain both material and agent because it was not a specific material.

Students of the *Inner Canon*, then, found some distinctions unimportant, but put great effort into delineating others. They followed their priorities, not ours. Given the potential for confusion in the *Canon of Problems'* "equation" of *ying* and *hsueh*, it is impressive that we do not find confusion in medical writers before recent decades.

The potential for confusion could not be activated until familiarity with Western medicine encouraged authors to see *hsueh* and *ch'i* as materials with distinct compositions. One of the most fundamental ideas of modern science is that in order to comprehend change it is essential to understand the physical and chemical identity of what takes part in change. This conviction may or may not suit the assumptions of a given classical tradition—that is, one which is willing to reinterpret its canons but not to reject their authority. Classical Chinese medicine is decidedly not built on assumptions about physical and chemical individuality. If such notions are applied willy-nilly, equations such as the one I have been discussing become statements that certain materials are the same.

Today it is not hard to find discussions that bear no resemblance to the traditional understanding as we have reviewed it. See, for instance, a 1983 Chinese-English dictionary defining what I have called constructive *ch'i*. "*Ying* (the nutrient principles): (1) Usually referring to the nutrients derived from foods, as a constituent of the

---

[52] *Huang ti nei ching ling shu chu cheng fa wei* 黃帝內經靈樞注證發微 , *55* (18): 53b; *Lei ching, 8* (23): 25b. Porkert notes that in LS *hsueh mai* may refer to two related structive energies (P174, 207), but here I suspect a textual error. Comparison with related statements by Chang indicates that he is referring merely to the production of *hsueh*.

blood (*hsueh-yeh* 血 液). (2) Sometimes referring to the blood circulating in blood vessels. (3) Sometimes referring to blood vessels
[*sic*] as the dwelling place of Qi [i.e., *ch'i*] and Blood." This is not
obviously a Westernized reading—to some extent it is an eccentric
one—but Western influence is perceptible in its attempt to reduce
body processes to a clear-cut, relatively simple set of materials and
structures.[53]

    This definition is not similar to what one finds in the better all-
Chinese dictionaries. The *Unabridged Dictionary of Chinese
Medicine*, for instance, gives only one physiological sense of *ying
ch'i*: "The essential *ch'i* that circulates in the vessels. It is
produced from liquid and solid food, originates in the splenetic and
stomach systems, and exits from the medial *chiao*. It has the functions of producing blood through metamorphosis and of nourishing
the whole body." This definition goes on to quote chapter 71 of the
Divine Pivot as translated above. It is functional from beginning to
end.[54] The *Glossary of Selected Chinese Medical Terms*, a
predecessor of the *Unabridged Dictionary* compiled during the Cultural Revolution, characteristically does not quote the *Inner Canon*.
It paraphrases the *Divine Pivot* in modern language, and adds an
odd conclusion: "Thus from the physiological viewpoint 'constructive *ch'i*' refers to the functions of blood." That assertion is not entirely incorrect. What makes it odd is that the *Glossary* fails in its
definition of *hsueh* to point out that it too refers to the functions of
blood; in fact there it does not even mention blood! Odder still, its
definition of *ying-hsueh* (i.e., constructive *ch'i* and *hsueh*) reads in
full: "From the physiological viewpoint '*ying-hsueh*' refers to blood."
One is not surprised to find that this confusion has been removed
from the post-Cultural Revolution versions.[55]

---

[53] Shih Hsueh-chung 帅 学 忠, et al. 1983: 105. See also the
    pertinent sense of *ch'i*: "Referring to the refined materials which
    are highly nutritious and circulate in the body. It is analogous to
    'Essence Principle' or 'Virtue Principle'" (page 107).
[54] Chung-i yen-chiu-yuan et al. ed. 1982: 273a, sense 1. The defini-
    tion of *hsueh* (page 120a, sense 1) identifies it with fluid blood,
    but is otherwise completely functional.
[55] Chung-i yen-chiu-yuan 1973: 70–71, 67; 1979: 769a-69b, 317a.
    The 1979 definition of *ying ch'i* is identical to the 1982 version;
    hsueh is not identified with blood but called "a material."

We see two conflicting tendencies in all three publications of the same project: the functional emphasis of the classics is preserved, and the materialist emphasis of modern physical science is juxtaposed with it. The 1973 version mixes these two tendencies in an incoherent way. The 1979 and 1982 versions segregate them as the *Revised Outline* does. *Hsueh* and *ch'i* are identified at the outset as material substances, but everything else said about them describes functions.

The theory of metabolism did not stop evolving when the *Inner Canon* and the *Canon of Problems* were compiled. In the *Inner Canon* all of the visceral systems were involved in the assimilation of food. Passages on this topic do not mention the constructive and defensive *ch'i* and *hsueh*. But here and there brief statements allow linkage; for instance, a passage on repletion and depletion in the yin visceral systems (7.3), and their consequences for acupuncture therapy, lists the storage functions of the visceral systems. Among them, "the pulmonary system stores *hsueh* . . . the splenetic system stores constructive *ch'i*."[56] As time passes, we find the theory drawing together these pieces of the functional picture and building on greater coherence to discuss more complex interactions among functional systems.[57]

We also find developing mechanical analogies for processes (although not, as I have noted, for organs). The *Origins and Symptoms of Medical Disorders* (610) explains functionally the yin-yang pairing of the splenetic and stomach systems (2.1.3.3): "The splenetic system is a yin system, and the stomach system is the reservoir of food and drink. Its major function is to accept and be filled with whatever is eaten and drunk. The splenetic *ch'i* grinds and digests it." Note that the splenetic system or its underlying spleen is not said to be a mill or a digesting vat; the metaphor concerns function, and as usual *ch'i* is the actor. Grinding is not an isolated metaphor for splenetic function. Eleven hundred years later it has become familiar, and can be mentioned in passing, as in *The Transmission of the Lamp of Medical Studies* (1700): "Most of all to be avoided is going to sleep right after eating. Since the ears have

---

[56] TS, *5* (1): 75 = LS, *2* (8): 21. A wide-ranging discussion of the distribution of nutritional essences that does not mention *hsueh* or *ying-wei* is SW, *7* (21): 121–24 = TS, *16* (3): 31–71, in TIZ only.

[57] See, for instance, Chang Chieh-pin's commentary on LS, *4* (18) in *Lei ching*, *8* (23): 25b.

nothing to hear, the splenetic system stops its grinding, and the pulmonary *ch'i* thereby is no longer distributed throughout, the inevitable result is medical disorder brought about by a static congelation (*yü-chieh* 鬱 結)."[58]

Also among the body's vital substances are the dispersed body fluids (*chin-yeh*). The distinction in the passage above (pages 149–50) seems to be clear enough. The fluids that leave the surface of the body are *chin*, naturally yang because of their centrifugal motion. The juices that are moved within the body by the flexure and extension of the joints are *yeh*. As much because of their nutritive role as because they remain within the surface of the skin, they are relatively yin.

That is a neat picture, but it ceases to be neat when we look further, even in the *Inner Canon*. The quotation just examined gives only one example of *chin*, namely sweat. A chapter of the *Inner Canon* on Five Phases correspondences of the visceral systems associates five such excretions with the yin systems: "The *yeh* transformed by the five yin systems of functions: that of the cardiac system is sweat; that of the pulmonary system is nasal mucus; that of the hepatic system is tear fluid; that of the splenetic system is oral mucus (*hsien* 涎); and that of the renal system is saliva (*t'o* 唾). These are called the five *yeh*."[59] In this passage the excretions are clearly not *chin* but *yeh*. It is of course impossible to make an absolute distinction between the fluid that keeps the skin moist and what seeps from it when it is warmed. The better annotators do not quibble, but take recourse to the flexibility of yin-yang relationships.[60]

---

[58] *Chu ping yuan hou lun, 21*: 116a; *I hsueh ch'uan teng* 醫 學 傳 燈, *1*: 2. "Static congelation" is a general term for *ch'i* that has "knotted up" in one place and blocked circulation. It is signalled by such symptoms as nodules, lumps, and sensations of fullness.

[59] SW, 7 (23): 132; the order and wording differ in TS, 6 (4): 88. Each item there is of the form "the cardiac system governs [that is, is responsible for] sweat." Neither version is obviously superior. The basic difference between *hsien* and *t'o* is in viscosity. A good deal of scholarship has been devoted to more elaborate distinctions, but I suspect that *hsien* was originally a word for thick spittle.

[60] See the quotation from Chang Chih-ts'ung 張 志 聰 in P191.

The word *hsien* in the quotation designates only normal oral mucus. Mucus connected with pathological processes is *t'an-yin* 痰 飲, another yin-yang pair which differ with respect to vicosity (3.5).

Not only is there no consensus in classical medicine about the demarcation of yin and yang dispersed body fluids, but the senses we have reviewed fall into two areas of meaning, well expressed in the best of the recent dictionaries of traditional medicine when it defines *chin-yeh:*

1. A nutritive substance formed when alimentary essences are subjected to the functions of the stomach, splenetic, pulmonary, triple *chiao,* and other visceral systems. That within the circulation vessels is a component of blood; that outside them is distributed throughout the interstices of the tissues. . . .

2. A general term for all body fluids and their metabolic products. *Basic Questions,* chapter 8: "the urinary bladder system is the office of the prefectural capital; the *chin-yeh* is stored there"; *Divine Pivot,* chapter 30: "when the interstices between skin and flesh leak, sweat exudes freely from them. This is called *chin.*" Thus they explain that both urine and sweat are produced metamorphically by the dispersed body fluids, which also have the function of regulating body fluids.[61]

---

[61] Chung-i yen-chiu-yuan et al. ed. 1982: 238b-39a. For more detail see the definitions of *chin* and *yeh* on pages 238b and 287b. The first quotation is from SW, *3* (8): 49–50. The term that I have translated "prefectural capital" can be understood in several ways. See, for instance, the quotations in Ch'eng Shih-te 1982: 135, note 25. The second quotation is given in context above, page 150.

The addition of urine to the list of fluids (identified as yang *chin* in the article on that word) is inferential. It is based on the association of the urinary bladder system with dispersed body fluids in the *Basic Questions'* list of civil service offices to which the visceral systems functionally correspond.

This is a useful definition, attentive to the diversity of meanings in basic medical writings—but note that attention has shifted from the flesh layer near the surface of the body to the circulation vessels as the border between *chin* and *yeh*.

Metabolism and *Ch'i*

This whirlwind tour of the body contents has at least suggested that classical medicine's doctrine of metabolism stressed function over substance, and saw the body fluids not as chemically distinct materials but as aspects of one generalized fusion of vitality and vital substance, namely *ch'i*. It was possible to discuss each fluid, or each pair, as though it were a species, but its activity as *ch'i* was more often the topic of discourse.

There is no question that before the emergence of medicine as an activity of specialists the body fluids were thought of concretely. Through the centuries they remained concrete for physicians closer to popular than to classical medicine. But they were transformed by the *Inner Canon* and its immediate predecessors to form the theoretical entities we have reviewed. This was a permanent metamorphosis.

Blood, breath, semen, sweat, and the other concrete materials that flowed into, through, and out of the body were not forgotten. They remained the roots of classical medicine's theories. These theories were too abstract for concrete fluids to serve also as their trunk. Their trunk was *ch'i*, an abstraction on the highest level—as high as any in the world's premodern scientific traditions—that drew on all known physiological and pathological functions.

Classical writings on vital substances, despite their divergences, are consistent in their areas of agreement. Let me summarize the premodern consensus with respect to body contents, beginning with the fluids. For the sake of simplicity, and acknowledging that there is a cost in rigor to be paid, these remarks will deal only with entities discussed substantially in the *Revised Outline*.[62]

Ch'i, as the sum of bodily energies, is partly inborn and partly extracted from food and drink. *Ching* is the indeterminate aspect of *ch'i*. It is *ch'i* in transition from one determinate form to another:

---

[62] See the more comprehensive discussion in P166–96, and the schematic overview in Porkert's table 19, page 195.

the semen that carries form and life from parents to offspring, the essence that the body takes from food pending assimilation to the individual's vital processes, and so on. *Ching* is what one calls *ch'i* when it is no longer the specific *ch'i* of the eggs in the omelet, and before it has become the characteristic *ch'i* of the eater. This is not a light in which *ching* would naturally be seen as yin or yang, for such judgments must pair it with something else. *Ching* may pair with other aspects of *ch'i* involved in transition, but because of the protean character of *ching*, the precise yin-yang correspondences tend to vary between contexts and thinkers.[63]

Ch'i and *hsueh* represent a division of the genetic *ch'i* into yang and yin aspects. It is not the only such division. This one is used, as we have seen, when the topic of discussion is the overall character of the circulation within the tract system. It is derived from the primordial distinction betweeen the two basic life-sustaining substances, breath and blood, but far abstracted from it. The emphasis on *hsueh* suits this combination to discourse concerned with the nurturant, conservative, yin aspect of vital process. The combination expresses a balance between this aspect and the yang activity that gives life, induces change, and sets processes in motion—the *ch'i* within the *ch'i*. The distinction between *hsueh* and *ch'i* is consistently so characterized. The difference between liquid and gas is practically ignored, although blood as the substratum of *hsueh* was by no means absent from physicians' minds.

The constructive and defensive *ch'i* are even more obviously yin and yang aspects of active *ch'i*. Like *ch'i* and *hsueh* they are derived from essences (*ching*). In this sense they are an aspect on the same level as *ch'i* and *hsueh*. They are useful when the topic is yang activity such as the formation of *hsueh* from genetic *ch'i*. Because they are on the same level, their exact role in that process can be understood in various ways, which few authors felt a need to sort out. Even the recent confusion of constructive *ch'i* with blood is an understandable consequence, since both separate in similar ways from the same source, and circulate in the same tracts. *Ying* and

---

[63] See Porkert's discussion of the many meanings of *ching-ch'i* (P176–80). In alchemical theory *ching-hua* 精 華 is a more clear-cut pair of yin-yang aspects. *Hua* is essence seen emerging from something else without yet being determined; *ching* is the essence seen as forming something else but not yet determined. See Sivin 1980: 229.

wei were assigned a range of activities that make them relatively yin and yang. The basic traditional distinction, as we have seen, is not in their substance but in their area of activity. The constructive *ch'i* remains within the circulation tracts (relatively yin). The defensive *ch'i* travels outside the tracts (relatively yang). Neither of these vital substances penetrates the surface of a healthy body.

The dispersed body fluids are another aspect of *ch'i*, derived from essences. They come up when the topic is the diverse fluids that do not circulate. The yin fluids (*yeh*) are diffused by the motion of the skeleton; the yang fluids (*chin*) are excreted, but their motion before they appear on the surface of the skin is indeterminate. In their diversity they differ from the defensive *ch'i*, the importance of which lies in its protection of the body surface, and which therefore is not divided into specific fluids such as sweat, saliva, and tears. The defensive *ch'i*, unlike the yin dispersed fluids, circulates.

We have seen that even in the *Inner Canon* the identification of particular body fluids as *chin* or *yeh* is not consistent. Generally the distinct, named fluids all fall into one category, and the fluid in the other category is neither named nor associated with an everyday substance (such indeterminacy is a sign of relatively yang character). The overt distinction between *chin* and *yeh* is of a different kind, and consistent in texts that try to distinguish them. As in the distinction between constructive and defensive *ch'i*, the criterion is spatial. The relatively yang *chin* escape from the body, and the yin fluids do not.

Once we understand that all these terms are aspects of one substance, *ch'i*, we can understand the reasoning behind many otherwise enigmatic statements about connections.

The *Inner Canon* states, for instance, that "the defensive *ch'i* is what warms the divisions of the flesh, fills out the skin, enriches the interstices and pores (*ts'ou-li* 腠理), and controls their opening and closing. . . . When the defensive *ch'i* is in harmony [with other aspects of *ch'i*] . . . the openings are tight and impenetrable."[64] Why should one fluid be regulating the openings that keep another fluid from flowing out? What is the mechanism of regulation? Such questions are not asked because only one fluid, namely *ch'i*, is involved. Prevention of pathological leakage is most readily discussed in relation to one pair of aspects, constructive and defensive *ch'i*; the seepage of *chin* at the surface of the skin as sweat is a different

---

[64] TS, *6* (2): 76 = LS, *7* (47): 74–75.

aspect (and thus is not mentioned in this passage, but rather taken up in writings on the dispersed fluids).

We have seen that some writers include the oral and nasal mucus among the yin dispersed fluids. They evidently see no conflict in the fact that mucus as *t'an-yin* is both yin and yang. There is no conflict. *T'an-yin* is a pathological aspect, whereas dispersed body fluids are mainly (but not exclusively) discussed in connection with normal body processes. Pathological mucus is divided into yin and yang types according to viscosity (which implies divergent functions) and not according to which type is evidenced inside the body and which outside.

We also find in the *Revised Outline* a purely pathological division of the body from periphery to center into four "sectors" named for *ch'i, hsueh,* and constructive and defensive *ch'i.* These are aspects of orthopathic *ch'i* involved at various stages of disease in the encounter with heteropathy (9.1).

Conclusions

The internal contradictions I have noted about details of the body contents within the *Inner Canon*, and between later writings, are not the weaknesses they appear to be from the modern medical viewpoint. They are useful data about basic differences between that viewpoint and the one that evolved classical medicine.

We can document over the centuries an increase in breadth of reference and precision, despite a shift of emphasis from physiology to therapy. This was a cumulative dialogue, in the sense that authors were aware of their predecessors. Because medical schools and organizations did not greatly evolve, despite some interesting initiatives the dialogue did not become cumulative in another important sense. Despite the efforts of individuals to resolve discrepancies by careful, documented argument, within the world of medicine no collective mechanism came into being for adjudging such arguments and declaring issues settled. There were no colleges of physicians; the medical elite were not inclined to take guilds seriously; the imperial medical service, although it shared the charisma of imperial ritual, had no intellectual prestige. Discrepancies were overcome to the extent that individual intellect and the prestige of schools could overcome them.

We have seen that classical discourse about the circulation tracts has been no less functional and aspectual than that about *ch'i.* Among the terms we have encountered above for circulation pathways are "vessel" (*mai*), "tract" (*ching* and related words), and "conduit" (*sui*). Another common term, sometimes used for specific pathways, is "*ch'i* thoroughfare" (*ch'i chieh* 氣 街).[65] The last two refer only to the cardinal network and its affiliated tracts (4.2). They were always less common than *ching* and *mai*, and are not used in the *Revised Outline* and other recent handbooks.

The complete circulation system exists on three structural levels, the cardinal tracts (*ching* or *ching mai* in their specific senses), the reticular tracts (*lo* or *lo mai*), with affiliates on both levels, and the capillary "third-generation tracts" (*sun mai, sun lo*), which the superficial discussion of the *Revised Outline* omits.

"Vessel" and "tract" are in some respects interchangeable and in others distinct. They are interchangeable in referring to structures; I have mentioned that there was no attempt from the oldest extant writings to modern times to identify them with different networks. They are distinct in the functions they emphasize. "Vessel" emphasizes the physical, pulsating carrier of vital substances. "Tract" emphasizes the articulation of the network and the regularity of flow. Etymologically and in rigorous usage it implies neither physical tubes nor pulsation. The choice of terminology for the traditional system depended, in other words, on the aspect of circulation being examined. When neither of these stresses was mandated, the terms became interchangeable.

For the visceral systems we are confronted with only one set of terms, although we have seen that set vary in size and membership. Aspect is thus not an issue.

The Chinese conception of visceral systems of functions was from first to last an attempt to understand the workings of physical organs. Nothing in historians' or anthropologists' current understanding of the origins of medicine supports the old prejudice that early curers thought of the body in an empirical way unaffected by preconceptions. Archaic Chinese preconceptions are obvious enough. In the pre-Confucian classics the heart and liver appear more often as loci of emotions than as innards, to give only one example. This granted, we do find in such writings a more concrete approach to the viscera than in the high medical tradition or even in the philosophy of 100 B.C., simply because by 500 B.C. overarching philosophic schemes did not yet exist.

---

[65] The *locus classicus* is TS, *10* (7): 159 = LS, *8* (52): 84.

From organs to visceral systems was one of the more striking leaps of abstraction in Chinese intellectual history. The outcome was well adapted to predominantly functional thought about vital processes. Traditional physicians gave remarkably little attention, early or late, to structure, location, and lesion. This emphasis on function is perhaps the most fundamental difference between classical medicine in China and Europe.

Where do recent handbooks of traditional medicine stand on the functional and aspectual character of the body contents? They do not address the issue specifically, but neither did their predecessors. What they say about the body contents is consistently functional, as was true of their predecessors. But when one of them happens to define the body's systems and vital substances, the influence of modern medicine, and of scientific materialism generally, becomes apparent. The result is often the lack of coherence I have already noted with respect to the visceral and circulation systems.

The results of Western influence can be seen in discussions of vital substances. The treatment of *hsueh* is typical. The *Outline of Chinese Medicine* (1958) does not find it necessary to define *hsueh* or to relate it to blood. Its discussion of constructive *ch'i* and *hsueh* is solidly based in the classics that it quotes. It is, in fact, as good a synthesis of late classical doctrine as one could hope for. The vagueness and inconsistency of the early sources we have examined is conspicuously missing. Defensive *ch'i* "is formed when ingested food and drink . . . has been digested by the splenetic and stomach systems, and its essential, subtle part (*ching*) assimilated and transformed. Thus the constructive *ch'i* is originally the essential *ch'i* within food. Its distribution is from stomach system to pulmonary system, and from pulmonary system to the *hsueh* vessels, in which it circulates unceasingly through the whole body." *Hsueh*, "concretely speaking, is formed when the medial *chiao* [connected with the splenetic and stomach systems] assimilates the subtle essence of food and drink, and volatilization has formed constructive *ch'i*; the fluid secreted by the latter flows into the pulsating vessels and becomes *hsueh*. The *hsueh* travels through the *hsueh* vessels along with the constructive *ch'i*, flowing into the visceral systems and outward to nurture the extremities and bones. . . . Although constructive *ch'i* and *hsueh* move together in the pulsating vessels, they are not simultaneously produced, and there are certain differences in their forms and qualities."[66]

The Cultural Revolution encouraged more materialist and modernized interpretations than this one. They have become the norm. *Basic Knowledge about the Fatherland's Medicine* (1971), a popular handbook, took the bull by the horns: " '*Hsueh*' in Chinese medicine refers in part to blood, but the two are by no means equivalent. For instance, the Chinese physician believes that anemia is due to depletion of both '*ch'i*' and '*hsueh*'; but the Chinese physician's '*hsueh*' depletion is not necessarily anemia.' "[67]

Later publications, the *Revised Outline* among them (3.0, 3.2), treat *hsueh* as blood, often without dwelling on definitions. Those that quote the classics usually give priority to the *Inner Canon's* statement about extracting and reddening of juices, which supports this identification (see above, page 150). Definitions, when they occur, do not suggest room for discrepancy. The post-Cultural Revolution *Outline of Chinese Medicine* (1978), a textbook for pharmacy students, defines *hsueh* simply as "a red liquid that circulates in the blood vessels." This book nevertheless retains in Westernized language traditional ideas that do not square with this definition, for instance, "blood is also the material basis of mental activity." Why this should be true of blood is explained only by a questionably relevant line from the *Inner Canon*. The *Unabridged Dictionary* of 1982 defines *hsueh* as "blood, which is transformed from alimentary essences and moves in the blood vessels." But this is still not the modern physician's blood pumped by the heart: "Blood depends on propulsion by *ch'i* in order to provide for the viscera and tissues of

---

[66] Nan-ching Chung-i hsueh-yuan ed. 1958: 63–64. The diction of this passage is almost entirely traditional. Exceptions are "digest" (*hsiao-hua* 消 化), "assimilate" (*hsi-shou* 吸 收), and "volatilization" (*ch'i-hua* 气 化). In classical medicine *hsiao-hua* is used for unblocking pathological stases, and *ch'i-hua* for transformation by *ch'i*.

[67] Shang-hai ti-i i-hsueh-yuan 上 海 第 一 医 学 院 1971: 29, quotation marks in the original. In some books such quotation marks are the only hint that their "blood" is not exactly blood. For an example in English see Academy of Traditional Chinese Medicine 1975: 33. Such books do not use quotation marks when they are referring to blood in the modern sense.

the entire body, maintaining their normal functions and activities."[68]

Hsueh is now, in other words, no longer officially distinguished from blood, although the way it is described remains very different. Recent textbooks and handbooks are consistently inconsistent because identifying *hsueh* and blood has consequences for the overall understanding of vital processes that have not yet been faced. It is difficult to see how those consequences, or the consequences already visible in recent writings on the circulation and visceral systems, can be avoided. Once they are faced, it is difficult to see whether traditional medicine will long remain more than a grab-bag of therapeutic techniques.

---

[68] Hu-pei Chung-i hsueh-yuan ed. 1978: 27, 29; Chung-i yen-chiu-yuan et al. ed. 1982: 120–21, and similarly in Nan-ching Chung-i hsueh-yuan ed. 1983: 31. "Blood vessels" in the first quotation is *mai-kuan* 脉管 , a term used in modern medicine.

Chapter V

CLINICAL CONCEPTS

Diagnosis

Whether one thinks of its goal as naming the disease or determining its cause or appropriate treatment, diagnosis is a matter of relating particulars to a system of classifications. It depends on nosologies such as those I have discussed in connection with medical disorders. Diagnosis is not only an act of classifying, but a process of determining what counts as evidence. Here I will consider how that process was carried out in classical medicine, and what changes are already perceptible.

In chapter 6 of the *Revised Outline* we find a detailed account of diagnostic methods. This chapter calls for coordinated interrogation of the patient, visual inspection, auditory and olfactory examination, and palpation of the radial pulse and certain parts of the body.

The point of diagnosis in the early classics is not so much naming the disease as determining its manifestations—that is, what functions it is interfering with—and the dynamic character of pathological changes under way. We find a profusion of diagnostic techniques, with emphasis on signs and the pulse. Again we are dealing with a system that does not separate practice from high theory, organized around yin-yang, the Five Phases, and other concepts.

In the formative phase of traditional medicine, diagnostic examination was by no means the fully formed system that it has seemed to commentators. To give only one example, in the *Inner Canon* "the nine readings on the three sections" (*san pu chiu hou* 三 部 九 候) refers to nine different pulses distributed over the head, hands, and feet, each read to detect pathological changes in one of the visceral systems of function or their associated sense organs. According to this approach, the radial pulse provides a single reading that indicates the condition of the pulmonary system. Elsewhere the radial pulse vaguely reflects alterations in all the visceral *ch'i.*[1]

This method shortly gave way to much more elaborate reading of the radial pulse, alone or principally. In the *Canon of Problems*, "the nine readings on the three sections" was given its definitive sense, namely readings at three different finger pressures each on the three sections of the radial pulse alone, as described below (6.4.1.1). Prognosis depends on the radial pulse alone, we are told in the first sentence of the book, but pulses elsewhere in the body— including those felt along each circulation tract—still have their diagnostic uses.[2]

Palpation and other diagnostic methods were ordinarily used in combination, since it is often not the individual datum but the relation between data that makes detailed evaluation possible. The *Inner Canon* makes this point:

> The response of facial coloration, pulse, and inner forearm skin tension (*ch'ih* = *ch'ih-fu* 尺 膚) to each other is [as direct] as that of drum to drumstick, of shadow or echo [to object or sound]; there should be no discrepancy. . . . If the facial color is gray (*ch'ing* 青) the pulse should be strung [6.4.2.1.6; and so on]. . . . When you see a certain coloration but do not detect the corresponding pulse, but instead the pulse related to it in the mutual conquest order (P52), the patient will die. If you detect the pulse related in the mutual production order (P51), the disorder will remit. . . . When the pulse is hurried (*chi* 急 = *chin* 緊 ?, 6.4.1.2.6), the skin should be tense [*chi*, and so on]. . . . Thus one skilled at evaluating skin tension need not pause

---

[1] TS, *14* (1) = SW, *6* (20), illustrated in Porkert 1976: 166 (English translation, 1983: 203). See also TS, *14* (5): 266 = SW *3* (11): 67–68. The "nine readings" are actually taken at eleven locations, including two on the thigh associated with the foot locations. Traditional diagnosis is treated at length in Porkert's book.

[2] *Nan ching, 1*, Problems 18, 1, and 10 respectively. Porkert 1983: 205 remarks on current use of pulses other than the radial.

over the radial pulse, and one skilled at evaluating the radial pulse need not pause over facial coloration; but one who in practice is able to combine all three can become superior in this art.[3]

Gradually we find emerging elaborate new techniques and, toward the end of imperial China, the comprehensive and balanced doctrine of diagnosis described in the *Revised Outline*. An important statement of this doctrine came in the *Selection of Subtleties in Diagnostic Technique* of 1723: "From the *Records of the Grand Historian* on, authors have emphasized the pulse and dealt cursorily with interrogation and visual, auditory and olfactory examination. Latter-day [physicians] therefore ignored these methods, straying far from the Sage's instruction to consider both coloration and pulse. . . . In the end not one [of the four methods of diagnosis] can be omitted, any more than humans can do away with walking, standing, sitting or lying down."[4]

The approach to diagnosis reflected in the *Revised Outline* was not fully formed even in the eighteenth century. For instance, changes in tongue tissues and coatings were first generalized and systematized (as below, 6.2.2) late in the nineteenth century. One book that contributed to this clarification was Chou Hsueh-hai's 周 學 海 *Simplified Study of External Diagnosis* (1894), so-called because it emphasizes methods other than palpation: "Our predecessors' discussions of tongue examination were greatly detailed, but dealt only with tongue coating. It was not that they

---

[3] TS, *15* (2): 280–82 = LS, *1* (4): 10–11. See also *Nan ching, 1* (13): 12–14.

[4] *Ssu chen chueh wei* 四 診 抉 微 , author's preface. What I translate above as "Records of the Grand Historian" (*Shih chi*) is actually *Tien-wu shih* 典 午 氏 , a synonym of the author's surname. The allusion is to the biography of Ch'un-yü I (see page 138, note 28 above), in which the pulse indeed plays a disproportionate role in diagnosis. "The Sage" refers to the Yellow Lord, and thus to the above passage and related passages. The *Inner Canon* was considered by most eighteenth-century writers to be much older than the *Records* (100/90 B.C.), although in the light of recent research that seems unlikely.

ignored the tongue tissues, but they were too inexact to distinguish the two."[5]

Diagnostic innovations in the twentieth century came, of course, overwhelmingly from modern medicine, with its concepts of cell, lesion, microorganism, and infection (although laboratory tests are not nearly as frequent in China as in Europe and the United States). The crucial question to consider about current practice, in fact, is not how modern medicine has influenced traditional diagnosis but how quickly the latter is falling out of use.

During the Cultural Revolution, in chapters on diseases in textbooks and handbooks of traditional medicine, modern diseases frequently replaced those previously listed. This is true of the *Revised Outline*, as appendix B shows. More recent medical-school textbooks for foundation courses have returned to traditional categories.[6] Nevertheless there is reason to believe that more advanced training in diagnosis, including clinical training, concentrates on Western diseases.[7] Examination of case records in traditional hospitals and clinics in 1978 indicates that the diagnoses overwhelmingly used Western entities.[8] The *Revised Outline* also reflects traditional doctors' use of scientific data generated by laboratory tests (for instance, in 7.5 and 10.6).

This tendency is not surprising, considering that so many patients are treated by a combination of traditional and modern means. Two separate diagnoses are apparently thought too great a luxury for China's health care resources, and a diagnosis compatible with modern treatment is an inevitable choice when a choice must be made. I have already argued that a modern diagnosis cannot be

---

[5] *Hsing se wai chen chien mo* 形色外診簡摩 , 2: 80. This statement is not entirely correct; see Ch'en Tse-lin 陈泽霖 1982.

[6] Pei-ching Chung-i hsueh-yuan ed. 1978, for students of traditional medicine, has no separate chapter on diseases, but uses traditional entities in its section on diagnosis (chapter 5). There is a section on diseases in Hu-pei Chung-i hsueh-yuan ed. 1978, for pharmacy students (section 2).

[7] Personal communication from Dr. Fu Xiaoyan, trained at Hubei College of Medicine and Beijing College of Traditional Chinese Medicine, and Dr. Shen Yu, a graduate of the latter. See also Kleinman 1980: 270–71 on points of similarity in Taiwan.

[8] See chapter I, note 23.

an adequate guide to traditional therapy, for there is too little overlap in the definitions of medical disorders; but many young traditional doctors obviously do not find this objection decisive. More important in their eyes are the unequivocality and concreteness of modern diagnosis.[9] At the same time there is no evidence that a rational system of traditional therapy based on modern diagnosis is being developed. The focus of therapeutic reasoning remains, rather, manifestation type determination. Whether it will be standardized and reconciled with diagnostic reasoning derived from the European tradition remains an open question.

Therapy

The specifics of therapy lie outside the scope of this book, but the broad principles on which treatment are based are outlined in chapter 10 of the *Revised Outline* and translated below. Here I will merely supplement chapter 10 with a few remarks on the general character of therapy and the organization of its basic ideas, with due attention to past and contemporary change.

Looked at most schematically, traditional therapy is based on two approaches (10.3), strengthening the body's own order-maintaining vitalities ("reinforcing the orthopathic *ch'i*," *pu cheng* 補正 or *fu cheng* 扶正 , 7.1) and attacking the opposing forces responsible for disorder, whether of external or internal origin ("expelling the heteropathic *ch'i*," *ch'ü hsieh* 祛邪 , also called "attacking," *kung* 攻 , 10.3.2). Drugs and other means restore balance (the basis of order) by opposing the dynamic character of the disorder. Cooling drugs, for instance, counteract hot heteropathy which has tilted the metabolic balance in favor of yang activity.

As chapter 10 makes clear with a plethora of subsidiary principles, examples, and an extended account of medical treatment,

---

[9] Porkert, in 1982a and elsewhere, believes that the disuse of traditional diagnostic entities must interfere decisively with the effectiveness of traditional therapy. That is plausible, although we still lack a systematic assessment of effectiveness. In view of the proclivity of patients for recovery without—sometimes despite—medical intervention, questions of effectiveness cannot be settled by anecdotes or appeals to history.

this principle of opposition therapy is not used in a simple-minded way. The need to apply it flexibly and often indirectly (10.2.1), to counter it when there is reason to do so (inverse therapy and use of inverse collaterals, 10.4.2), to reason subtly on priorities (10.4.1), and to fit medication to circumstances and cases (10.5), make exceptional demands on clinical judgment shaped by training and experience.

The purpose of chapter 10 is to demonstrate the application to therapy of dialectical method. It emphasizes two linked aspects of clinical reasoning, the need to consciously employ dialectical relations (that is, complementary but opposed concepts), and the necessity to encompass the entire situation of which dialectical contradictions are aspects. Although the language of the chapter is in many respects that of modern Chinese philosophy of science (called "the dialectic of nature," *tzu-jan pien-cheng-fa* 自 然 辩 证 法 , after Engels), the examples of holistic approach and yin-yang complementarity are typical of classical medicine. The emphasis on struggle and battle as metaphors for therapy (e.g., 10.3) is Maoist, but the old ideas of attacking and expelling the heteropathy, not nearly as prominent an image in discourse before modern times, provide a precedent for it.

Chinese therapy combines a broad range of techniques (10.3.1). Even in the earliest surviving handbooks of remedies we find a great many kinds. *Prescriptions for Fifty-two Ailments*, a text possibly as old as the third century B.C., includes drugs of plant, animal, and mineral origin in simple and composite prescriptions; moxibustion and other kinds of cauterization; fumigation; hot and cold compresses; massage; simple surgery without incision; lancing with stone probes and horns; dietary regulation; and a variety of magical and religious practices. The medical prescriptions on bamboo slips and wooden tablets from Wuwei 武 威 , Gansu, in northwest China, buried in the first century A.D., use drugs, acupuncture with unspecified instruments, moxibustion, fumigation, and what is almost certainly exorcism or interdiction.[10]

---

[10] *Wu-shih-erh ping fang* 五 十 二 病 方 . Therapy is analyzed by Harper 1982: 22–42. *Wu-wei Han tai i chien* 武 威 漢 代 醫 簡 , Japanese translation in Akahori 1978b. The original titles of both these collections are lost; these were given by their modern editors. Neither published text can be considered a definitive edition.

This is not to say that all major classical sources were equally eclectic. Of the two great classical traditions, that of the *Inner Canon of the Yellow Lord* and that of the *Treatise on Cold Damage Disorders*, we have seen that the first emphasizes acupuncture and the second, drug presciptions, although neither is entirely specialized. Of all the important therapies acupuncture was most often dispensed with in classical times. As important a therapeutic handbook as *Arcane Essentials from the Imperial Library* (752) rejects it outright as dangerous, although the book includes moxibusion, which would seem to carry no less danger of serious infection. Lu and Needham note that acupuncture was "rather a lost art" by the mid-eighteenth century, and its teaching was proscribed in 1822.[11] Although the *Revised Outline* devotes the preponderance of its space to drugs, its discussions of particular diseases (those of Western, not traditional medicine) recommend not only acupuncture but various "new therapeutic methods" such as drug injections at acupuncture loci.

The most important resource of traditional therapy was undoubtedly drugs. From earliest times they were derived from animals and minerals as well as plants. The latter were at first found wild, but were increasingly cultivated after the first millennium A.D.[12]

It was possible within limits, before the era of laboratory analysis, to control the concentration of active ingredients in drugs of vegetable origin. A given alkaloid, desirable in one application and not in another, could not be distinguished from other constituents of the plant in which it occurs, nor could its effect be separated from theirs. Still its comparative strength could be more or less standardized by choosing plants from certain places with certain environments and climates, by gathering them at a certain time of day and season, by drying them in the sun rather than in the shade or vice versa, by processing a certain part of the plant, or by preparing the prescription in a certain way. These details were all matters of great concern in the handbooks of materia medica.

The diversity of drugs was remarkable. The oldest treatise on medical simples, the *Divine Husbandman's Materia Medica* (*Shen nung pen-ts'ao* 神農本草 , late first or second century A.D.)

---

[11] *Wai t'ai pi yao* 外臺祕要 ; see, among other sources, Lu and Needham 1980: 127–28 and, on official rejections of acupuncture, page 160.

[12] Hu Tao-ching 1963.

includes 365 drugs. The classical source most commonly used today, the *Systematic Materia Medica* (*Pen-ts'ao kang mu* 本 草 綱 目) of 1596, contains 1892 drugs, and its sequel (*Pen-ts'ao kang mu shih i* 本 草 綱 目 拾 遺 , ca. 1803) adds another 716. The most authoritative modern reference work on simples lists 5,767 types. The *Revised Outline* itself lists 973 plant names, of which perhaps a quarter are synonyms.[13]

How, then, are so many drugs and disorders matched as patients are cared for? The matching must, of course, reflect accumulated clinical results. But the notion that therapy of such complexity can be built upon simple empiricism is unlikely to survive acquaintance with the literature. The matching of symptoms to a limited number of prescriptions in the *Treatise on Cold Damage Disorders* cannot be far removed from the experiential roots of traditional drug therapy. But the basic prescriptions and their modifications are organized by the highly abstract Six Warps concept, as we have already seen (page 84). Does this theoretical thrust strengthen or weaken the effectiveness of the prescriptions? The question can hardly be answered until the prescriptions have been clinically evaluated in a rigorous way.

Recent studies of an analogous issue, various acupuncture techniques for replenishing and draining, indicate that these "are not empirical procedures but the results of artificial processing" of experience.[14] In this instance critical trials reveal little value in clinical applications despite centuries of use. This may also be true of

---

[13] *Pen-ts'ao kang mu* often treats more than one physiologically active part of a plant in one article, so the number of distinct drugs included is well over two thousand. A count of drugs in nine classical compilations of materia medica is given in Yuan Han-ch'ing 袁 翰 青 1956: 239. For mineral drugs in Chinese and European compilations see Needham 1954- : III, 647. The modern reference work is Chiang-su hsin i-hsueh-yuan 江 苏 新 医 学 院 ed. 1977–78.

[14] Shang-hai shih chen-chiu yen-chiu-so ed. 1970: 187–92. Replenishing (*pu* 補) and draining (*hsieh* 瀉) are explained (as "reinforcing and reducing") in Beijing College of Traditional Chinese Medicine et al. 1980: 307–9. The discussions of acupuncture in the *Revised Outline* ignore these concepts. The common translation of *pu* and *hsieh* as "tonification and sedation" is extremely misleading.

the Six Warps; or they may prove to be an efficient framework for a complex structure of proven knowledge. Only testing will tell.

In the earliest classics we find more than one classification of drug functions. The best known, that by which the three hundred and sixty-five drugs of the *Divine Husbandman's Materia Medica* was organized, transcends the bounds of medicine:

> Drugs of the higher sort, one hundred twenty kinds, used as principal drugs [literally, "monarchs," in prescriptions]; for nurturing life; corresponding to heaven [among the Three Powers, heaven, earth, and man]; without toxic principles. When taken in large amounts or for long periods they are not harmful. Those who want to lighten their bodies, augment their *ch'i*, and increase their longevity without growing old will use drugs in the higher canon.
>
> Drugs of the middle sort, one hundred twenty kinds, used as adjuvants (literally, "ministers,"); for nurturing the nature; corresponding to man; with or without toxic principles, so that appropriate usage must be considered. Those who wish to check medical disorders and replenish depleted energies will use drugs in the middle canon.
>
> Drugs of the lower sort, one hundred twenty-five kinds, used as collaterals and guides (literally, "assistants and emissaries"); for treating medical disorders; corresponding to earth; mostly toxic. May not be taken for long periods. Those who wish to expel cold or hot heteropathic *ch'i*, to break up accumulations [of *ch'i* in the body], or to cure diseases will use drugs in the lower canon.

This classification is too catholic to be very useful to physicians preoccupied with curing disease, its lowest priority. Drugs within each of these three broad classes were further characterized in three ways, the first two of which were further developed by later authors on materia medica: "For drugs there are five sapors [*wu wei* 五 味 , literally, 'flavors,' P193]—sour, salty, sweet, bitter, and pungent—and four *ch'i*—chilling, heating, warming, and cooling—and they may or may not contain toxicity." When we look up the first two drugs in the *Divine Husbandman's* "higher canon" of immortality agents, we find "Jade: Sapor sweet, [*ch'i*] neutral

... Cinnabar: Sapor sweet, [ch'i] slightly chilling." It is obvious that something more than sense impressions is involved. As the primitive meaning of *wei* indicates, the sapors must have originated in ordinary tastes. In cooking *wu wei* refers precisely to sour, salty, sweet, bitter, and pungent flavors. But cinnabar (HgS) is insoluble, and has no taste, nor is it possible to see how jade could taste sweet. In the *Inner Canon* (probably a little earlier than the materia medica just quoted) we are given lists of foods that provide each sapor. Some correspond well to culinary flavors, some poorly. Among those that correspond poorly, wheat and lamb or goat are given for "bitter," and soybeans, pork, and chestnuts for "salty." Common sense tells us these are abstractions made to fit the fivefold schema.[15]

As for the primitive significance of *ch'i*, there is no point in guessing precisely what warm or cold feelings in the body once underlay this concept. The example again alerts us that we are dealing with concepts, not simple, direct sensations: cinnabar's physiological effect is described not as cooling but as slightly chilling, which should be the same thing but patently is not.

"Sapor" and "*ch'i*" are concepts related only indirectly to flavors and warm or cold feelings; they relate directly to the Five Phases and yin-yang theory. The primary function of the *wu wei* concept in its specialized, medical form ("five sapors") is to express Five Phases correspondences, and thus to relate drugs to disorders of the

---

[15] *Shen nung pen-ts'ao, 1:* 5a-5b (page 9), 7a (page 10), *3:* 1a-2a (page 27); TS, *2* (4): 17 = SW, *7* (22): 129. In the first quotation, for *chih* 執 read *han* 寒 ; this is a copyist's error, not seen in the extant Six Dynasties or T'ang MS of *Pen-ts'ao ching chi chu* 本 草 經 集 注 . "Toxicity" does not refer to poisonous properties pure and simple, but to utility for "attacking poison with poison" (*i tu kung tu* 以 毒 攻 毒). The literature emphasizes that drugs considered toxic in this sense do not harm patients if they are correctly prescribed, but should not be used longer than necessary. "Warming" and "cooling" refer to milder effects than "heating" and "chilling."

The most concrete historical outline of drug classification in traditional medicine known to me is in Nan-ching Chung-i hsueh-yuan ed. 1964: 10–12. For interesting comparisons between the understanding and use of materia medica in the medical systems of various cultures see Porkert 1978: 15–34.

five yin visceral systems of function, and related entities. A sixth class, "neutral" (*tan* 淡), was added to extend the system of sapors to correspond as well to the Six Warps, the six yang visceral systems of function, and so on. It was essential for that purpose that "neutral" not be strictly neutral, but be considered alongside the pungent and sweet sapors as yang. The Four *Ch'i* correspond to the four gradations, immature and mature, of yin and yang. This set of correspondences was furnished with its own term for "neutral," *p'ing* 平 , as the balance point. The Four *Ch'i* make it possible to express with some precision the applicability of a drug to disorders expressed as yin or yang.

The five sapors and four *ch'i* together could thus rather flexibly match the effects of drugs to symptoms analyzed according to manifestion types, and they were supplemented by other classifications to make them even more comprehensive. The most important of these, the rubrics "rising, descending, floating, and sinking" (*sheng chiang fu ch'en* 升 降 浮 沉), express the tendency of a given drug's action toward, respectively, the upper, lower, outer, and inner aspect of the body. These activities enrich the major pathological and pharmacological theories through the usual yin-yang associations.[16]

Such classifications are important to those actively exploring and extending the materia medica, but are hardly essential to therapists who merely apply pharmaceutical knowledge; traditional physicians of the new type are increasingly consumers in this sense. No doubt it was always possible to find half-educated doctors for whom *wei* is simply the flavor of a drug, and *ch'i* no more than its subjective warming or cooling effect in the stomach or in the body as a whole.

In recent handbooks and textbooks meant for public education and the general training of traditional physicians, *wei* and *ch'i* are defined briefly and without nuance. For instance, in the *Revised Outline*, the four *ch'i* are "four characteristics," listed but undefined, and the five sapors are "five types of flavor" (11.1.1; I translate *wu*

---

[16] The term appears without clear discussion in *I-hsueh ch'i yuan* 醫 學 啟 源 (late 12th century), 2 (11): 155–58, and a full account is given in *Pen-ts'ao kang mu*, 1: 54–55. For modern discussions see Nan-ching Chung-i hsueh-yuan ed. 1958: 215–17 and Kan-su sheng hsin i-yao-hsueh yen-chiu-so 甘 肅 省 新 医 药 学 研 究 所 ed. 1982: 17–24.

wei as "five flavors" below to reflect this understanding). When we move on to specialist writings on traditional pharmacy, of course, we find due qualifications. "These 'flavors' are in the main those detected with the organs of taste or those determined on the basis of the results of clinical therapy."[17]

Whether the Five Sapors are simplified to equate them with flavors has thus become largely a matter of educational level and degree of specialization. In the most discriminating writing the difference is still quite clear, as in the magisterial little introduction to yin-yang and Five Phases theory by Jen Ying-ch'iu: "the so-called sour, bitter, sweet, pungent, and salty are not actually like the sour and salty flavors of food, but instead simply represent the *ch'i* and characteristics corresponding to the Five Phases."[18]

The abstract character of the five sapors and four *ch'i*, no matter how deeply ingrained in classical medicine, is not at all certain to survive when it is not generally understood by practitioners. The specializations of modern science can maintain vast accumulations of highly technical knowledge that only a few comprehend. Traditional medicine, however, has hardly begun to develop in this direction.[19]

---

[17] Ibid., 18. Such qualifications do not appear in all specialized writings, especially not in those meant for secondary rather than higher education, such as Li Hsiang-chung 李相中 1964: 62, which concentrates on relating taste to modern knowledge of chemical composition.

[18] Jen 1960: 30, explicating SW, 2 (5): 30–34.

[19] Historians of medicine frequently write of "specialization" in early European or Chinese medicine, but the evidence shows a situation that has little in common with modern specialization. Chinese doctors generally considered treatises on particular diseases, and medical careers devoted to particular kinds of patients (e.g., women and childbirth), by comparison with unspecialized activity, a lower rather than a higher qualification, and a sign of deficient medical education. Two assumptions underlay this attitude: that full competence requires command of the integral art of medicine—which entails an understanding of Nature, society, and the individual besides—and that the physician is ethically obligated to respond to every patient in need of help. Both assumptions were influentially stated in the opening pages of *Pei chi ch'ien chin yao fang* 備急千金要方 (650/659), *1* (1–

In addition to this classification of therapeutic drugs by yin-yang and Five Phases functions, the *Divine Husbandman's Materia Medica* offers another that relates them directly to type of disorder: "Cold heteropathy disorders are treated with heating drugs; hot heteropathy disorders with chilling drugs; indigestion with drugs for disgorging or bringing down [*t'u hsia yao* 吐下药 , equivalent to emetics and purges]; possession by ghosts and *ku* 蠱 poisoning [a kind of witchcraft] with toxic drugs; abscesses, ulcerations, swellings, and surface growths with drugs for lesions (*ch'uang yao* 瘡藥); and wind and moist heteropathy disorders with Wind drugs, as appropriate in each case."[20]

This is not a systematic classification, since by classical standards some types of activity are very general and some specific; that is, some are directed toward a particular heteropathy, and some toward effects that may be caused by more than one sort of heteropathy. This scheme was eventually modified in the light of drug functions implicit in the *Treatise on Cold Damage Disorders*, even though the latter described prescriptions and not simples. The definitive version (although not the last) was the "eight basic methods of drug therapy," systematized in *The Awakening of the Mind in Medical Studies* (*I hsueh hsin wu*, 1732) and discussed in the *Revised Outline* (10.3.2): sweating, disgorging, bringing down, mediating, warming, clearing, dispersing, and replenishing.

This set of eight actions does not exhaust the classical repertory of therapeutic tactics; but the more elaborate approaches can generally be understood as built on this basis, even though the terminology may vary. To choose one among the many complex therapies recommended in the *Revised Outline*, "flushing the outer aspect and clearing the active *ch'i* sector" (9.1.2.5), a specific technique for dealing with heteropathies passing into the inner aspect of the body, would be considered a combination of sweating and clearing—that is, a specific technique using sudorifics and (roughly) antipyretics to drive out a heteropathy located partly in the outer aspect but partly passed into the inner aspect.

---

2): 1a-2a. There is a partial translation in Lee 1943. The full translation of Section 2 in Unschuld 1979: 29-33 contains many errors.

[20] *Shen nung pen-ts'ao, 1*: 8b (page 11). The understanding of *ku* at roughly the time this work was compiled is discussed in Loewe 1974: 81-90.

If we compare this list of eight basic methods with the familiar therapeutic rubrics in European pharmacognosy—the desiccants, astringents, laxatives, lithagogues, etc.—a pattern of differences becomes obvious despite the wide scope of both classifications, which leads to much overlap. The Western nomenclature reflects the use of drugs to manipulate specific symptoms, specific body fluids (and, in an earlier day, humors), and specific abnormalities in tissues. They could, of course, have very general applications, such as the use of sudorifics to precipitate the crisis in febrile diseases when perspiration has stopped. Still the Chinese classifications are often only superficially similar. They are based on response to heteropathy, a pathological vector that interferes with normal body functions and may be directly or indirectly responsible for a given constellation of symptoms. A particular symptom may fall under more than one Chinese category; constipation may be treated by "bringing down" or "dispersing," using an unblocking purgative, lubricant, or moistening prescription, depending on the origin and character of the constipation (types of prescriptions will be discussed below).

So far I have introduced ways of classifying individual drugs and basic therapeutic methods. This is not the whole story. Even in the earliest medical compendia we find drugs being used in combination.

Blending drugs does not, for the traditional physician, raise problems of their chemical or, within limits, physiological interaction. The engaging eighteenth-century physician Hsu Ta-ch'un makes this point in his *Topical Discussions of the History of Medicine* when discussing the use of drugs with replenishing and attacking functions in the same prescription:

> A doubter objected: "If two drugs of opposed characters are decocted in the same liquid, they will cancel each other out, so that the one that is supposed to attack will not attack, and the one that is supposed to replenish will not replenish. One might as well not take the medicine. And if they do not cancel each other out, and each goes its separate way, then it may well happen that what was meant to be attacked will be strengthened instead, and vice versa. If so, not only will the prescription not help, it will do harm. These possibilities call for reflection."

This is quite wrong. It would seem that drugs by nature carry out their functions. A drug the function of which is to attack will attack [heteropathic *ch'i*] that is too strong. One whose function is to replenish will replenish [orthopathic *ch'i*] that is too weak. This is just as, when you dig a pit in the earth and water flows down from a high place, it is bound to fill the pit before flowing onward, and in any case will not turn and flow back up to the high place.

For example, when rhubarb rhizome and ginseng root are used together, the rhubarb will certainly serve to get rid of hard accumulations [as in constipation], and in no instance will harm the orthopathic *ch'i*; the ginseng will serve to increase the level of orthopathic *ch'i*, and in no instance will replenish the heteropathic *ch'i*.

The ancients, when they worked out the techniques of compounding, distinguished the tracts and visceral systems [in which each simple specifically acts] ... In Cassia Twig Infusion (page 86 and 9.1.1.5), the cassia travels along the circulation path of the defensive *ch'i* in order to expel the wind heteropathy, and the peony root, along that of the constructive *ch'i* in order to stop the perspiration. Here too each drug reverts to its proper part of the circulation.[21]

Even though drugs used in combination do not interfere with each other, composite medicines must be governed by unified therapeutic goals. But the functions of prescriptions eventually were seen as too diverse to be encompassed by a few categories. By the middle of the sixth century we find the Ten Prescription Types (*shih chi* 十 劑). There is some question whether these labels originally pertained to simples or compound prescriptions, but they were taken up from the eleventh century on to analyze the activity of prescriptions in a way that relates it to the gamut of physiologi-

---

[21] *I hsueh yuan-liu lun* (1757), pages 103–4. See also the discussion in Jen Ying-ch'iu 1978: 72.

cal states, referring more directly than the Eight Methods to psychological states as well:

1. dispersing (*hsuan* 宣), for stasis of circulation due to heteropathy that congeals when orthopathic *ch'i* resists its inward transmission

2. unblocking (*t'ung* 通), for obstructed circulation due to moist or hot heteropathy in the *ch'i* sector (9.1.2), and interference with elimination

3. replenishing *(pu)* 補 , for debilitation and *ch'i* depletion generally

4. purgative (*hsieh* 泄 , 瀉), for obstructions due to repletion, especially but not only those related to constipation

5. unburdening (*ch'ing* 輕 , literally, "to make lighter in weight"), for heteropathy in the skin and flesh, mainly sudorific prescriptions

6. restraining (*chung* 重 , literally, "to make heavier"), for repressing instability, especially of emotions

7. lubricating (*hua* 滑), for eliminating substances abnormally retained in the body, expelled in such forms as urinary calculi, urethral discharges, and purulence of abscesses

8. roughening (*se* 澀), for stopping abnormal loss of body substances in such forms as spermatorrhea, chronic diarrhea, and chronic coughs

9. desiccating (*tsao* 燥), for the effects of moist heteropathy (5.1.4)

10.   moistening (*shih* 濕, *jun* 潤), for the effects of dry heteropathy (5.1.5).[22]

Although the Ten Prescriptions saw service for a millennium, with minor modifications from time to time, this classification remained far from comprehensive. It did not reflect the specific character of some important prescriptions, such as those proven effective for external lesions and for parasites. Disorders peculiar to women and children, although classical physicians considered them distinct, were also not reflected.

A considerably more comprehensive set of associations between prescriptions and types of disorders became the basis of classification in Wang Ang's 汪 昂 *Collected Explanations of Medical Prescriptions* (1682). Wang combined aspects of the *Eight Methods* and the Ten Prescriptions with new categories.[23]

1.   replenishing and strengthening (*pu yang* 補 養): prescriptions for *ch'i* and *hsueh* depletion and general tonic functions (= replenishing, # 3; 12.16)

---

[22] This set of categories is generally but not universally considered to come from the lost *Lei kung yao tui* 雷 公 藥 對, attributed to Hsu Ts'ai or Hsu Chih-ts'ai 徐 之 才, a prominent statesman and medical author. This work is cited in Sung compilations of materia medica such as the *Ching shih cheng lei Ta-kuan pen-ts'ao* 經 史 證 類 大 觀 本 草 (1108), *1*: 27a–27b (page 35) and *Sheng chi ching* (1118), *10*: 153–55. Later commentaries, which treat this as a classification of prescriptions and also reflect changing understanding of the categories, are gathered in *Pen-ts'ao kang mu* (1596), *1*: 43–49. Examples of composite prescriptions for each category are given in Nan-ching Chung-i hsueh-yuan ed. 1964: 11.

[23] *I fang chi chieh* 醫 方 集 解. Wang added to his 21 rubrics short sections on acute emergencies and life-lengthening hygiene. In the list that follows, overlaps with the Eight Methods (by name) and the Ten Prescriptions (by number, preceded by "#") are indicated, as well as section numbers for corresponding categories in the *Revised Outline*. A slightly different system of twenty heads is used in chapter 12.

2. venting the outer aspect *(fa piao)* 發表 : prescriptions for driving out heteropathy in the skin and flesh (= sweating, # 5; 12.1)

3. emesis *(yung t'u* 涌吐): prescriptions for leading heteropathy upward and out (= disgorging; 12.8)

4. attacking in the inner aspect *(kung li* 攻裏): prescriptions for relieving constipation due to stasis of elimination processes in the stomach and intestines (= bringing down, # 4; 12.9)

5. outer and inner aspect *(piao li)* 表裏 : prescriptions for blockages due to repletion heteropathy in both aspects (a combination of agents for sweating and bringing down)

6. mediating and flushing *(ho chieh* 和解): prescriptions for heteropathy of external origin, especially of epidemic disorders, in both aspects, for which attack therapy of the last category is not appropriate; also for circulation stasis due to certain internal causes (= mediating; 12.7)

7. reordering the *ch'i* (*li ch'i* 理氣): prescriptions directed at defects in the circulation of *ch'i* (not the vitalities in general, but the yang counterpart of *hsueh;* 12.12)

8. reordering the *hsueh* (*li hsueh* 理血): prescriptions directed at defects in the circulation of *hsueh* (the yin aspect of *ch'i* in the general sense), including blockages due to coagulation of blood (12.13)

9. expelling wind heteropathy *(ch'ü feng* 祛風 ; 5.1.1; 12.3)

10. expelling cold heteropathy *(ch'ü han* 祛寒 , = warming; 5.1.2, 12.4)

11. clearing heat heteropathy *(ch'ing shu* 清暑 , = clearing; 5.1.3; 12.2)

12. freeing moist heteropathy (*li shih* 利濕): prescriptions that expel moist heteropathy through the skin or in the urine or stool (= # 9; 5.1.4, 12.5)

13. moistening dry heteropathy (*jun tsao*)潤燥= # 10; 5.1.5, 12.6

14. draining Fire Heteropathy (*hsieh huo* 瀉火): prescriptions directed against intense hot heteropathy of external and internal origin; includes antipyretics and prescriptions that conserve body fluids (5.1.6, 12.2)

15. eliminating mucus (*ch'u t'an* 除痰): prescriptions directed against pathological mucus (3.5, 12.11)

16. dispersing and leading out (*hsiao tao* 消導): prescriptions for dispersing blockages that interfere with the splenetic and stomach functions (= dispersing, # 1; 2.1.3, 12.10)

17. astringents (*shou se* 收濇): prescriptions for stopping abnormal loss of body substances (= # 8; 12.17)

18. vermicides (*sha ch'ung* 殺蟲): prescriptions that kill or expel parasites infecting the alimentary and urogenital tracts and the skin (12.18)

19. improving eyesight (*ming mu* 明目): prescriptions for eye disorders in general

20. swellings and sores (*yung yang* 癰瘍): prescriptions for external lesions (12.19)

21. menstruation and childbirth (*ching ch'an* 經產): prescriptions for obstetrical and gynecological disorders in general.

Wang's scheme of twenty-one types of prescriptions is certainly more comprehensive than its predecessors, although still far from systematic. As the titles indicate, some classes are based on abstract principles of opposition therapy (for instance, mediating and flushing), some on straightforward physiological effects (emesis), and some on groupings of disorders by body function affected or by type of patient (improving eyesight, menstruation, and childbirth). Despite this catchall quality, the twenty-one types have been adapted in influential compilations of prescriptions, such as the *Practical Prescriptions* of 1761.[24] This system has also provided the basis for organizing prescriptions in handbooks and textbooks of the last quarter-century.

This is not to say, however, that it has become the common standard of organization. Its breadth made it attractive, but its lack of taxonomic rigor has led to endless piecemeal revisions, with no consensus. We can see this as early as *Practical Prescriptions*, which expanded Wang's twenty-one headings to twenty-four. We can see it as well in the twenty rubrics of the *Revised Outline*. The 1972 compilation rejected three of Wang's ad hoc categories (5, 19, and 21), combined the two categories of prescriptions directed against heat heteropathy (11 and 14), and added three new rubrics for prescriptions that treat mental confusion due to mucus blocking the orifices of the heart ("opening the passages," *hsuan ch'iao* 宣 竅 , 12.14), for prescriptions that treat emotional instability due to hepatic yang excess (8.2.2), internal wind heteropathy (5.1.1.2), and other causes ("yang latensification and sedation," *chen ch'ien an shen* 鎮 潛 安 神, 3.1.3, 12.15), and for drugs applied externally to treat external disorders ("external remedies," *wai chih* 外 治 , 12.20). This revision (based on that of the 1964 *Outline of Chinese Materia Medica* or an unavailable predecessor) modernizes the classification of drugs for mental disorders, which had been reflected in the old Ten Prescriptions fourteen centuries earlier under the head "restraining"; but it does not come to grips with the defects in systematic rigor.

Similar tinkering has been the rule in publications since 1958. The *Outline of Chinese Medicine* published in that year is the only recent work I have seen that uses Wang Ang's classification without significant modification.

Nineteen of the treatises listed below in appendix A arrange their discussions of prescriptions (or in some instances simples) under headings ultimately derived from the organization of *Collected Explanations of Medical Prescriptions,* and also draw on modifications by their recent predecessors. None uses a classification of independent origin.

---

[24] *Ch'eng fang ch'ieh yung* 成 方 切 用 by Wu I-lo 吳 儀 洛·

Nevertheless continuity is regularly undercut by changing the order of classes and modifying their names. It will not be obvious to the novice that, for instance, "freeing moist heteropathy," "freeing the Water" (*li shui* 利 水), "expelling moist heteropathy" (*ch'ü shih* 祛 濕), "freeing urination" (*li niao* 利 尿), and "inducing leakage of moist heteropathy and driving out Water" (*shen shih chu shui* 滲 濕 逐 水) refer to the same function. The number of rubrics in these nineteen books fluctuates between twelve and twenty-three.[25]

Considering all the textbooks and handbooks published since 1958 that I have been able to consult, a clear distinction of change in the classification of prescriptions is easy to see. That direction is away from the authority of *Collected Explanations of Medical Prescriptions*. There is no sign that it points toward a single taxonomy.

The significance of these findings should not be exaggerated. The variations and embellishments are, after all, on a single theme. One tends to expect of socialist nations feats of standardization that are difficult to achieve anywhere. The fact remains that the textbooks in question were compiled at different medical schools, and no national medical organization effectively controls the organization and content of medical nomenclature. Finally, given the pace and frequent abruptness of change in China, only a fool would extrapolate a decade's trend far into the future.

This has been a very incomplete sketch of therapeutic classifications, relating drugs to disorders. I have discussed only historically significant classifications, emphasizing those that lie at the roots of present-day practice. It is clear that these basic ideas about the natural classes of drugs did not spring full-blown from the brow of the Divine Husbandman (much less that of the Yellow Emperor, whose canon offers no taxonomy). They evolved gradually, and are still evolving.

Therapeutic agents themselves are rapidly changing in character and use. Acupuncture loci recommended for each application are being reduced in number on the basis of clinical effectiveness and scientific studies. In the last generation moxibustion has been transformed from a therapy that often produced blisters (and thence

---

[25] Nan-ching Chung-i hsueh-yuan ed. 1958: 265–96. The system of thirty rubrics in Chou Chin-huang 周 金 黃 ed. 1984: *passim* is for modern as well as traditional drugs.

infections) as a cone of punk burned down to the skin, to one that provides local but gentle warmth. The role of diet in hygiene and medical care has begun to change as the diet itself is changing. Twenty years ago the contents of the same drug prescription from city to city was anything but standardized, but this situation had already become a matter of administrative concern.[26] Standardized and purified extracts are used increasingly instead of crude natural drugs. Prescriptions are distributed more and more in factory-produced form—as compounded mixtures, capsules, etc.—rather than made up from simples by a pharmacist before use. Most important, a wide variety of drugs and methods of treatment have been adopted from modern medicine. They are being used without hesitation in traditional clinics, in clinics devoted to combined therapy, and especially in the less specialized domains of practice.[27]

One can think of many other important issues concerning change in therapy, change that has been perceptible throughout the tradition and is not accelerated. One is the frequency with which various drugs, singly and in combination, are prescribed. Another is dosage. A third is the coordination of drug remedies with other therapies. A fourth is the availability of simples and ready-to-take drugs in a rapidly developing nationwide and international commercial system. Still another is the cost of health care (remembering that health care until recently encompassed religious and magical curing and medical services at many different levels of society). All of these are poorly understood with respect to classical medicine as well as recent practice.

---

[26] Chung-i yen-chiu-yuan et al. ed. 1964, a survey of dispensing practices in 25 main cities.

[27] There are large sections on modern drugs in handbooks written for barefoot doctors and village physicians. The latter received more education than barefoot doctors and were responsible for production brigade clinics and similar facilities. See, for instance, Shang-hai Chung-i hsueh-yuan et al. ed. 1970: 679–739, a typical handbook for barefoot doctors, and Hu-nan i-hsueh-yuan ed. 1971: 1159–1225, for village physicians. Oddly, the English translation of a 1970 barefoot doctor's manual does not include such a discussion, although Western drugs are recommended throughout the chapter on therapy (Revolutionary Health Committee of Hunan Province ed. 1977: 64–184).

The only issue on which substantial research has been done is historical changes in the drugs of choice for certain medical disorders. In a remarkable series of short but compendious studies, Miyasita Saburō has discussed trends in the content of prescriptions for seven disorders in the most important formularies from early times to the present. He finds that for most but not all of the disorders studied, despite the continuity afforded by a cumulative written tradition, there were major shifts in patterns of drug use. The most frequent pattern was a change centered on the late eleventh and early twelfth century. Miyasita also suggests that from about the fourteenth century on there was an increasing emphasis on the use of replenishing drugs to enhance the body's resistance.[28] These are only tentative and partial findings, but they suggest that research questions can be intelligently defined and investigated to lessen our ignorance of therapeutic change.

There remains a larger and much less tractable difficulty. This is the abiding problem of medical pluralism, characteristic of most of the major Asian cultures. Chinese chose freely throughout history—as freely as their social and financial circumstances permitted—among priests, spirit mediums, magicians, itinerant herbalists and acupuncturists, classical physicians, and other healers. Even the penniless might have had access to acquaintances who knew how to administer herbs gathered in the vicinity, local families who dispensed certain prescriptions as a charity, Buddhist priests who cared for the sick, and so on. All of these choices are still available in Taiwan, and some in Chinese communities on the periphery of the mainland. In the People's Republic, most of them have been eradicated as superstitious, and the pluralism of the past has given way to the dualism of traditional and modern medicine.[29]

---

[28] Miyasita 1976, 1977, 1979, and 1980. Some very tentative estimates of health finance and expenditure have been made for the recent past in Hu Teh-wei 1974 and Jamison et al. 1984: 62–76 and annex E.

[29] I do not wish to imply that traditional medicine is uniform. Since the end of the Cultural Revolution some curers who do not practice in the classical tradition are allowed to practice privately—for instance, a doctor who cures with snake venom whose clinic I saw in Suzhou in 1982. On medical pluralism see Leslie ed. 1976: 184–316, Kleinman et al. ed. 1975: 177–280, and Kleinman 1980b. There is a great deal of variation in the quality

Just as the ubiquity of Western diagnosis casts the future of Chinese methods in doubt, the access of patients to both modern and traditional therapies makes it practically impossible to evaluate the effectiveness of the latter. Clinical evaluation, complicated enough in the best of circumstances, becomes additionally complicated when patients may be receiving medications from other doctors and may not be sure what they are. Physicians working in one tradition do not always inquire whether their patients are also being treated in another. Not many European or American doctors would know what to do with information about the precise acupuncture therapy that has been given for a case of arthritis under their care—if indeed they saw any point in asking about it. Conversely, Chinese acupuncturists are not the only acupuncturists who neglect to ask whether their arthritic patients have received cortisone, which decreases the body's adrenocorticotrophic hormone (ACTH) secretion and thus demands modifications in therapy.[30] If the future of Chinese therapeutic methods is to be affected by rational considerations, this difficulty will have to be surmounted.

---

of papers in the two collections. Most authors are unaware that pluralism was the norm in Europe and China before the twentieth century.

[30] A Chinese example of research obviously invalidated by such negligence is Wang Min-kang et al. 1970: 40–56 on adrenocortical activity in bronchial asthma; an English example is Mann et al. 1973 on intractable pain, also criticized in other respects. I am grateful to Hans Ågren for calling these publications to my attention.

Chapter VI

CONCLUSION

This survey of ideas about the body, health, and illness in traditional Chinese medicine yields two pointers for reading the *Revised Outline* and similar recent publications. One is that they are documents of a medical system in turmoil. The other is that they reflect not only contemporary change but ceaseless change over two thousand years. Over this two millennia the myth of an unchanging medical tradition has been maintained. Accumulating knowledge and new perspectives were always assimilated to ageless dicta from the *Inner Canon of the Yellow Lord*, the *Divine Husbandsman's Materia Medica*, and other canonical writings. Nevertheless some of the most fundamental organizing concepts of current Chinese medicine were born in periods that historians used to ignore as unoriginal—for instance, the twenty-one classes of prescriptions (1682).[1] Are recent developments simply the moving endpoint of a continuum of change, unacknowledged because innovation has always been unacknowledged?

What we have seen in one reinterpretation after another over the last quarter-century—of the etiology of jaundice, of the anatomical meaning of the triple *chiao* and the Heart Envelope, of the circulation tract system, of *hsueh* and other vital substances—is a move away from the hard-won coherence of classical medical doctrine. Underlying every case, and revealed when recent ex-

---

[1] "A decline in Chinese Medicine was perceptible from the Ming dynasty reaching its lowest ebb in the Ch'ing period," according to Wong and Wu 1936: 141 (echoes for acupuncture in CL160). This view has been corrected in the best of the recent histories, Chia Te-tao 賈 得 道 1979, Ma Po-ying 马 伯 英 1982, and Chao P'u-shan 赵 璞 珊 1983.

197

planations are compared with old ones, is Western influence. Sometimes this influence is specific, as when the mechanism of jaundice
is clarified, and sometimes general, as when the materialistic discourse of modern medicine satisfies the Marxist-Leninist demand for
an entirely materialistic explanation of all vital functions.

What we see in the *Revised Outline* is not the replacement of the
old coherence by that of modern medicine, but—at least for the time
being—an increase of incoherence. By "incoherence" I mean merely
that the improvements desired by those who make the changes are
achieved by replacing assertions in the old tissue of explanation according to the criteria of a different medical system, without being
guided by an overall plan of alteration. Traditional medicine translated purely into the terms of modern medicine becomes partly non-
sensical, partly irrelevant, and partly mistaken; that is also true the
other way round, a point easily overlooked. In the midst of all this
subtle change, there is no indication over the past two innovative
decades that a well-knit new fabric is emerging. Bits and pieces of
modern medicine are merely being patched onto the traditional
structure. The result increasingly fails to hold together.

Only a limited number of explanations have been revised. The
patches have been chosen because a modern explanation is clear-cut
and happens to discredit claims on which the traditional account is
based. It is easy enough to say, as a number of commentators on
contemporary medicine have done, that this replacement should be
automatic because it provides for the first time an accurate description of somatic reality. Obvious though that may seem to the
modern physician proud of his science, it becomes obvious only after
the most basic assumptions of traditional medicine have been called
into question. Modern scientific knowledge does not merely correct
facts. I have demonstrated that traditional and modern medicine
are seldom directly concerned with the same facts, even when they
are contemplating what would seem to be the same activities in the
same parts of the body. Modern medicine replaces parts of reality.
It creates new facts, and destroys the facticity of old ones. The new
explanations could not have been adopted, of course, until influential
traditional physicians and teachers knew enough about modern
medicine and found its assumptions plausible enough to take its
claims seriously. Once those assumptions are granted, can the new
reality remain enclosed in neat little compartments here and there
in the interstices of the old?

The present situation is clearly transitional, but toward what
new dispensation? One hypothesis is that classical theory will be

revised systematically to incorporate modern ideas that strengthen it, minimally disturbing established concepts and methods of reasoning. A second is that piecemeal "improvements" will accumulate until finally an increasingly fragmented classical theory is abandoned altogether. A third hypothesis is that traditional physicians will at some point throw off Western influence and return to their pristine tradition.

One might indeed argue that the public would best be served by a truly dual system in which the proven strengths of modern medicine are complemented by the superiority of unreconstructed Chinese medicine in holistic approach, emphasis on caring for as well as treating patients, and responsiveness to the cultural and social environment. Despite such abstract merits of a return to the "separate but equal" policy of the 1950s, it is impossible to read sources such as the book translated below without being convinced that the point of no return has been reached. Reading them in the light of the classical tradition reminds us that this fateful set of changes is part of a history of incessant change. There is no static norm to return to. We are left, then, wondering which of the first two outcomes is more likely.

Both of these trends have dedicated constituencies in China. The resolution will depend, as in any society, on the competition and accommodation of these interest groups as well as on the abstract merits of each course. The challenge is to avoid a succession of political compromises that ignore what in the long run will be best for the health of the public. So far little attention has been paid to the way traditional medicine has been changing. It is not even clear how to determine what will be best for the health of the public. The future of traditional Chinese medicine depends on how intently these problems are faced.

PART II

REVISED OUTLINE OF CHINESE MEDICINE

Revised Outline of Chinese Medicine

(For Use of Western Physicians Studying Chinese Medicine)

Organizations organizing the editing:

Public Health Section, Rear Support Unit, Guangzhou
Command, People's Liberation Army

Public Health Bureau, Guangdong Provincial
Revolutionary Committee

Public Health Bureau, Hunan Provincial
Revolutionary Committee

Public Health Bureau, Guangxi Zhuang Autonomous Region
Revolutionary Committee

Organizations participating in the editing:

Units of the Guangzhou Command

Guangdong College of Chinese Medicine

Guangdong Provincial Hospital of Chinese Medicine

Hunan College of Chinese Medicine

Guangxi College of Chinese Medicine

College of Military Medicine, People's Liberation Army

Zhongshan Hospital

Guangdong Provincial Medicine and Public Health
Research Institute

Hunan Hospital

Guangxi Hospital

People's Health Publishers
Beijing, 1972

1. Yin-yang and the Five Phases

Yin-yang 陰 陽 and the Five Phases (*wu-hsing* 五 行) are ancient Chinese philosophical ideas. They are spontaneous, naive materialist theories that also contain elementary dialectic ideas. More than two thousand years ago they were applied in Chinese medicine and combined with practical therapeutic experience to form its fundamental theory. They were used to explain the physiological functioning of the human body and the laws of the occurrence and development of medical disorders, and to guide clinical diagnosis and treatment. Not only did they serve an active function in the historical development of medicine, but they have been used up to the present day in the Chinese doctor's clinical practice. Of the two, the yin-yang theory was applied more broadly.

1.1. Yin-yang

1.1.1. Basic concepts

The yin-yang theory proceeds from a naive viewpoint based on contradiction to explain every sort of physiological and pathological phenomenon in the human body, and even the principles of therapy and pharmacology. It holds that every part of the body is constituted of two opposed yet unitary kinds of matter and function—yin and yang. Medical disorders occur and develop when the normal relation between the opposed faces of yin and yang is broken.

With respect to the structure and functions of the human body, the system of yin and yang attributes is indicated by the examples in table 1.1. Yin-yang attributes are not absolute but relative, and often change under given circumstances. For instance, considering the relation of chest and back, the chest is yin and the back yang, but when associating chest and abdomen, the chest, being above, is assigned to yang, and the abdomen below to yin.

Table 1.1

Correspondences of Yin and Yang

Yang	Yin
Outer part or exterior aspect	Inner part or interior aspect
Upper part or aspect	Lower part or aspect
Back, dorsal part or aspect	Abdomen, ventral part or aspect
Six yang visceral system of function (fu 腑 , 2.1)†	Five yin visceral systems of function (tsang 脏)
Ch'i (3.1)	Hsueh (3.2)
Vital function	Materials substratum
Stimulation (excitation, etc.)	Restraint (inhibition, sedation, etc., 1.2.1)
Activity	Quiescence
Increase, growth	Decrease, decline
Ascent	Descent
Outward orientation	Inward orientation

†Numbers in this form are cross-references to sections of this translation.

Thus yin and yang can be used as equivalents for the dual, opposed aspects of the structure and functions of the interior and exterior of the body. Even more important, they can be used to explain their complementary relations, the most important manifestations of which are the following.

1.1.1.1. The mutual roots of yin and yang

Traditional physicians believe that "yin is born of yang, and yang of yin," and that "yin alone cannot be born; yang alone cannot mature." That is to say, each depends on the other for its subsistence, and without one the other cannot be. It is also said that "the basis of life is rooted in yin and yang" and that "when yin and yang are sundered the vital energies expire." Human life from beginning to tend is a process of mutual connection and mutual struggle between yin and yang, and when their relation ceases life ends. This viewpoint of Chinese physicians is summarized as "the mutual roots of yin and yang." As an example from physiology, the functions of the entire body belong to yang and its material substratum to yin. Functional activity must depend on material entities to serve as substratum, while at the same time the continuous replenishing of material substratum must depend upon function (for example, assimilation, digestion, absorption, metabolism, and blood circulation as a system of activities). In pathology, if the yin aspect of the cardiac system of functions is insufficient, a condition may ensue in which the cardiac yang becomes insufficient.

1.1.1.2. The interdependent growth and diminution of yin and yang

Chinese doctors believe that "as the yin diminishes the yang grows; as the yang diminishes the yin grows," which is to say that they alternate in growth and diminution within constant change. Because in the body every organ and tissue is ceaselessly active, and the material substratum is endlessly used up and replaced, this diminution and growth within definite limits is normal. But if one aspect "diminishes" or "grows" excessively, pathological changes may occur. Thus yin depletion (*hsu* 虛 , excessive diminution) may lead to yang excess (*k'ang* 亢), and yang depletion may lead to yin preponderance (*sheng* 盛). On the other hand, yin preponderance (excessive growth) may lead to yang depletion, and yang excess to yin depletion (7.3). For instance, the symptoms of one type of high blood pressure disorder are headache, dizziness, insomnia and a tendency to dream, an agitated and irritable disposition, tongue red and dry, and pulse strung, small, and accelerated (6.4.1.2); it is produced when yin depletion brings on yang excess. In acute hot heteropathy disorders, often great heat (over-preponderance of yang) impairs the yin and brings about symptoms of yin body-fluid loss (3.4); this is yin depletion brought on by yang preponderance.

1.1.1.3. The inversion of yin and yang

Chinese doctors believe that "the yin doubled must become yang; the yang doubled must become yin." This is to say that under certain conditions each can be transformed by inversion into the other. In clinical practice one can often see, as a result of various causes, such changes as penetration of heteropathy (*hsieh*

邪) from an outer (yang) to an inner aspect (yin; 7.1),[1] inversion from repletion (shih 实 , yang) to depletion (yin, 7.3), and transformation from hot manifestation type (yang) to cold (yin; 7.2). For example, wind heteropathy of cold outer manifestation type (5.1.1.1), if not flushed out by perspiration, may change to hot type and penetrate inward. A heteropathic preponderance of repletion manifestation type, if treated in a way detrimental to the orthopathic energies, may invert to depletion manifestation type. A yang preponderance of hot manifestation type, if too much chilling or cooling medicine is used, may transform into a cold type. Alterations in the opposite direction are also seen.

1.1.2. Clinical applications

1.1.2.1. Application in the study of the development of disorders (nosogeny)

Traditional physicians believe that "if yin and yang are in balance[2] the vitalities and spirits (ching-shen 精 神) will be in a well-ordered state," for only when they are in a condition of balanced opposition in the body can normal physiological activity be maintained. When this balance is upset, medical disorders may ensue; thus the latter are simply the result of an unbalanced preponderance or deficiency (shuai 衰) of either yin or yang ch'i. The interdependent growth and diminution of yin and yang is often

---

[1] Heteropathy or heteropathic ch'i is any agent that brings about disorder in the body, as opposed to orthopathic ch'i which maintains and renews normal body processes. See introductory study, pages 49 and 102.

[2] Yin p'ing yang mi 阴 平 阳 秘 , more literally, "if the yin is equable and the yang maintains the body's impregnability." This text is from a passage in the Huang ti nei ching 黄 帝 内 经 , which indicates that these characteristics are requisite to the dynamic balance between yin and yang ch'i. See SW, 1 (3): 19, no parallel in TS, 3 (2): 40. For this form of citation see the introductory study, note 3. A thorough technical discussion of ching-shen appears in Porkert 1974: 193–96 (hereafter abbreviated in the form P193–96). On classical significances of yin-yang theory see the introductory study, pages 59–70.

observed in clinical practice, as when yin preponderance brings on yang deficiency. This can cause the appearance of such symptoms of yang *ch'i* insufficiency as sensitivity to cold, chilly extremities, pale face, perspiration without external cause, protracted voiding of clear urine, tongue pale in color, and empty pulse (6.4.1.2). Another example is when pulmonary system yin depletion (in pulmonary tuberculosis) brings on such symptoms of yang excess as insomnia due to agitation, excessive sexual desire, dry mouth, red tongue, and accelerated pulse.

Also, due to the mutual roots of yin and yang, the attenuation to a certain degree of either regularly brings about an insufficiency of the other, as in "yang diminished affects yin; yin diminished affects yang." The frequent development of both yin and yang depletion in the last stages of certain chronic disorders is due to this reason.

1.1.2.2. Diagnosis

When Chinese doctors mention that "in the examination and in therapy yin and yang must be considered first," they mean that when analyzing a medical condition one regularly reasons inductively with yin and yang, generalizing the observed signs under the major categories of yin and yang manifestation types (7.4). After clarifying whether a repletion manifestation type is a matter of yin preponderance or yang excess, or whether a depletion manifestation type is a matter of yin or yang depletion, one can proceed a step further in classifying the manifestation type and determining the principles of therapy.

1.1.2.3. Therapy

When Chinese physicians mention "carefully observing the presence of yin or yang and regulating until balance is achieved," they are saying that the principle of therapy is to proceed through treatment to alter the condition of unbalanced preponderance or deficiency of yin or yang, and by regulating the yin-yang relation to reach the goals of restoring the complementary balance and doing away with the disorder. Thus when one uses yin drugs for yang preponderance and yang drugs for yin preponderance, the goal is to level off the surplus; when one uses yang drugs for yang depletion and yin drugs for yin depletion, the goal is to replenish the insufficiency.

The energetic character and flavor (*hsing-wei* 性 味) of medical substances are also divided according to yin and yang.[3] For instance, warming and heating drugs are assigned to yang, and chilling and cooling drugs to yin. Drugs of pungent, sweet, and neutral flavor belong to yang, and those of sour, salty, and bitter flavor to yin. Again, drugs of buoyant or diffusing function belong to yang, and those of sinking or draining (emetic and purgative) function to yin (11.1.2).

1.2. Five Phases

1.2.1. Basic concepts

Anciently in philosophy it was believed that wood, fire, earth, metal, and water were the fundamental materials of which the universe is constructed. Each has its own definite character. All the many sorts of things and events in the universe can be compared with these five kinds of fundamental matter on the basis of their characters, classified and assigned to one of the five great categories Wood, Fire, Earth, Metal, and Water (*mu huo t'u chin shui* 木 火 土 金 水). This classification system, used to explain the mutual relations between phenomena, is collectively called the "Five Phases" (*wu hsing*).[4] Chinese physicians have adapted the Five Phases theory to explain relations within the human body and relations of the body to its environment. For example, they associate the seasons, the Five Climatic Configurations (*wu ch'i* 五 氣), and other elements of nature with the visceral systems (2.1), and assign them to the Five Phases according to the special characteristics of each. Here set out in a table (see table 1.2) is a portion of the Five Phases classification as used in Chinese medicine.

---

[3] There is a discussion in the untranslated portion of the *Revised Outline*, Section 11.1.1. In classical medicine *wei* refers to "sapor," an abstract quality only indirectly related to flavor; see the introductory study, pages 181–84.

[4] P43–54. Compare the introductory study, page 94, on the materialist character of the Five Phases.

Table 1.2
Correspondences of the Five Phases†

Phenomenon	Wood	Fire	Earth	Metal	Water
Five yin visceral systems	Hepatic (2.1.2.1)	Cardiac (2.1.1.1)	Splenetic (2.1.3.1)	Pulmonary (2.1.4.1)	Renal (2.1.5.1)
Yang visceral systems	Gall bladder (2.1.2.2)	Small intestine (2.1.1.2)	Stomach (2.1.3.2)	Large intestine (2.1.4.1)	Urinary bladder (2.1.5.2)
Sense organs	Eyes	Tongue	Mouth	Nose	Ears
Tissues	Sinews (2.1.2.1.4)	Circulation Tracts (4.0)	Flesh	Hair	Bone
Emotional states	Anger	Joy	Ratiocination	Sorrow	Apprehension
Colors	Virid	Red	Yellow	White	Black
Flavors	Sour	Bitter	Sweet	Pungent	Salty
Climatic configurations	Wind	Hot	Moist	Dry	Cold
Seasons	Spring	Summer	Midsummer	Autumn	Winter

†The reader is reminded that the yin and yang visceral systems do not correspond to the Western anatomical entities, and that the distribution of functions between them differs considerably from that between the organs of the same names in modern medicine. In Chinese medicine the organs are merely the most prominent part of the material substrata on which the systems of function are based. A comparison of the visceral systems with Western organs is given in sections 2.1.1.3, 2.1.2.3, and so on, and a summary of the distribution of functions between systems is provided in section 2.3. The Five Climatic Configurations are the Six Climatic Configurations (5.1) minus Fire, into which any of the other five may change (5.1.6). "Virid" is ch'ing 青 , a term that covers a variety of saturated colors in the vicinity of green and blue, and that was also applied to gray animals and gray facial coloration in humans.

Taking the Wood column as an example, since the hepatic functions tend to produce a well-ramified and free-flowing distribution of *ch'i*, and have the life-sustaining function of upward dispersion, the hepatic system is associated with spring, in which plants sprout and grow, with wind, with virid color, and similar natural phenomena. The yang visceral system, sense organ, tissue, psychic state, and so on, related to the hepatic system are entered into the Wood column, and analogously for the other phases.

According to the Five Phases theory, the five yin visceral systems have relations of production (*sheng* 生) and conquest (*k'o* 克).[5] "Production" means facilitation [by one function of the next in the series], and "conquest" means restraint.

The mutual production pattern for the five yin systems is that a facilitating function is exerted by the hepatic system on the cardiac system, by the cardiac system on the splenetic system, by the splenetic system on the pulmonary system, by the pulmonary system on the renal system, and by the renal system on the hepatic system. That is, Wood produces Fire, Fire produces Earth, Earth produces Metal, Metal produces Water, and Water produces Wood. In these relations of mutual production, each of the phases has relations by which it is produced and by which it produces. The phase that produces it is called its "mother"; the phase it produces is called its "child." For example, since Fire produces Earth, Fire is the mother of Earth; since Earth produces Metal, Metal is the child of Earth.

The pattern of mutual conquest is that a function of restraint is exerted by the hepatic system on the splenetic, by the cardiac system on the pulmonary, by the splenetic system on the renal, by the pulmonary system on the hepatic, and by the renal system on the cardiac system. That is, Wood conquers Earth, Fire conquers Metal, Earth conquers Water, Metal conquers Wood, and Water conquers Fire. In these relations of mutual conquest, each of the phases has relations by which it is conquered and by which it conquers. The phase it conquers is called "what is overcome"; the phrase that conquers is called "what is not overcome." For example, since Wood conquers Earth, Earth is "what Wood overcomes"; since Metal conquers Wood, Metal is "what Wood does not overcome."

---

[5] Needham et al. 1954- : 253–61; Eberhard 1970: 11–100.

In addition there is "reverse checking" (*fan k'o* 反 克 , or "violation," *hsiang hui* 相 侮).[6] For instance, originally the Earth of the splenetic system conquers [i.e., checks] the Water of the renal system, but in medical disorders the renal Water may flood and reverse-check the splenetic functions, giving rise to thin stool.

In this way each visceral system facilitates the functioning of one system and restrains the functioning of another. Facilitation and restraint combine to support normal relations between each of the visceral systems and maintain the normal physiological activity of the body.

1.2.2. Clinical applications

The Five Phases come into play in clinical examination as well as therapy. For instance, in the visual phase of examination one often determines the visceral system manifestation type of the disorder from facial coloration and sheen (6.2.1.1). Gray coloration [classed with virid, *ch'ing* 青] is mostly associated with hepatic system wind type, red with cardiac Fire [i.e., hot] type, yellow with splenetic moist type, white with pulmonary cold type, and black with renal depletion type. When treating visceral system disorders one may prescribe medication according to the selectivity of the five yin systems for the Five Flavors (*wu wei* 五 味). It is generally said that drugs of sour flavor enter the hepatic system, those of bitter flavor the pulmonary, and those of salty flavor the renal.

In the past the clinical use of Five Phases production and conquest ideas was comparatively mechanical and over-elaborate, and in some respects did not correspond to reality, so eventually there was some selectivity [literally, "sublation," *yang-ch'i* 扬 弃] in their application. Some examples in relatively common use follow.

Since according to the mutual production relations of the five yin systems, each exerts a facilitating function on another, one often uses this relation to treat certain disorders. For instance on the basis of the relation by which Earth produces Metal one sometimes uses the technique of cultivating the splenetic system and its associated stomach system to treat pulmonary tuberculosis; this is called "cultivating Earth to produce Metal" (*p'ei t'u sheng chin* 培

---

[6] P53 and Jen Ying-ch'iu 任 应 秋 1960: 27–28.

土 生 金). Again, when treating the manifestation type in which hepatic yang rises in excess, since Water produces Wood one often uses the technique of nourishing the renal yin; this is called "nourishing Water to culture Wood" (*tzu shui han mu* 滋 水 涵 木).

Although according to the mutual conquest relations of the five yin visceral systems, each exerts a restraining function upon another, under normal circumstances this restraint is not harmful, but rather can perform a regulating function. For instance, the conquest relation of the cardiac (Fire) and renal (Water) systems under normal conditions is called "reinforcement of Water and Fire" (*shui huo hsiang chi* 水 火 相 济). But when the mutual conquest relation exceeds the normal level,[7] pathological changes ensue in the system subject to conquest. When the coordination of the cardiac and renal systems is broken, such symptoms as worry and mental upset, throbbing of the heart, insomnia, forgetfulness, and aching and weak loins and knees, occur. This is called "cardiac and renal systems not in contact" (*hsin shen pu chiao* 心 肾 不 交) or "Water and Fire not reinforcing" (*shui huo pu chi* 水 火 不 济). Therapy uses techniques for reestablishing communication between the cardiac and renal systems. As another example, a preponderance of the hepatic Wood *ch'i* can bring on an unbalanced condition of the splenetic Earth *ch'i* and produce such symptoms as abdominal pain with loose bowels. This manifestation type is called "Earth conquered by Wood" or "Hepatic Wood encroaching upon the splenetic system" (*kan mu ch'eng p'i* 肝 木 乘 脾). The therapy relaxes the hepatic functions and strengthens the splenetic functions.

---

[7] Porkert (ibid.) refers to this situation as "accroachment."

2. The Visceral Systems of Function

The doctrine of the visceral systems is an important constituent of the basic theory of Chinese medicine. This doctrine, proceeding from a holistic viewpoint, holds that the physiological and pathological activity of the human body proceeds as the five yin systems (*wu tsang* 五 脏) and the six yang systems (*liu fu* 六 腑) connect the tissues and organs of the entire body, through the medium of the circulation tract system (*ching-lo* 经 络), into a single organic whole. Physiologically the visceral systems are interdependent and interact with each other; when medical disorders occur they influence and transmit pathological changes to each other.

The five yin visceral systems are the cardiac (*hsin* 心), hepatic (*kan* 肝), splenetic (*p'i* 脾), pulmonary (*fei* 肺), and renal (*shen* 肾). The six yang visceral systems are those of the gall bladder (*tan* 胆), stomach (*wei* 胃), large intestine (*ta ch'ang* 大 肠), small intestine (*hsiao ch'ang* 小 肠), urinary bladder (*p'ang-kuang* 膀 胱), and the triple *chiao* (*san chiao* 三 焦).[1]

Traditional medicine's conceptions of the functions of some of the visceral systems are basically similar to those of Western medicine, but some other conceptions differ greatly, and still others have no analogue in the organs of Western medicine (e.g., the triple *chiao* system). We therefore cannot simply impose Western medicine's conception of the internal organs.

The doctrine of the visceral systems of function was developed on the basis of long clinical experience. Because of this it has an important guiding significance for the diagnosis and treatment of ill-

---

[1] On the triple *chiao*, a system with no determinate substratum, see the introductory study, pages 124–27, section 2.1.6 below, and P158–62. Needham renders *shen* into English as "renal and urinogenital system," which does justice to the scope of the concept (e.g., 1970: 306). My more concise "renal system" should be understood in this broad sense.

213

ness in Chinese medicine. Nevertheless, its character, problematic in several respects, must await a more systematic understanding.

2.1. Essential Physiology and Pathology of the Visceral Systems

The human body is a whole in which there exist complex associations between the five yin systems and the six yang systems. There is a division of labor between them, but at the same time they are complementary. Generally speaking, the difference between the yin and yang visceral systems is that the former have the function of storing *ching-ch'i* 精气 [nutritive essence refined from food, 3.1, sense 2], and the latter have the functions of fermenting food (*shui ku* 水谷), separating the pure product (*ching-ch'i*) from the impure (2.1.1.2), and transporting the residue to be excreted. In addition there are the cerebral (*nao* 脑), medullary (*sui* 髓), bone (*ku* 骨), circulation vessel (*mai* 脉), (gall bladder, *tan*, 2.1.2.2), and womb (*nu-tzu p'ao* 女子胞) systems. Since their functions are both similar to and different from those of the visceral systems, they make up a separate category called the "auxiliary yang systems of function" (*ch'i heng chih fu* 奇恒之腑).[2]

2.1.1. Cardiac and small intestine systems of function (and associated Cardiac Envelope Junction system of function)

The cardiac system is the master of the body's vital activity, and holds the chief place among the visceral systems. The other visceral systems are unified and coordinated by the cardiac system as they carry on their activities.

---

[2] The gall bladder system is listed in parentheses because it is also one of the regular yang visceral systems. On the complementarity of the yin and yang systems see P164–65 and, on *ching-ch'i*, pages 169, 179–80. Porkert systematically describes the visceral systems on pages 112–14. Early commentators do not agree on the literal meaning of *ch'i heng chih fu*. See P111–12 and Needham 1970: 49–51.

Table 2.1
The Visceral Systems of Function

Type of System	Type of Functions	Typical Functions
Five Yin Visceral Systems	Common	Storage of *ching* and *ch'i*
	Individual	**Cardiac system:** controls mental state and blood channels; is vented in the tongue **Hepatic system:** controls upward and outward dispersion, stores blood; controls sinews; is vented in the eyes **Splenetic system:** controls transmission and assimilation, is in charge of blood distribution; controls flesh; is vented in the mouth **Pulmonary system:** controls *ch'i* respiration; keeps liquid channels open and regulated; controls skin and body hair; is vented in the nose **Renal system:** stores *ching*, controls water; controls bone; produces marrow; connected to brain; controls Fire of the Gate of Life; is vented in the ears, anus, and urethra
Six Yang Visceral Systems	Common	Reception, digestion and assimilation, transmission, excretion
	Individual	**Stomach system:** receives food **Gall bladder system:** stores gall bile **Small intestine system:** digests and assimilates; separates pure from impure **Large intestine system:** transmits residues **Urinary bladder system:** stores and excretes urine **Triple *chiao* system:** allocates liquid nutriments and excretes waste
Auxiliary Yang Systems	Common	Concurrent storage of *ching* and *ch'i*
	Individual	**Gall bladder system:** as above (belongs to both types of system) **Cerebral system:** serves as medullary reservoir **Medullary system:** fills out and nourishes the bony structure **Bony system:** serves as the body's framework **Circulation tract system:** transports blood **Womb system:** controls menstruation and reproduction

2.1.1.1. Physiology and pathology of the cardiac system

2.1.1.1.1. *Controls state of mind.* The cardiac system is responsible for mental, conscious, and ratiocinative activity, corresponding to higher nervous activity. If this function is normal, general vitality is at a high level and the mind is clear. If it is impeded, various manifestations of disorder may occur, such as throbbing of the heart, fearfulness, forgetfulness, insomnia, manic behavior, compulsive and protracted laughter, coma, and raving.

2.1.1.1.2. *Controls the circulation of blood.* The cardiac system and circulation vessels are joined; the circulation of blood in the blood vessels depends entirely on its propulsion by the *ch'i* of the cardiac system. The degree of strength of this *ch'i* directly affects the circulation of the blood, as may be ascertained from the pulse beat. When the *ch'i* of the cardiac system is insufficient, the pulse is small, weak, and debilitated; when the *ch'i* does not come steadily the rhythm of the pulse is irregular (called a hurried, hesitant, or intermittent pulse, 6.4.1.2.7).

2.1.1.1.3. *Its shining (i.e., luster) is in the face; it is vented in the tongue.* The blood vessels in the facial region and the tongue are comparatively thickly distributed. The normality or abnormality of the cardiac function is readily ascertained from the color and luster of the face and tongue. When normal, the face is pink and lustrous, and the tongue pale pink. When the *ch'i* of the cardiac system is insufficient and the circulation not free, the face is pale, greyish, or purplish, without luster, and the tongue is purplish, darkened, and dull. When the cardiac Fire is excessively intense (i.e., there is a yang excess in the cardiac system, 8.1.6), the tip of the tongue is reddish or scarlet, or sores form in the mouth or on the tongue. When phlegm clogs the openings of the heart (*hsin ch'iao* 心 竅 , 8.5.5), one observes the tongue to be stiff and incapable of speech. Thus it is also said that "the tongue is the outward sprouting of the cardiac system."

2.1.1.1.4. *Relation of the cardiac system and perspiration.* There is an intimate connection; it is said that "sweat is the dispersed fluid (*yeh* 液 , 3.4) associated with the cardiac system." When in illness diaphoretics are used excessively, or when as a result of other causes there is profuse sweating, it is possible to damage the cardiac yang, even to the point of bringing about the serious phenomenon called "loss of yang *ch'i* through profuse sweating."

2.1.1.1.5. Addendum on the Cardiac Envelope Junction. This system (*hsin pao* or *hsin pao lo* 心 包 络) is peripheral to the cardiac system. Because the heart is the most important of the internal organs, there is a peripheral organ to protect it. Usually when external heteropathies encroach on the cardiac system they must first invade the Cardiac Envelope Junction system. For instance, mental confusion and raving in Heat Factor Disorders (9.0) are evidence that "hot heteropathy has entered the Cardiac Envelope Junction system." Thus "Cardiac Envelope Junction system of functions" mainly refers to a portion of the activity of the higher nervous system.[3]

2.1.1.2. Physiology and pathology of the small intestine system

The main function of the small intestine system is to receive food transported to it from the stomach system, continue the digestive process, and separate the clear from the turbid. "Clear" refers to the refined portion of the food (*ching* 精 , 3.3), which after assimilation by the small intestine system is transmitted to the splenetic system.[4] "Turbid" refers to the residual portion which pours from the small intestine system into the large intestine system or is transferred to the urinary bladder system. When the small intestine system is disordered, not only are the functions of digestion and assimilation affected but urinary abnormalities may occur.

2.1.1.3. Interrelations

The cardiac and small intestine systems, through their interconnection by the circulation tracts, form an "inner-outer" (*piao li* 表

---

[3] On the Cardiac Envelope Junction system see the introductory study, pages 126–31.

[4] For *ching* see the introductory study, table 2, page 148 and accompanying discussion, and P176–77.

里) relation [of complementarity in a yin-yang pair].[5] For instance, when the cardiac Fire is excessively intense, one may observe the tip of the tongue red and painful; erosions in the mouth, and possibly ulcerations; and urination brief, urine tinged scarlet or even bloody. These pathological phenomena are called "cardiac system passing hot heteropathy to the small intestine system."

From the physiology and pathology described above, it may be seen that what Chinese medicine calls the cardiac system essentially encompasses the functions and pathology of what Western medicine calls the heart and part of the central and vegetative nervous systems.

2.1.2. Hepatic and gall bladder systems of function

2.1.2.1. Physiology and pathology of the hepatic system

2.1.2.1.1. Controls upward and outward dispersion. The hepatic system has the function of upward and outward dispersion (*sheng fa t'ou hsieh* 升 发 透 泄 or *shu hsieh* 疏 泄), and is responsible for free-flowing distribution of *ch'i* throughout the body. If the hepatic system is remiss in this ramified distribution function, dispersion is no longer normal, the *ch'i* no longer flows freely, and various manifestations of disorder may eventuate. If there is a static congelation (*yü chieh* 鬱 結) of the hepatic *ch'i*, one may observe such symptoms as irritability, headache, swelling and pain in the chest and flanks, and irregular menstruation. If the upward dispersal of the hepatic *ch'i* is excessive— "hepatic yang rising in excess" (*kan yang shang k'ang* 肝 阳 上 亢)—one observes headache and disturbances of equilibrium. If the hepatic yang in great excess turns to Fire (5.1.6), headache pain becomes intense, sometimes with reddened or painful eyes, ringing in the ears, or

---

[5] P114; note that the sense of "inner" and "outer" in section 7.1 below is quite different. Inner and outer aspects are purely relational. As in this instance, "outer" does not imply the surface of the body or anything more directly observable than what is "inner." For this reason the explanation of *piao-li* in Lu and Needham 1980: 43 is not applicable to the full range of usage. That monograph is hereafter abbreviated in the form CL43.

deafness. If the hepatic yang excess reaches its limit, turning to Fire and giving rise to [internal] wind heteropathy (5.1.1.2), then the series of symptoms (e.g., paralytic strokes) which go with the Wind Attack (*chung feng* 中 风) manifestation type (3.5) may occur. Insufficient upward dispersion of the hepatic *ch'i* may bring on vertigo, faintness, or dizziness; insomnia; a tendency to be easily frightened; mental vagueness [e.g., confusion of reality and unreality]; and other symptoms.

2.1.2.1.2.   Controls the storage of blood. The hepatic system has the function of storing the blood and regulating its quantity.[6] When the body is active, the blood stored by the hepatic system is supplied to all the tissues and organs. When the body is at rest or asleep, the blood returns to be stored in the hepatic system. An implication of storing blood is preventing its loss; when the storage function is impeded it is likely that hemorrhage will occur, as in vomiting blood or nosebleed.

2.1.2.1.3.   Is vented in the eyes. The hepatic system and the eyes are intimately related. Impairments of the hepatic system often affect the eyes. *Ch'i* depletion in the hepatic system results in blurred vision and night blindness; a flaming upward of the hepatic Fire (5.1.1.2) results in inflamed eyes.

2.1.2.1.4.   Controls the sinews (chin 筋 *[i.e., muscles, tendons, ligaments, nerve tissue, etc.]) and is manifested outwardly in the nails.*[7] The hepatic system is responsible for muscular activity, controlling the motion of the whole body's flesh and joints. The sinews depend on the hepatic system's blood for nourishment; if it is insufficient, pain in these tissues, numbness, difficulty in moving the joints, or cramps may appear. If hot factors reach their limit and activate hepatic wind heteropathy, muscle spasms may occur. "The nails are the outcrop of the sinews"; when the hepatic blood is at an adequate level the nails are pink and shiny, and when inadequate the nails are desiccated and tend to become thin or soft.

---

[6] This sentence uses the modern word for blood, *hsueh-yeh* 血液 , lit., "*hsueh* fluid." The *Revised Outline's* discussion of blood diverges greatly from discourse about *hsueh* in classical medicine, on which see the introductory study, pages 51–52, pages 147–62.

[7] On relationships of this kind see P115, 121–23.

2.1.2.2. Physiology and pathology of the gall bladder system

The function of the gall bladder system—storing the bile—is quite different from that of the other yang visceral systems, which is why it is also considered an auxiliary system (2.1). Because the gall bile is a clear, pure fluid, the gall bladder system is classically called "the yang system whose contents are clear" [in contrast to the heterogeneous, impure residues stored in the other yang systems pending excretion]. The main manifestations of its disorders are pain in the ribs, yellow jaundice, a bitter taste in the mouth, vomiting a thin bitter liquid, and so on.

2.1.2.3. Interrelations

The hepatic and gall bladder systems, through their interconnection by the circulation tracts, form an "inner-outer" relation, and are also directly joined. In medical disorders they regularly affect each other, and so are usually treated together.

It may be seen that what Chinese medicine calls the hepatic and gall bladder systems essentially encompass the functions and medical disorders of what Western medicine calls the liver, gall bladder, and parts of the central nervous system, vegetative nervous system, locomotor system, and blood circulation system, as well as the visual organs.

2.1.3. Splenetic and stomach systems

2.1.3.1. Physiology and pathology of the splenetic system

2.1.3.1.1. Controls transmission and assimilation. The splenetic system is responsible for digestion, assimilation, and transport of food. Whatever is eaten or drunk enters the stomach and undergoes preliminary digestion, and then the digestion proceeds a step further under direction of the splenetic system. At the same time the refined substance is assimilated and distributed to every part of the body, where it can be used by every tissue as nourishment. In addition, the splenetic system transmits and assimilates moisture, and in concert with the pulmonary and renal systems maintains the liquid balance within the body. When these functions are proceeding normally and the digestion and assimilation metabolism is healthy, the *ch'i* and blood flourish and the bodily vigor is at capacity. When there is a depletion in the splenetic system, the transmission and assimilation functions become abnormal. Digestion and absorption may be impaired, giving rise to deficiency in the stomach's ability to receive food (2.1.3.2), abdominal distension, and thin stool. Impediment of liquid transmission and assimilation may lead to blockage of moisture and bring on dropsy, mucus formation, and so on.

2.1.3.1.2. Is in charge of the blood. The splenetic system has charge of the whole body's blood supply. Impediment of this function by splenetic system depletion can bring on all sorts of hemorrhage symptoms, such as vomiting blood, nosebleed, irregular and excessive menses, and blood stool. In addition, because the relation of the splenetic system to the production of blood is also intimate, splenetic depletion can decrease the blood production and assimilation functions and bring on anemia.

2.1.3.1.3. Control the limbs and flesh; is vented in the mouth, and is manifested outwardly in the lips. When the splenetic system is normally transporting and assimilating the refined portion of food and nourishing the entire body, the appetite is strong, the flesh full and healthy, the limbs vigorous, and the lips red and moist. When the *ch'i* of the splenetic system is debilitated and the transmission and assimilation functions become abnormal, the appetite is poor, the flesh becomes emaciated, the limbs lack strength, and the lips become pale or faded brown and lose their luster.

2.1.3.2. Physiology and pathology of the stomach system

The main function of the stomach system is to receive food; another is to ferment it. Thus it is said that "the stomach system is the sea for food."[8] Disorders of this system can bring about the

---

[8] Scholars have often understood the word "sea" in this passage from the *Huang ti nei ching ling shu* 黃帝內經靈樞 (hereafter LS) to mean "reservoir" (which does not imply fermentation). This interpretation is reflected in P155. Actually the passage does not discuss the function of the stomach system as a

appearance of such symptoms as painful distension of the upper abdomen, diminution of the appetite, and nausea and vomiting.

2.1.3.3. Interrelations

The splenetic and stomach systems, through interconnection by the circulation tracts, form an "inner-outer" relation. The stomach system, in charge of reception, and the splenetic system, in charge of transmission and assimilation, together discharge the responsibility for digestion, absorption, and transport of nutriment, and so on. But the two systems differ in character. For instance, the *ch'i* of the splenetic system controls upward motion; it tends toward dry heat and abhors moisture. The *ch'i* of the stomach system controls downward motion; it tends toward moisture and abhors dry heat. The two are opposite but complementary. Only when carried downward by descent of the stomach *ch'i* can food descend as required for digestion; only when carried upward by the ascent of the splenetic *ch'i* can the refined alimentary essence move upward to the pulmonary system and be sent on throughout the other visceral systems of the body. When the stomach *ch'i* does not descend, but rather backs upward (*ni* 逆 ["contravection," P170 (9)]), such symptoms appear as nausea and vomiting, belching and hiccups, and stomach pains. When the splenetic *ch'i* does not ascend, but rather sinks downward (called "sinking of the medial *ch'i*" [*chung ch'i hsia hsien* 中 气 下 陷], 3.1.2), lack of energy shown in drawling or slurring speech, chronic diarrhea, rectal prolapse, abdominal droop, prolapse of the uterus, and other symptoms appear in which internal organs hang downward.

The splenetic system belongs to yin, and thus easily gives rise to moist impairments (occlusion of moisture within the body when the transmission function is not sound), and is also easily invaded by moist heteropathy. When this sort of invasion occurs, one may

---

reservoir, but is concerned with the unlimited extent of the distribution system which it supplies. The original metaphor is: "The stomach system is the sea of drink, food, *ch'i* and *hsueh*. Where the clouds set in motion by the sea move is the whole world. Where the *ch'i* and *hsueh* are sent out by the stomach system are the cardinal conduits (*ching sui* 経 隨)" (LS, 9 (60): 91, no parallel in TS).

observe fever, a heavy feeling in the head, body pains, a heavy feeling in the limbs accompanied by bodily languor, fullness and distress in the stomach cavity, a soft, moderate pulse, a thick whitish coating on the tongue, and so on. The preferred therapy is "warming the splenetic system to dry up the moisture" (wen p'i tsao shih 温 脾 燥 湿, 12.5). The stomach system belongs to yang, and the general run of its complaints have to do with hot heteropathy or Fire of the stomach system, producing such signs as dry mouth with desire to drink (hsi yin 喜 飲 ; cf. 9.1.2.4), disinterest in eating, and sometimes toothache, bleeding gums, vomiting blood, or nosebleed. Preferred therapy is to "clear the hot factors and bring down the Fire" (ch'ing je chiang huo 清 热 降 火 , 12.2).

It may be seen that physiologically and pathologically the stomach system of Chinese medicine and the stomach of Western medicine are on the whole similar, but what Chinese medicine calls the splenetic system, encompassing the functions and pathology of digestion, assimilation, material metabolism, balance of bodily fluids, and a fraction of the blood circulation, differs greatly from what Western medicine calls the spleen.

2.1.4. Pulmonary and large intestine systems

2.1.4.1. Physiology and pathology of the pulmonary system

2.1.4.1.1. Controls the ch'i. On the one hand this refers to the pulmonary system's governance of respiration. It carries on gas exchange to maintain the vital functions. On the other it refers to the role of the pulmonary system—which "encounters every circulation tract" in the circulation of blood and the distribution of refined alimentary essence throughout the body.[9] In addition, Chinese doctors believe that the pulmonary system controls the ch'i of the whole body, and that variations in the state of the ch'i in the visceral systems and the tracts are closely related to the state of the

---

[9] The quotation is *fei ch'ao pai mai* 肺 朝 百 脉 , literally, "the pulmonary system gives audience to the hundred vessels" (just as the emperor meets his massed officials). It comes from a famous passage in the *Inner Canon* on the distribution of alimentary essence, SW, *7* (21): 122 = TS (TIZ ed. only), *16* (3): 296.

pulmonary system. When this *ch'i-* controlling function is impeded, the main manifestations are disorders of the respiratory system, frequently giving rise to such symptoms as coughing, labored and noisy breathing, lack of vigor, low and weak voice, or lack of energy shown in drawling or slurring speech.

2.1.4.1.2. Controls clearing away and carrying downward, and keeps the liquid drainage channels open and regulated. Downward clearing is the normal direction of the pulmonary *ch'i;* upward backflow produces labored and noisy breathing, coughing, and so on. Transport and elimination of body fluids not only require initial transmission and assimilation and subsequent distribution by the splenetic system, but depend on clearing and carrying downward (*su chiang* 肅 降) by the pulmonary system to keep the liquid channels to the urinary bladder system open and regulated. If the pulmonary system is remiss in these functions, the fluid metabolism will be affected, bringing on occlusion of moisture and subsequently difficult urination or edema. Thus it is said that "the pulmonary system is the upper source of Water." Remissness on the part of the pulmonary *ch'i* is sometimes related to a blockage; in certain cases of asthma and of dropsy one often includes in prescriptions drugs that unblock the pulmonary *ch'i* (ephedra [*ma-huang* 麻 黃 , E. sinica or E. equisetina, 12.1.1.1], Chinese wild ginger rhizome [*hsi-hsin* 細 辛 , Asarum heterotropoides or A. Sieboldii, 12.1.1.1], or apricot kernel [*k'u-hsing* 苦 杏 , Prunus armeniaca, 12.11.1.1]).

2.1.4.1.3. Controls the skin and body hair. The pulmonary system is intimately related to the skin and the external part of the flesh. When the pulmonary system's defensive *ch'i* [*wei* 衛 , which undergirds the skin] is up to strength, the outer part of the flesh is firm and tight, the skin is lustrous, the bodily defenses are vigorous, and invasion by external heteropathy is not easy. But when the pulmonary *ch'i* is not steadfast, the pores relax and the body is easily invaded; in serious circumstances the external heteropathy advances and encroaches upon the pulmonary system. In addition, if the exernal part of the flesh is not firm, the dispersed body fluids leak away; this can produce such symptoms as perspiration without external cause and nocturnal sweating [*tao han* 盜 汗 , a common sign of yin exhaustion].[10]

2.1.4.1.4. Is vented in the nose. The nose, connected with the pulmonary system, is the doorway of respiration. In disorders of the pulmonary system, the nose often runs or is stopped up, and breathing is difficult; in serious conditions there is spasmodic quivering of the wings of the nose (*alae nasi, pi i shan tung* 鼻 翼 煽 动).

2.1.4.1.5. Relation of the pulmonary system and the voice. The production of sound is related to the functioning of the *ch'i* of the pulmonary system. When the pulmonary *ch'i* is adequate the voice is resonant and clear, but when there is a depletion the voice is low and indistinct. When wind or cold heteropathy invades the pulmonary system and its *ch'i* is blocked up, the voice is hoarse. Pulmonary Consumption Disorder [*fei lao ping* 肺 癆 病 , which includes modern pulmonary tuberculosis, some lung cancer, etc.] due to heteropathic damage or overconsumption of pulmonary *ch'i* can bring about loss of voice.

2.1.4.2. Physiology and pathology of the large intestine system

The main function of the large intestine system is transmission of residues and elimination of excrement. Disorders of this system influence elimination, whether as constipation due to desiccant congelation [of hot heteropathic *ch'i, tsao chieh pien mi* 燥 结 便 秘], diarrhea accompanied by abdominal pain, or purulent bloody diarrhea.

2.1.4.3. Interrelations

The pulmonary and large intestine systems, through their interconnection by the circulation tracts, form an "inner-outer" relation.

---

[10] On the defensive *ch'i* see section 3.1.3 below, P188–90 and 215–16, and the introductory study, pages 147–61 above. The dispersed body fluids are discussed in section 3.4, P190–91, and the introductory study, pages 162–63.

When the pulmonary *ch'i* is "clearing away and carrying downward" the excretory function of the large intestine system is normal, but an accumulation in the latter, impeding the flow, can influence pulmonary activity. In clinical therapy one sometimes can treat one system to cure disorders in the other. For instance, in certain cases of constipation one uses for improved results not only laxatives but pulmonary moistening drugs or drugs which cause the pulmonary *ch'i* to descend. For certain pulmonary system repletion hot manifestation types (7.3.2), when one adds laxatives to drugs for clearing pulmonary hot factors (12.2) the outcome is better.

It may be seen that physiologically and pathologically the pulmonary and large intestine systems are essentially similar to the lungs and large intestine of Western medicine. The Chinese pulmonary system, however, in addition to respiratory functions, encompasses part of the functioning of blood circulation, fluid metabolism, and body temperature regulation.

2.1.5. The renal and urinary bladder system

2.1.5.1. Physiology and pathology of the renal system

2.1.5.1.1.   *Controls storage of ching.* The renal [or renal-urogenital] system's function of storing the *ching* (3.3) can be divided into two categories. One is storing the *ching* of reproduction [female as well as male semen]—and thus governing human reproduction and fertility. The other is storing the *ching* of the visceral systems of function [i.e., the essence that they extract from food and *ch'i*], and thus governing the body's growth, development, and other important vital activity. Clinically most renal disorders are depletion manifestation types (7.3); disorders of the reproductive system and a number of those of the endocrine system may be cured by replenishing (*pu* 补) the renal system.[11]

2.1.5.1.2.   *Controls water.* The kidneys are the organ of importance for regulating the internal water metabolism; therefore the renal system is called the "storehouse of water." Disorders of the

---

[11] Replenishing is the same as "reinforcing the orthopathic *ch'i*," on which see the introductory study, page 177.

renal system may bring about abnormalities in the distribution of water; one may observe such symptoms as difficult urination, stasis of dispersed body fluids, edema in all parts of the body, and in some cases urinary incontinence, excessive ingestion of liquids with excessive urination, or nocturnal or other enuresis.

2.1.5.1.3. Controls bone, produces bone and medulla, and is connected to the brain. The renal system stores the *ching*, which produces medulla (*sui* 髓).[12] This system is also related to the brain. When the renal *ching* is at an adequate level, bone, marrow and brain are all strong and healthy, the limbs move easily and vigorously, motion is responsive, vitality at capacity, and sight and hearing acute. When the renal *ching* is inadequate, movement is often sluggish, the bones weak and debilitated, with anemia or dizziness, forgetfulness, retarded development of intelligence in children, and other symptoms. In addition, "the teeth are the outcrop of the bone"; teeth and bone are related, and when the *ch'i* of the renal system is debilitated the teeth readily loosen and fall out.

2.1.5.1.4. Controls the "Fire of the Gate of Life." The renal system is the "storehouse of water," but it also stores the Fire of the Gate of Life (*ming men huo* 命 門 火 ; the renal yang is the main power which maintains life, hence the name).[13] This Fire and the renal Water (i.e., renal *ching*), adjusted to each other as yang to yin, maintain the body's normal power of reproduction, growth, and development, as well as the functioning of the visceral systems. Weakening of the Fire of the Gate of Life can bring on impotence and premature ejaculation; if it is impossible to "warm the renal system" (*wen shen* 温 肾 , 12.4.1.2) predawn or chronic loose bowels may appear. When the Fire of the Gate of Life is intense it may produce such symptoms as nocturnal emission accompanied by

---

[12] The scope of the word *sui* is similar to that of "medulla" (*OED* sense 1): the substance of the brain, the spinal cord ("spinal marrow"), and the marrow of bones. *Sui* is not, however, the permanent solid material, but a moistening and revitalizing component which must be continually renewed by the renal and urinary bladder systems of function.

[13] The term "Gate of Life" has had many denotations in various classical sources, on which see Jen Ying-ch'iu, ed. 1980: 181–86 and the introductory study, pages 126–29 above.

erotic dreams, excessive sexual desire, and Depletion Agitation Disorder (*hsu fan* 虚 烦 [general agitation, anxiety, insomnia, etc., in yin depletion that has given rise to internal hot heteropathy, 7.4.3]).

2.1.5.1.5. Controls reception of ch'i. Although respiration is controlled by the pulmonary system, there must be mutual adjustment with the renal system. The latter aids the former's function of inspiring *ch'i* and carrying it downward; this is called "admission of *ch'i* (na *ch'i* 纳 气)." Failure of the renal system to admit *ch'i* can produce difficulty in breathing due to *ch'i* depletion (*hsu ch'uan* 虚 喘) or shortness of breath.[14] The special feature of this depletion breathing is that expiration exceeds inspiration. Clinical therapy should proceed from replenishing the renal system.

2.1.5.1.6. Is vented above in the ears and below in the two yin openings. The ears are related to the renal system and serve as its upper body opening. When the renal *ch'i* is at an adequate level, hearing is normal; when it is depleted, there is ringing in the ears or deafness. The "two yin openings" (*erh yin* 二 阴) refers to the anus and urethra, the renal system's lower body openings. Thus elimination of feces and urine is related to the renal system. Depletion of the renal system may bring about urinary incontinence or strangury. Insufficiency of renal yin may bring about constipation. Debilitation of the Fire of the Gate of Life may bring on predawn loose bowels, and so on.

2.1.5.1.7. Is manifested outwardly in the hair of the head. The growth and amount of hair being shed constantly reflects the strength of the renal *ch'i*. If the latter is vigorous, the hair is thick, black as a raven, and lustrous; if debilitated, the hair is thin and shreds or turns white and lusterless.

2.1.5.2. Physiology and pathology of the urinary bladder system

Among the functions of the urinary bladder system the most important are to store and excrete urine. Disorders can bring about

---

[14] *Ch'uan* is a general term for labored and noisy breathing and other asthmatic symptoms.

frequent urination, excessive urge to urinate, painful excretion of urine, and similar symptoms.

2.1.5.3. Interrelations

The renal and urinary bladder systems, through their interconnection by circulation tracts, form an "inner-outer" relation. Abnormality of the urinary bladder system's urine excretion function sometimes is related to disorders of the renal system. If in cases of renal depletion it is impossible to keep control over the retentive function intact (*ku she* 固 攝),[15] urinary incontinence or enuresis may appear. If renal depletion leads to inadequate *ch'i* transformation (*ch'i hua pu chi* 气 化 不 及 [a lowered level of vital function that interferes with digestion and respiration and thus gives rise to systemic disorders]), inability to urinate or impaired urination appear.

It may be seen that physiologically and pathologically the renal system of Chinese medicine basically encompasses what Western medicine calls the functions and disorders of the urogenital system and parts of the hematogenic, endocrine, and nervous systems. The urinary bladder system of Chinese medicine and the urinary bladder of Western medicine are on the whole similar.

2.1.6. The triple *chiao* system

The triple *chiao* system (*san chiao*), one of the six yang visceral systems, includes a superior, medial, and inferior *chiao*. To this day there has been no definitive explanation of the configuration and

---

[15] Keeping substances that belong within the body from escaping was seen as a single activity of the healthy body and thus, to some extent, treatable by the same methods regardless of the substance involved. Chung-i yen-chiu-yuan 中 医 研 究 院 ed. 1982: 188a includes under this rubric "astringent" remedies for excessive perspiration, chronic coughing (irregular loss of *ch'i*), diarrhea, involuntary loss of semen, and urethral discharges.

functioning of this system.[16] Most people believe that the superior *chiao* refers to the cardiac and pulmonary systems and corresponds to the functioning of the thoracic organs, the medial *chiao* refers to the splenetic and stomach systems and corresponds to the functioning of the upper abdominal (*wan* 脘) organs, and the inferior *chiao* refers to the hepatic, renal, urinary bladder and intestinal systems and corresponds to the functioning of the lower abdominal (*fu* 腹) organs.

With the reference to physiological functions, the superior *chiao* is likened to mist, referring to the [pervasive] nutriment-allocating function of the cardiac and pulmonary systems; the medial *chiao* is likened to a bubble, referring to the [refined essence borne along freely by the] transmission and assimilation functions of the splenetic and stomach systems; and the inferior *chiao* is likened to a ditch, referring to the excretory function of the renal and urinary bladder systems.[17]

In the theory of Warm Factor Disorders (9.5), manifestation type is determined using the triple *chiao* system as a rubric for classification of symptoms and therapeutic reasoning. This meaning is not identical with that discussed above and should not be confused with it.

In sum, the functioning of the triple *chiao* system is a generalization for the physiological functions of several of the visceral systems within the body cavity. The manifestations of pathological change in the triple *chiao* system are on the whole related to the transport of fluid nutriment and the excretion of wastes.

2.1.7. The womb auxiliary system

The womb auxiliary system is also called that of the "womb palace" (*p'ao kung* 胞 宮); it encompasses the womb and its appendages. Its functions are control of menstruation and governance of reproduction. Its relation to the renal system and to the concep-

---

[16] Nor of the basic meaning of *chiao*. See the introductory study, pages 124–29, especially page 125, note 13.

[17] This enigmatic passage is from the *Huang ti nei ching*, LS, *4* (18): 44. The parallel passage in TS, *12* (1): 205 is a great deal more corrupt than it appears in Chinese editions; compare the TIZ edition, *12* (1): 18 (I, 504).

tion (*jen mai* 任 脉) and highway (*ch'ung mai* 冲 脉)[18] tracts is extremely close; the three jointly ensure the normality of menstruation, reproduction, and childbirth. When the *ching* of the renal system suffers loss and there is depletion in the two tracts, menstruation becomes irregular and in serious cases infertility ensues.

2.2. Relations between the
Visceral Systems of Function

The relations between one yin system and another, between yin and yang systems, and between one yang system and another are extraordinarily close. Some have been discussed briefly above. Here relations often clinically observed between yin systems will be discussed.

2.2.1. Cardiac and pulmonary systems

The cardiac system controls the blood and the pulmonary system controls *ch'i*; they aid each other in governing the circulation of blood in the body. When the blood associated with the cardiac system is sufficient, the *ch'i* of the pulmonary system is at capacity, and the blood circulation is thus normal. Conversely, when the pulmonary *ch'i* is inadequate, the blood circulation is affected; when the functioning of the cardiac system is not good, respiration is affected.

2.2.2. Cardiac and renal systems

The cardiac system occupies the superior *chiao* and belongs to Fire; the renal system occupies the inferior *chiao* and belongs to Water (1.2.2).

---

[18] Below, 4.0; P283–84; Lu and Needham 1980: 48–51 et passim. The latter source is cited below in the form CL48–51.

2.2.3. Cardiac and hepatic systems

The cardiac system controls the blood vessels of the whole body, and the hepatic system's function is to store and regulate the blood. Their relation is thus close. Inadequacy of the cardiac blood can bring about hepatic depletion. This initiates a condition in which "blood does not nourish the sinews." One may observe such symptoms as sinew and bone pains, muscle spasms, and cramps.

2.2.4. Cardiac and splenetic systems

Transmission and assimilation by the splenetic system requires nourishment by the cardiac blood [carrying yin energy] and propulsion by the cardiac yang. The functioning of the cardiac system also requires nutrition by refined alimentary essence which the splenetic system allocates. Secondly, the cardiac system controls the transport of blood, while the splenetic system is in charge of its distribution. Therefore their relation is close. Clinically one often observes "depletion in both cardiac and splenetic systems," the manifestations of which are throbbing of the heart, forgetfulness, insomnia, faded yellow facial color, diminished appetite, thin stool, and similar symptoms.

2.2.5. Hepatic and splenetic systems

Both excessive hepatic *ch'i* and depleted splenetic *ch'i* easily give rise to "hepatic Wood encroaching upon the splenetic system" (1.2.2) or "hepatic and stomach systems not in harmony," the manifestations of which are pain in the flanks or stomach, or abdominal distension.

2.2.6. Hepatic and pulmonary systems

Under normal conditions the pulmonary system "conquers" [i.e., precedes in the Five Phases conquest order] the hepatic system, but under pathological conditions the hepatic system reverse-checks it (1.2.1). For example, if the pulmonary *ch'i* is originally depleted and cannot constrain the hepatic system, the hepatic *ch'i* may back upward. The pulmonary *ch'i's* work of clearing away and carrying downward then becomes blocked, and one observes discomfort from distension of the chest and diaphragm. If the hepatic Fire is overintense it "burns" the pulmonary system, giving rise to irritability, pain in the chest and flanks, dry cough, coughing up phlegm or blood, and other so-called "Wood and Fire punish Metal" (*mu huo hsing chin* 木 火 刑 金) manifestations.

2.2.7. Hepatic and renal systems

The relation between the hepatic and renal systems is so close that Chinese doctors say "the hepatic and renal systems have a common source." The hepatic system relies on the renal Water (renal yin *ch'i*) for nourishment. If the latter is inadequate the hepatic yin will also be inadequate. Because of this yin depletion the hepatic system will be unable to hold in balance its yang *ch'i*, and it will be possible for the hepatic yang to rise in excess, bringing on such symptoms as dizziness, headache, and high blood pressure.

2.2.8. Splenetic and pulmonary systems

The pulmonary *ch'i* depends for nourishment on the refined alimentary essence transmitted and assimilated by the splenetic system. In disorders involving pulmonary *ch'i* depletion one can sometimes proceed therapeutically with the method of "replenishing the splenetic system to augment the pulmonary system" (*pu p'i i fei* 补 脾 益 肺 , 12.16).

2.2.9. Splenetic and renal systems

Transmission and assimilation by the splenetic system depend for assistance upon the Fire of the Gate of Life (2.1.5.1.4). Inadequacy of the latter may lead to weakened functioning of the splenetic system and bring about loose bowels. In addition, the splenetic system has the ability to restrain the renal Water, but if *ch'i* depletion weakens its transmission and assimilation function so that it can no longer do so, the renal Water floods and produces edema.

2.2.10. Pulmonary and renal systems

The pulmonary system controls *ch'i*, and the renal system controls reception of *ch'i*; the renal system can aid in the pulmonary *ch'i's* work of clearing away and carrying downward. If because of yang depletion the renal system is unable to receive *ch'i*, one observes labored and noisy breathing. Treatment of asthmatic symptoms brought on by renal depletion must proceed from replenishing the splenetic system.

2.3. Conclusion

As an aid in comprehending the functioning of the visceral systems of function, below we compare them with the physiological and anatomic systems of Western medicine:

2.3.1. Digestion and assimilation

The stomach system controls reception; the splenetic system controls transmission and assimilation; the small intestine system separates clear from turbid; the large intestine system transports the residues. In addition, the hepatic system's upward and outward dispersion and the Fire of the Gate of Life are relied upon to aid these processes.

2.3.2. Respiratory activity

The pulmonary system governs respiration and controls gas exchange; the renal system controls reception of *ch'i* and aids the pulmonary system's function of clearing away and carrying downward.

2.3.3. Blood circulation

The cardiac system controls the blood vessels and is the driving force of the circulation; "the pulmonary system encounters every circulation tract," participating in vascular circulation; the hepatic system stores blood and can regulate its quantity; the splenetic system takes charge of blood circulation and can make the blood circulate through the vascular system without escaping.[19]

2.3.4. Hematogenic functions

The splenetic and stomach systems are "the root of the postnatal vitalities" (*hou t'ien* 后 天 , 3.0) and the source of assimilation of nutriment and production of blood. The renal system is "the root of the prenatal vitalities" (*hsien t'ien* 先 天); production of blood also relies on its nurture [i.e., depends not only on inborn vitality but on that drawn from the environment].[20]

2.3.5. Water metabolism

The splenetic system controls the transmission and assimilation of moisture; the pulmonary system governs keeping the liquid channels open and regulated; the renal system controls elimination of water; the triple *chiao* system controls *ch'i* transformation (2.1.5.3); the urinary bladder system controls storage and excretion of urine.

---

[19] In classical medicine it is not the heart but the cardiac vitalities (*ch'i*) that power the circulation. See appendix C. On the quotation see note 9 above.

[20] *Hsien t'ien* and *hou t'ien* are philosophical terms with a broad range of meaning, particularly developed in connection with Neo-Confucian cosmogony. They stand for the primordial state of undifferentiation and the hierarchically differentiated world of experience, corresponding states of mystical experience and normal cognition, prenatal and postnatal endowments of *ch'i*, etc. The association of inherited and environmental energies with the visceral systems of function is detailed in a famous essay by Li Chung-tzu 李 仲 梓 in his *I tsung pi tu* 醫 宗 必 讀 (1637), *1*: 6–7.

2.3.6. Nervous functions

Part of the cardiac system's function corresponds to that of the cerebrum as center of emotional and intellectual activity. All the other yin visceral systems incorporate nervous and mental activity.

2.3.7. Locomotive functions

The renal system governs the bones and keeps movement correctly adjusted so that physical activity is dexterous and responsive; the hepatic system controls the sinews, and is responsible for the flexibility of the joints; the splenetic system governs the limbs and is responsible for the flesh of the whole body.

2.3.8. Endocrine and reproductive functions

These are related to the renal and hepatic systems and to the womb auxiliary system and its two associated circulation tracts.

3. *Ch'i*, Blood, *Ching*, and Dispersed Body Fluids

Ch'i 气 , blood (*hsueh* 血), *ching* 精 , and dispersed body fluids (*chin-yeh* 津液) are the indispensable material foundation of the body's vital activities.[1] They originate in the prenatal endowment of vitality (*ching-ch'i* 精气) as well as in air and food obtained from the postnatal environment. They are produced through processes of transformation by the visceral systems, which control their distribution. On the other hand, they nurture the visceral systems and the tissues of the whole body, in order to ensure normal physiological activity.

3.1. *Ch'i*

Ch'i has two senses; one is physiological function or motive force and the other is subtle, refined matter which has a nutritive function. Generally speaking, the functions of *ch'i* include producing the blood by metamorphosis, propelling it, and strengthening the functions that retain it within the body; warming and nurturing the tissues of the whole body; resisting external heteropathy; and promoting the activity of the tissues and the visceral systems of function.

The *ch'i* in the human body may be summarily characterized according to its various functions as follows:

3.1.1. Primordial *ch'i*

Also called "orthopathic *ch'i*" (*cheng ch'i* 正气) or "true *ch'i*" (*chen ch'i* 真气), this is a collective manifestation of the body's

---

[1] This account, although typical of recent writing, differs considerably from the classical understanding. Cf. the introductory study, pages 117–71 (especially pages 147–63), and P167–91.

potential for vital activity, and represents its power of resistance.[2] When the general primordial *ch'i* (*yuan ch'i* 元 气) is up to strength, one does not easily develop medical disorders; even when one does, speedy victory over the heteropathy and complete recovery follow appropriate treatment [see also 5.7].

3.1.2. *Ch'i* of the visceral systems

This is the *ch'i* that promotes the activity of the visceral systems, for instance the *ch'i* of the cardiac and stomach systems. The *ch'i* of the splenetic and stomach systems together is called the "medial *ch'i*" (*chung ch'i* 中 气), the function of which is to further digestion and assimilation and to maintain the normal positions of the abdominal organs. When the medial *ch'i* is inadequate, such symptoms appear as weakening of digestion and assimilation, mental fog (*ching-shen pu chen* 精 神 不 振), and low and indistinct voice, as well as abdominal or renal droop [ptosis], prolapse of the uterus, and prolapse of the anus or anal mucosa. For therapy the technique of "replenishing the medial aspect to strengthen the *ch'i*" (*pu chung i ch'i* 补 中 益 气 , 12.16) is used. The cardiac and pulmonary *ch'i* together are called the "genetic *ch'i*" (*tsung ch'i* 宗 气), the function of which is to promote the respiratory and circulatory capacities. When it is inadequate, the respiration and the heartbeat are weakened. Therapy uses the technique of "replenishing the *ch'i*" (*pu ch'i* 补 气 , 12.16).

3.1.3. Defensive *ch'i* and constructive *ch'i*

What is distributed outside the tract system and circulates alongside it is called the defensive *ch'i* (*wei ch'i* 卫 气). It disperses in the chest and abdomen, where it is able to warm and nurture the visceral systems; it circulates between the skin and the flesh, where it is able to do the same for both. Its functions are fortifying

---

[2] P166–67 discusses the many varieties of *ch'i* in the *Huang ti nei ching* tradition. See *cheng ch'i*, no. 25, *chen ch'i*, no. 20, and *yuan ch'i*, no. 27. In classical medicine these differ in respect to function, not substance, and primordial *ch'i*, orthopathic *ch'i*, and true *ch'i* are distinct.

the outer aspect (7.1) and resisting the invasion of exogenous heteropathy. What is distributed and circulates within the tract system and has the functions of producing the blood by metamorphosis and nourishing the whole body is called the constructive *ch'i* (*ying ch'i* 营 气).[3] It and the defensive *ch'i* act in concert to nourish the body and resist heteropathy that causes medical disorders.

Among *ch'i* disorders the most important are *ch'i* depletion (*ch'i hsu* 气 虚), *ch'i* stasis (*ch'i chih* 气 滞 or *ch'i yü* 气 郁), and *ch'i* backflow (*ch'i ni* 气 逆).

Ch'i depletion. These manifestation types are usually thought of as energetic insufficiencies in the five yin visceral systems, but the preponderance of clinical cases involve the splenetic and pulmonary systems. The most frequent symptoms are lack of energy shown in drawling or slurring speech, low and indistinct voice, dizziness and mental exhaustion, perspiration without external cause, poor appetite, or in some cases downward displacement of the internal organs, empty and soft pulse, pale and tender tongue, thin coating on the tongue, and so on. Therapy uses the technique of "replenishing the *ch'i*" (12.16).

Ch'i stasis. When the *ch'i* of the visceral systems loses its mobility or its circulation is impeded, *ch'i* stasis manifestations appear. Pulmonary, splenetic and stomach, and hepatic stasis are seen comparatively often; common symptoms are distension and pain in the chest, flanks, and abdomen. In pulmonary *ch'i* stasis one observes a sensation of fullness in the chest, chest pain, rapid breathing, and excessive phlegm; in splenetic and stomach *ch'i* stasis one observes abdominal fullness, distension and pain, and poor digestion; in hepatic *ch'i* stasis one observes such symptoms as emotional tension, fullness, distension, and pain in the flanks and abdomen, and painful or irregular menstruation; in *ch'i* stasis of the circulation tracts there is pain in the flesh and joints of the extremities. Therapy uses the technique of "reordering the *ch'i*" (*li ch'i* 理 气 , 12.12).

Ch'i backflow. The proper motion of the *ch'i* of the pulmonary and stomach systems is downward. When this is impossible an upward backflow develops. In addition, excessive upward and outward dispersion due to the hepatic system can bring on disorders marked by backup of hepatic *ch'i*. In pulmonary *ch'i* backflow one

---

[3] P170, nos. 8, 10; CL28–29.

observes asthmatic cough and other symptoms; in stomach system *ch'i* backflow one observes such symptoms as dizziness, fainting, or vomiting blood. If the backflow is associated with the stomach system, the technique of "bringing down the *ch'i*" (*chiang ch'i* 降气, 12.12) is used; if with the hepatic system, the technique of "yang latensification" (*chen ch'ien* 鎮潜, 12.15) is used.[4]

From these considerations, *ch'i* to a very large extent represents nervous functions and all sorts of internal energies.

3.2. Blood

Blood (*hsueh*) is metamorphosed from food by the functions of the splenetic and stomach systems.[5] Its characteristic functioning is unceasing circulation to nourish the whole body and maintain its normal physiological functioning. The saying that "the eyes receive blood and are able to see, the feet receive blood and are able to walk, the hands receive blood and are able to grasp," and so on, asserts that all the tissues and organs of the body—visceral systems, bones and sinews, hair, etc.—in the absence of nurture by blood would be unable to maintain their normal physiological functions. If for various reasons the motion of the blood is impeded and the skin does not receive adequate blood, there may be numbness. If the supply to the extremities is inadequate, the hands and feet may lack warmth, or even become useless (as in paralysis).

The relation between *ch'i* and blood is extremely close, and they are often combined in a single term.[6] *Ch'i* and blood constitute an interdependent yin-yang pair. "The *ch'i* is the commander of the blood, and the blood is the mother of the *ch'i*" means that the motion of the blood depends upon propulsion by the *ch'i*. If the *ch'i* moves the blood moves, and if the *ch'i* is static the blood coagulates.

---

[4] "Yang latensification and sedation" (*chen ch'ien an shen* 鎮潜安神) includes specific therapies for "hepatic yang rising in excess" and similar manifestations (8.2.2). The traditional notion of sedation does not greatly overlap that of modern medicine.

[5] The reader is reminded that in classical medicine *hsueh* was a functional as well as material concept, and did not refer simply to blood; see the introductory study, pages 52, 150.

[6] P27, 175 (no. 6), writes of the combination as "individually specific physiological energy."

On the other hand, the functions and activities of all tissues and organs depend upon the blood for nourishment; in this sense it is the mother of the *ch'i* (the material foundation [of physiological function]).

Among blood disorders the most important are hemorrhage, blood depletion, and coagulation of blood (*hsueh yü* 血 瘀).

Hemorrhage. Fire or heat repletion heteropathy which forces the blood into uncontrolled motion; depletion which makes the *ch'i* unable to control (*she* 攝) the blood; failure of the hepatic system to store blood and of the splenetic system to govern it; loss of renal yin *ch'i* and internal development of Depletion Fire Disorder (*hsu huo* 虛 火 [hot sensations and associated symptoms due to yin depletion of this sort]), with ill effects extending to the circulation tract system; or mental stimulus under which emotion is transformed into Fire (5.1.6), and so on: all of these can lead to hemorrhage. Treatment of hemorrhage manifestations cannot be restricted to use of hemostatic drugs, but determination of manifestation type and treatment should be directed toward the parts in which the above causes have concurred to bring about hemorrhage. If stomach system Fire has eventuated in vomiting blood, it is best to use the technique of "clearing the hot heteropathy and bringing down the Fire" (*ch'ing je chiang huo* 清 热 降 火 , 12.2). If splenetic exhaustion has led to excessive menstruation or failure of the menses to terminate, the technique of "replenishing the medial aspect to strengthen the *ch'i*" (*pu chung i ch'i* 补 中 益 气 , 12.16) should be used.

Blood depletion. Excessive loss or insufficient production of blood can produce this condition. Its common symptoms are face faded yellow in color; lips, tongue, and nails pale and without luster; throbbing of the heart; dizziness and disturbances of vision; fatigue or lack of vigor; or in some cases numbness in the hands or feet; pulse small and soft, and so on. In therapy the technique of "replenishing the blood" (*pu hsueh* 补 血 , 12.16) is usually used. On the principle that "the *ch'i* is the commander of the blood," the technique of "replenishing the *ch'i*" (12.16) is often applied concurrently.

Blood coagulation. This condition may develop when external injury causes hemorrhage and the blood collects in tissues or organs; when *ch'i* stasis causes a halt in the blood flow; when cold heteropathy in the blood vessels congeals the blood; when a predominance of hot heteropathy compels uncontrolled motion of the blood, so that it leaves the vascular passages and collects outside as a coagulation; and when hot heteropathies reach extreme intensity, damaging the yin *ch'i* and the blood, which also causes a blood stasis and results in coagulation. The manifestations depend on location. A coagulation in the cardiac system may bring about throbbing palpitations or pains of the heart, and so on. A coagulation in the pulmonary system may bring about spitting of phlegm and blood, chest pains, and so on; if in the womb system, a coagulation may result in irregularities in the highway and conception tracts (4.0); it may bring about irregular or blocked menstruation (*pi ching* 閉 經 [amenorrhea]), swellings (for instance, that of extrauterine pregnancy), tumors, and so on. A coagulation in the flanks or abdomen may bring about twinges or dull cutting pains, as well as fixed pains and in some cases swellings, and so on. A coagulation in the extremities may bring about pain or lack of sensation there, or in some cases loss of motor response, paralysis, and so on. Therapy for blood coagulation may use such techniques as "dispelling the coagulum" (*ch'ü yü* 祛 瘀 , 12.13) or "replenishing the *ch'i* and vivifying the blood" (*pu ch'i huo hsueh* 补 气 活 血 , 12.16).

3.3. *Ching*

Ching means on the one hand the male or female reproductive essence [as in semen], the origin of life, and on the other the essence produced by metamorphosis from alimentary nourishment, the material basis of physical growth and development.[7] Under normal conditions storage of the essence associated with all the visceral systems is the responsibility of the renal system; a portion of this *ching* is transformed in turn into the semen of reproduction.

In sum, the *ching* is the foundation of life; it is a fundamental substance that shapes the human body and maintains every kind of vital activity, directly affecting growth, development, aging, and death. If it is at capacity, it is possible for the body to be strong, vitality high, and the resistance of the organism powerful; if it is debilitated, the body may be weakened, the vitality inadequate,

---

[7] In classical medicine, *ching* is *ch'i* seen as in transition from one determinate form to another. See the introductory study, pages 164–65, and P176–80. Porkert translates *ching* as "unattached structure energy" or "structure potential."

development retarded, aging accelerated, and the power of resistance weakened.

3.4. Dispersed Body Fluids

"Dispersed body fluids" (*chin-yeh*) is a general term for all normal moisture and fluids in the body [excluding blood and semen], important substances for the maintenance of vital activity. These fluids originate in alimentary nutrition. After transmission and assimilation by the splenetic and stomach systems, distribution throughout the body and excretion proceed as regulated by the pulmonary, renal, urinary bladder, triple *chiao*, and other visceral systems.

The terms *chin* and *yeh* are generally used in combination, but there are differences between them. What are dispersed within the tissues and organs and between the flesh and skin, moistening and nourishing them, are called *chin* [and considered relatively yang]. What are dispersed in the hollows of the joints, brain and marrow, sense organs, and so on, moistening them and maintaining circulation, are called *yeh* [and considered yin]. In addition, the term "dispersed body fluids" is used generally for sweat, normal nasal mucus, tear fluid, saliva, gastric juice, and every sort of glandular secretion.[8]

The relation of dispersed body fluids to *ch'i* and blood is close; it is said that "body fluids come from the same origin as blood." Loss of body fluids can often bring on *ch'i* or blood depletion or debilitation. For instance, often when body fluids have been lost as a result of profuse vomiting, diarrhea, or sweating, there appear such manifestations of debility as respiration in short, hurried breaths, accelerated heartbeat, subtle and small pulse, and cold extremities. After great loss of blood such manifestations of body fluid inade-

---

[8] This account greatly simplifies the picture of dispersed body fluids given in classical sources, and of course departs from it in the interest of a modern, materialist interpretation. Note in particular that no attempt is made to explain the inconsistency between the two definitions, one as "what are dispersed" in different parts of the body to perform a nutritive function, and one which consists of a list of secretions. See the introductory study, page 166.

quacy appear as thirst, scanty urination, and hardened feces. Clinically loss of blood and loss of body fluids are often noted together; as early as the *Treatise on Cold Damage Disorders* (*Shang han lun* 傷 寒 論 , A.D. 196/220), the principle that "a chronic bleeder (*wang hsueh chia* 亡 血 家) should not be made to perspire" was mentioned, and later there was a saying that "by nourishing the blood one can protect the blood."[9] Both quotations point out the intimate relation between dispersed body fluids on the one hand and *ch'i* and blood on the other.

Manifestations involving the body fluids are mainly divided into two types: "damage to body fluids by Fire or hot heteropathy" and "body fluid loss."

Damage to body fluids by Fire or hot heteropathy. These disorders are mainly stimulated by the heteropathic *ch'i* of the Six Excesses (*liu yin* 六 淫 , 5.1) metamorphosing into Fire (5.1.6). Onset is generally abrupt. One may observe high fever; worry and mental upset, or even manic agitation with raving; great thirst and copious perspiration, or in some cases constipation; scorched appearance of the lips; tongue dry and spiky [i.e., hairy, 6.2.2.1]; pulse either swollen and accelerated or sunken and accelerated; and other signs of violence to the body fluids. Therapy uses the techniques of "clearing the hot heteropathy and draining the Fire" (*ch'ing je hsieh huo* 清 热 泻 火, 12.2), or "draining and bringing down" (*hsieh hsia* 泻 下 , 12.9), in order to preserve the body fluids—an important principle in Heat Factor Disorders (9.0).

If the damage is due to a preponderance of hot heteropathy in the visceral systems, such manifestations may appear as fever, dried, solidified stool, reddened eyes, dry mouth with thirst, and tongue coat yellow and dry. It is necessary to proceed a step further and determine which visceral system's dispersed fluid has been damaged, carrying out therapy accordingly.

Body fluid loss. This is a depletion manifestation type, unlike the proceding repletion type (7.3). Body fluid loss is brought about when pulmonary, stomach, or renal system depletion causes inadequacies in the sources of dispersed body fluids. Common symptoms include low body temperature or hectic fever, intermittent fever, agitation accompanied by hot sensations in the Five Hearts (*wu hsin fan je* 五 心 烦 热 [i.e., cardiac region, palms of the hands, and

---

[9] This passage is not accepted by Ōtsuka in his edition of the *Shang han lun*, but see the Shanghai reprint, *3*: 21a.

arches of the feet]),[10] deficient appetite, mouth dry with temporary relief from hot drinks, or in some cases increased thirst in the early evening or late at night, loss of weight and vigor, tongue red with scanty saliva and thin or absent coat, and pulse small and accelerated. Therapy should use the technique of "nourishing the yin and moistening the dry factors" (*yang yin jun tsao* 养 阴 润 燥, 12.6).

3.5. Appendix: Mucus

Mucus (*t'an* 痰) is the product of pathological changes, and can become the cause of many types of medical disorder. The concept of mucus is relatively broad, and is not confined to sputum. Chinese doctors say "As water accumulates it becomes watery mucus; as watery mucus congeals it becomes phlegm" (the clear and thin is watery mucus [*yin*, lit., "swallowed fluid"] and the thick and turbid is phlegm [*t'an*, but the latter term can be used in the collective sense "mucus" to stand for both]). The point is that when heteropathic influence or pulmonary *ch'i* depletion interferes with the free flow of pulmonary *ch'i* so that the latter is remiss in "clearing away and carrying down," liquid stasis may give rise to phlegm or watery mucus. In addition, debility of the splenetic system's transmission function, or overeating of rich food, may make it impossible for food and liquids to be normally transmitted and assimilated. Moisture then flows into the pulmonary system and collects there to form mucus. Thus it is said that "the splenetic system is the wellspring of mucus production, and the pulmonary system the utensil in which it is stored." When the renal yang *ch'i* is inadequate, liquid vapors are not metamorphosed, but instead condense and flood upward; they too may develop into mucus.

Most of the pathological changes involving mucus take place in the pulmonary system, but some are located in the cardiac system and some in the peripheral parts of the circulation tract system.

Mucus in the pulmonary system. One may observe coughing, labored and noisy breathing, inability to lie horizontally, fullness and pains in the chest, and so on. Therapy, in addition to use of

---

[10] *Fan* actually covers a variety of what Western physicians would consider somatic as well as psychological upset, feelings of oppression and depression, etc. (Kleinman 1980b: 140).

mucus-eliminating drugs (12.11), should employ other medicines in accord with etiology. A knowledge that does not extend beyond "see phlegm, eliminate phlegm" is not comprehensive enough.

Mucus in the cardiac system. One may observe regular throbbing of the heart, irregular heart rhythm, and other symptoms. Other nervous and mental disorders such as epilepsy in adults and children (*tien hsien* 癲 癇), manic behavior, sudden unconsciousness, and Wind Attack Disorder manifestations (*chung feng* 中 风 [including strokes, apoplexy, etc.]) may be brought about when phlegm clogs the openings of the heart. Therapy uses the technique of "opening the passages and eliminating the mucus" (*hsuan ch'iao ch'u t'an* 宣 窍 除 痰 , 12.13).

Mucus in the peripheral parts of the circulation tract system. One may observe such symptoms as tuberculous lymphadenitis (*lei li* 瘰 疬), stony carbuncles (*shih chü* 石 疽 [i.e., hard growths, lymph system neoplasms, etc.]), goiter, and migrating sores due to mucous moist heteropathy (bone tuberculosis, cold abscesses, or tuberculous fistulas). Therapy may use the technique of "eliminating the mucus and freeing the circulation tracts" (*ch'u t'an t'ung lo* 除 痰 通 络 , 12.11).

3.6. Conclusion

Ch'i, blood, *ching*, and dispersed body fluids are all substances important to the vital activities within the human body. *Ching*, blood, and body fluids are all substantial liquid matter, and are able to interact; thus they may all be referred to as yin or as *ching* in the wide sense. The characteristics they share, besides yin quality, are their substantiality, their receptive [as opposed to active] nature, and the material foundation which they provide for functional activity.

Ch'i on the one hand refers to subtle matter which has a nutritive function, but more important is its use to refer to the functional activity of the tissues and organs of the visceral systems. Its characteristics, by contrast to those enumerated above, are yang status, insubstantiality (the subtle matter is invisible to the eye), active nature, and major manifestation in functional activity.

Ching (in the wide sense) forms an opposed but complementary yin-yang, receptive-active pair with *ch'i*. They support and complete each other, and are inseparable. If the *ching* is up to capacity the *ch'i* is adequate, and if the *ch'i* is debilitated the *ch'i* is lost. The *ch'i*, blood, *ching*, and dispersed body fluids [in sum, the body's vital resources] are not only the material foundation of the functional activity of the visceral and circulation tract systems, but also its concrete embodiment, remaining at capacity so long as that activity remains normal. Only in this situation is the body healthy.

Mucus and blood coagulum are products of pathological processes, and serve in turn as causes of other disorders. The concepts of "mucus" and "coagulum" in Chinese medicine are wider than those of expectorant phlegm and clotted blood [in modern usage].

4. The Circulation Tract System

The circulation tract system, like the visceral systems, is an important constituent part of the human body's structure and function. The tracts and visceral systems constitute an organic, interconnected whole, in which each visceral system has an associated tract. Interconnections between the yin and yang systems, as well as those between the visceral systems and other tissues, are provided by the circulation tracts.

The tracts are the pathways along which the *ch'i* and blood are transported within the human body. The main lines are called cardinal tracts (*ching* 经), and the branch lines are called reticular tracts (*lo* 络). They form a communication network of crosswise intersections, which permit flow outward and inward, upward and downward, connecting the whole body.

The tract system [excepting the reticular tracts] is divided into two types, the regular or cardinal tracts (*cheng ching* 正 经) and the extraordinary tracts (*chi ching* 奇 经).[1] The regular tracts

---

[1] In classical sources the eight extraordinary tracts are usually called *ch'i ching pa mai*, also transcribed *chi ching pa mo* 奇 经 八 脉 . The literal meaning of this term, and even the pronunciation of the first graph, are in contention (*mo* is merely a more literary reading for *mai*). The concept originates in the *Huang ti pa-shih-i nan ching* 黄 帝 八 十 一 難 经 (hereafter *Nan ching*), 1 (27–28): 33–35: "None of these eight vessels is constrained (*chü* 拘) by the regular tracts; thus they are called the eight extraordinary tracts. . . . The sages invented ditches to connect and ease [the flow of water in streams], to provide for the unexpected. When the rain falls the ditches may fill to overflowing. When that happens, the water spreads out and moves in an uncontrolled way, but the sages made no further provision. Similarly, when the [*ch'i* of] the reticular tracts [which serve as a kind of overflow sytem] overflows, the cardinal tracts are no

are twelvefold, each paired left and right. There are the three yin and three yang tracts for each of the hands and of the feet, called collectively the twelve cardinal tracts (*ching mai* or *mo* 经 脉). Each is associated with a yin or yang visceral system. There are eight extraordinary tracts: the superintendent tract (*tu mai* 督 脉), the conception tract (*jen mai* 任 脉), the highway tract (*ch'ung mai* 冲 or 衝 脉), the belt tract (*tai mai* 带 脉), the yin and yang ligative tracts (*wei mai* 维 脉), and the yin and yang

---

longer able to constrain it [, so that the body needs a second set of overflow channels to prevent 'flooding']. . . . Thus when the *ch'i* in the circulation vessels reaches an abnormally high level, entering these eight vessels and no longer circulating, the twelve regular tracts are no longer able to constrain them." There is a great leap of interpretation from this primary source—admittedly not a tight argument—to the way the extraordinary tracts are introduced by most modern authors: "they do not pertain to or connect with the *zang-fu* organs," i.e., the visceral systems of function (Beijing College of Traditional Chinese Medicine et al. 1980: 31–32, P213, and CL48–49).

That recent characterization is logical, but it is not the purport of the classical understanding. Nor do the main classical commentators on the *Canon of Problems* find it necessary to make such a leap. See, for instance, *Nan ching pen i* 難 经 本 義 (1361), *1*: 33–35, *Nan ching chi chu* 難 经 集 註 (1505), *3*: 49b–51b, *Nan ching ching shih* 難 经 经 釋 (1727), *1*: 20–22, and *Nan ching cheng i* 難 经 正 義 (1895), *2*: 46–51. The major premodern monograph on the supernumerary tracts, Li Shih-chen's 李 時 珍 *Ch'i ching pa mai k'ao* 奇 经 八 脉 考 (1578), follows the same tradition. For an excellent modern discussion that conveys and expands on the original meaning see Shang-hai Chung-i hsueh-yuan 上 海 中 医 学 院 ed. 1960: 34–35.

Porkert's translation, "Odd conduits," because of the ambiguity of "odd," does not seem as satisfactory as the translation used in Chinese publications, "extraordinary tracts," which conveys one original sense of the term. Porkert's interpretation of 奇 as "un-paired"—not involved in the pairing of tracts which are related as inner and outer aspects—reflects the consensus of the classical commentators, and implies the old pronunciation *chi*.

heel tracts (*chiao* 跷 or 蹻 *mai*). The twelve cardinal tracts are commonly combined with the superintendent and conception tracts under the term "fourteen cardinal tracts."

4.1. Physiology and Pathology of the Tracts

The physiological functions of the tracts are "to move *ch'i* and blood, to distribute yin and yang, to maintain the condition of the sinews and bones, and to keep the joints supple." They are associated inwardly with the visceral systems and connect outwardly to the joints of the limbs; they pass between the inner and outer aspects (2.1.1.3); they circulate *ch'i* and blood; they interconnect the whole body; thus they maintain the normal physiological functioning of the body's tissues and organs. The body's five yin and six yang visceral systems, the four limbs and hundred bones, the five sense organs and the nine orifices, the flesh and the sinewy and skeletal tissues, and so on: all must depend on irrigation and nutrition by *ch'i* and blood, and on interconnection by the circulation tract system, if they are to carry out their individual functions and coordinate them to form an organic whole.

In pathological circumstances, the tract system is associated with the occurrence of medical disorders, and with changes due to transfer of heteropathy from one visceral system to another (*ch'uan pien* 传 变). When external heteropathy invades the body, if there is an abnormality in the defensive function of the circulating *ch'i* (*ching ch'i* 经 气), the heteropathy will follow the path of the tracts and pass into the visceral systems. For instance, when wind-cold heteropathy (9.1.1.5) that has invaded the peripheral flesh is transferred inward, it may give rise to coughing, spitting of phlegm, distress and pain in the chest, and other pulmonary system manifestations. Further, because the large intestine and pulmonary systems are the inner and outer aspects of a configuration, this heteropathy sometimes also gives rise to abdominal pains, loose bowels, constipation, and other manifestations associated with the large intestine tract (IG). Conversely, when there is a disorder in a visceral system, it may follow the path of its associated tract and react upon the corresponding outer aspect of the body. For instance, in hepatic system disorders, pains in the flanks are often remarked; in renal system disorders, pains in the loins; and in pulmonary system disorders, pains in the shoulders and back. But these transfers of heteropathy via the tract system can only be rela-

Table 4.1
The Tract System and Its Associations†

Limb	Phase	Visceral System	Abbreviation	Reference	Orthopathic Order	Heteropathic Order
Hand	Mature yin (t'ai yin 太 陰)	Pulmonary	P	2.1.4.1	1	4
Foot		Splenetic	LP	2.1.3.1	4	
Hand	Attenuated yin (chueh yin 厥 陰)	Cardiac Envelope Junction	HC	2.1.1.1.5	9	6
Foot		Hepatic	H	2.1.2.1	12	
Hand	Immature yin (shao yin 少 陰)	Cardiac	C	2.1.1.1	5	5
Foot		Renal	R	2.1.5.1	8	
Hand	Yang brightness (yang ming 陽 明)	Large intestine	IG	2.1.4.2	2	2
Foot		Stomach	V	2.1.3.2	3	
Hand	Immature yang (shao yang)	Triple chiao	SC	2.1.6	10	3
Foot		Gall bladder	VF	2.1.2.2	11	
Hand	Mature yang (t'ai yang)	Small intestine	IT	2.1.1.2	6	1
Foot		Urinary bladder	VU	2.1.5.2	7	

†The order given here is the conventional one of the six yin-yang cardinal divisions of the circulation system, named for the Six Warps. Since this is a closed system, the initial point is arbitrary. This succession differs from the "empirical" order in which orthopathic ch'i circulates through the cardinal tract system, as outlined in section 4.2. I summarily indicate the latter in the "orthopathic order" column; cf. CL46. The conventional sequence of the tracts also differs from the order in which heteropathy is transmitted amongst the Six Warps (in the latter case physicians do not distinguish hand and foot branches); see the "heteropathic order" column.

The associated visceral system is shown for each tract, along with a cross-reference to the section in which its physiology and pathology are described. The standard European abbreviation, derived from the Latin designation of the viscus, is added for each tract here and below. For corresponding Chinese abbreviations see appendix E.

tive. Whether or not they will take place can be determined only in view of such factors as the character and strength of the disease heteropathy, the level of the body's orthopathic *ch'i* (3.1.1), and the appropriateness of previous therapy.

4.2. Courses and Therapeutic Functions of the Circulation Tracts

4.2.1. Peripheral courses and therapeutic functions of the twelve cardinal tracts

[Omitted from the translation.][2]

4.2.2. Courses and therapeutic functions of the Conception and Superintendent Tracts

[Omitted from the translation.]

4.2.3. Rules for the peripheral distribution of the twelve cardinal tracts

4.2.3.1. On the head

Since the yang tracts of the hands and feet converge on the head, it is said that "the head is the meeting-place of the yang tracts." The hand and foot yang brightness tracts (IG, V) are distributed on the face and the front of the head; the hand and foot immature yang tracts (SC, VF) are distributed on the sides of the

---

[2] Concise accounts greatly superior to that in these two sections are given in P216-82, with additional discussion in CL39-52. For details, see Academy of Traditional Chinese Medicine 1975: 33-69, and Beijing College of Traditional Chinese Medicine et al. 1980: 84-86, 96-286. The parts of this chapter that have been retained provide a useful summary of information pertinent to diagnosis and therapy.

head; the hand mature yang tract (IT) is distributed in the region of the cheeks; and the foot mature yang tract (VU) is distributed on the back of the head, the frontal region, and the top of the head.

4.2.3.2. The trunk

The yin tracts of the hands and feet are distributed on the ventral side. The three foot yin tracts are distributed on the chest and abdomen, and the hand yin tracts on the chest. Of the three foot yang tracts, the foot yang brightness tract (V) is distributed on the chest and abdomen, the foot immature yang tract (VF) is distributed laterally on the trunk, and the foot mature yang tract (VU) is distributed on the back.

4.2.3.3. The upper extremities

The three yin tracts of the hands are distributed on the palmar (medial) side, with the mature yin tract (P) in front, the immature yin tract (C) in back, and the attenuated yin tract (HC) in the middle. The three yang tracts of the hands are distributed on the dorsal (lateral) side, with the yang brightness tract (IG) in front, the mature yang tract (IT) in back, and the immature yang tract (SC) in the middle.

4.2.3.4. The lower extremities

The three yin tracts of the feet are distributed on the proximal side, with their arrangement back to front fundamentally the same as on the upper extremities; but in the lower part of the calves the positions of the attenuated yin (H) and mature yin (LP) tracts are interchanged. The foot yang brightness tract (V) is distributed on the anterior side, the foot immature yang tract (VF) on the outside, and the foot mature yang tract (VU) on the posterior.

A grasp of these approximate rules for distribution will be of definite aid in the diagnostic and therapeutic aspects of acupuncture.

4.2.4. Rules for the inner-outer relationships of the twelve cardinal tracts

The twelve cardinal tracts are associated with the visceral systems. The yin tracts, associated with the yin visceral systems (with reticular connections to the yang systems), constitute the inner aspect of the relationship; the yang tracts, associated with the yang visceral systems (with reticular connections to the yin systems), constitute the outer aspect. Because of these associations and reticular connections of the circulation tracts in their course through the body, yin-yang and inner-outer relationships are formed between the visceral systems and between the circulation tracts. Because the cardinal tracts in an inner-outer pair are linked by reticular tracts, their physiological and pathological aspects are associated and influence each other. A grasp of these rules often makes it possible in therapy to choose acupuncture loci according to the matching of inner-outer tract pairs.[3]

4.2.5. Rules for the therapeutic functions of loci on the fourteen cardinal tracts

4.2.5.1.   The route of a tract is the locus of its therapeutic functions. That is, the parts through which the course of a cardinal tract passes correspond to the [minimal] scope of its therapeutic functions.

4.2.5.2.   Generally speaking, the great majority of head and face loci are used to treat local manifestations. There are, however, a minority of such loci, such as *pai-hui* 百 会 (TM19), *jen-chung* 人

---

[3] The common translation "point" for *hsueh* 穴 is neither philologically nor scientifically defensible. *Hsueh* originally means "pit, cave," with no implications of position without size, "excessively small size," etc. Recent studies indicate the dimensions of acupuncture loci are commonly on the order of 1 centimeter; that is, insertion of the needle need be no more precise than that to produce a given result. "Locus" does not suggest perceptible pits, which seems to me an advantage in rendering the technical term, while leaving open the matter of size.

中 (TM25), *su-liao* 素 髎 (TM24), and *feng-fu* 风 府 (TM15), which also can be used to treat manifestations involving the whole body.

4.2.5.3. Generally speaking, loci on the trunk can be used not only to treat local manifestations, but also have functions involving the viscera and the body as a whole. For instance, loci on the chest and abdomen can be used to treat local disorders, disorders of the viscera, and acute disorders; loci on the loins and back can be used to treat local disorders, disorders of the viscera, and chronic disorders. Thus such loci as *shan-chung* 膻 中 (JM17), *kuan-yuan* 关 元 (JM4), *ch'i-hai* 气 海 (JM6), *ta-chui* 大 椎 (TM13), *ming-men* 命 门 (TM4), and *shen-shu* 肾 俞 (VU23) can also be used to treat disorders of the body as a whole.

4.2.5.4. Loci of the three hand and three foot yang tracts on the hands and feet can all be used to treat manifestations involving the head, face, and sense organs, disorders involving hot sensations, and disorders of consciousness. Loci in the forearms and lower legs can be used to treat disorders involving the visceral systems, including manifestations in the chest, abdomen, loins, and back. Most loci of the three hand yang tracts can also be used to treat manifestations in the shoulders, back, neck, head, and face. Loci on the upper arms and thighs are mainly used to treat local manifestations.

4.2.5.5. The loci of the hand and foot yin tracts distributed on the hands and feet can be used to treat manifestations in the throat, chest, and pulmonary system as well as disorders of consciousness; a portion of the loci on the three foot yin tracts can also be used to treat disorders of the urogenital system as well as of the hepatic, splenetic, and renal systems. Loci on the forearms and lower legs can be used to treat disorders of the visceral systems. Of these loci, those on the three hand yin tracts mainly treat disorders of the cardiac, pulmonary, and pericardial systems, and those on the three foot yin tracts mainly treat disorders of the hepatic, splenetic, and renal systems. Most loci on the upper arms and thighs are mainly used to treat local manifestations.

4.2.5.6. Loci on the tract associated with a given visceral system can be used to treat manifestations not only of that system but of the system associated with it in an inner-outer relationship.

4.3. Clinical Applications of the Tract System

4.3.1. Applications of the tract system in diagnosis

Diagnosis of pathological changes in the visceral systems may be aided by the appearance of pain or pressure or abnormal sensations, or the detection of nodular or ropy reactive corpuscles along the courses of the tracts or at places where the circulating *ch'i* concentrates, such as the dorsal transmission and ventral collection loci (4.3.3.3.1) or the primordial *ch'i* loci (4.3.3.3.2). If there is a disorder in the pulmonary system, there will be a painful reaction to pressure at the "pulmonary transmission locus" (*fei-shu* 肺 俞 , VU13 [on the urinary bladder tract]) or *chung-fu* 中 府 (P1); if in the stomach system, the same reaction at the "stomach transmission locus" (*wei-shu* 胃 俞 , VU21) or the "splenetic transmission locus" (*p'i-shu* 脾 俞 , VU20). In appendicitis, there is pain or pressure at the "appendix locus" (*lan-wei hsueh* 阑 尾 穴 [a spot just below V36]); in gall bladder inflammations, at the "gall bladder spot" (*tan-nang tien* 胆 囊 点 [the site of the gall bladder in the upper right quadrant of the abdomen]), and so on.

Next, diagnosis may also be aided by the rules for distribution of the tracts' courses. For instance, considering the course traced by the foot immature yang gall bladder tract (VF) on the surface of the body, one is led to reason that a patient with dizziness, deafness, bitter taste in the mouth, pain in the flanks, and so on, is exhibiting manifestations of an immature yang tract disorder. Again, according to the rules for distribution of the courses of the fourteen tracts over the head, among headache manifestations one can distinguish frontal pains, associated with the yang brightness tracts; lateral pains, associated with the immature yang tracts; occipital pains, associated with the mature yang tracts; and parietal pains, associated with the foot attentuated yin tract (H) or the superintendent tract (TM).

4.3.2. Applications of the tract system to drug functions

Traditional physicians believe that certain drugs are selective toward certain visceral systems or circulation tracts. Thus they have produced the theory of tract induction (*kuei ching* 归 经), which has definite applications as a guide to the clinical use of drugs. For instance, among drugs all of which cure headache,

Chinese lovage root (*kao-pen* 藁 本 [Ligusticum sinense or L. jeholense]) enters the mature yang tracts and cures headache due to their disorders; Chinese angelica root (*pai-chih* 白 芷 [A. anomala, etc.]) enters the yang brightness tracts and cures headache due to their disorders; and root of the hare's ear (*ch'ai-hu* 柴 胡 [Bupleurum falcatum or B. scorzoneraefolium)] enters the immature yang tracts and cures headaches due to their disorders. In addition, there are what are called "tract guide drugs" (*yin ching yao* 引 经 药). That is, certain drugs not only themselves enter certain tracts, they can also serve as guides for other drugs, leading them into those tracts. For instance, rhizome of chianghuo (*ch'iang-huo* 羌 活 [Notopterygium incisum]) is the tract guide drug for the foot mature yang urinary bladder tract (VU).

4.3.3. Applications of the tract system in acupuncture and the new therapies

Acupuncture and moxibustion therapies familiar in clinical applications, and the new therapeutic methods developed in recent years on the basis of the theories of the tract system and of acupuncture and moxibustion (e.g., those in which at certain loci strands or loops of catgut are surgically implanted below the skin, needle stimulation is applied following excision of a small amount of subcutaneous fatty tissue, or drug injections are given) have received a cordial welcome from the broad masses of workers, farmers, and soldiers; they are a happy harbinger of the integration of Chinese and Western medicine. For the sake of reference, we will merely provide some introductory remarks on the general rules for choosing loci.[4]

---

[4] The *Revised Outline* does not discuss the content of the new therapies, for which see Academy of Traditional Chinese Medicine 1975: 269-90. Interest in many of these techniques seems to have abated in the aftermath of the Cultural Revolution, but injection at acupuncture loci is taken up in Chang Sheng-hsing 张 晟 星 , ed. 1983: 23-25, along with electrical stimulation used independently of surgery (pages 20-23).

4.3.3.1. Local or adjacent locus selection

Based on the applicability of each locus to the treatment of local or adjacent sites of disorder, when pathological changes develop at a certain location one can select local or nearby acupuncture loci for treatment. For instance, for disorders of the eyes, ears, or shoulders, the choice of loci in those regions is called "local selection" (*chü-pu ch'ü hsueh* 局 部 取 穴). The choice of *feng-ch'ih* 凤 池 [VF20, below the occipital protuberance on the back of the neck] in eye disorders; of *yin-t'ang* 印 堂 [between the eyebrows] or *shang-hsing* 上 星 [TM22, a little above the anterior hairline] in nose disorders; or of *yang-ling-ch'üan* 阳 陵 泉 [VF34, in front of and below the small head of the fibula] in cases of knee pain, is called "adjacent locus selection" (*lin chin* 邻 近 *ch'ü hsueh*). If there is no local distribution of loci, the spot where painful response to pressure is most apparent may be selected as the locus, in which case it is called a "that's it" locus (*a-shih hsueh* 阿 是 穴).[5]

4.3.3.2. Distal locus selection

This method of choosing loci includes:

4.3.3.2.1. Selection of locus according to the path of the tract (tract course selection). For instance, since the yang brightness tract is distributed in the front of the head, for frontal headache *ho-ku* 合 谷 (IG4) on the hand yang brightness tract, or *nei-t'ing* 内 庭 (V44) on the foot yang brightness tract, is selected. The immature yang tract is distributed in the ear region, so for ear disorders *chung-chu* 中 渚 (SC3) on the hand minor yang tract, or *yang-ling-ch'üan* (VF34) on the foot immature yang tract, is chosen. Analogously, for back pains *wei-chung* 委 中 (VU54) or *yin-men* 殷 门 (VU51) on the foot mature yang tract, or for disorders of the urogenital system *san-yin-chiao* 三 阴 交 (LP6), is chosen.

---

[5] On locus selection see Academy of Traditional Chinese Medicine 1975: 218–26. CL52 gives historical citations for the "that's it" loci, which they call "pain points." C. Chung 1982 gives medical case histories involving *a-shih hsueh*.

4.3.3.2.2.   Selection of locus according to the relation between a tract and its assigned visceral system. For a disorder in a certain visceral system, a locus on the tract associated with it is chosen. For example, choosing *t'ai yuan* 太 淵 (P9), *lieh-ch'ueh* 列 缺 (P7), *k'ung-tsui* 孔 最 (P6), *yü chi* 魚 际 (P10), or *ch'ih-tse* 尺 泽 (P5) on the pulmonary tract for pulmonary system disorders which involve coughing and labored breathing or spitting blood; *tsu-san-li* 足 三 里 (V36), *nei-t'ing* 内 庭 (V44), *shang-chü-hsu* 上 巨 墟 (V37), or *liang-men* 梁 门 (V21) on the stomach tract for pains in the stomach cavity or hiccupping with abdominal distension; and *t'ai-ch'ung* 太 冲 (H3), *chung-feng* 中 封 (H4), *ch'i-men* 期 门 (H14), or *H14*, or *chang-men* 章 门 (H13) on the hepatic tract for hepatic disorders which involve pain in the flanks or jaundice, gives relatively good results.

4.3.3.2.3.   Selection of locus according to the inner-outer relation of tracts. A disorder affecting a certain tract is often treated by using loci on it and the tract paired with it in an inner-outer relationship (2.1.1.3). For example, for coughing or spitting blood, *ho-ku* (IG4) on the hand yang brightness large intestine tract is frequently used in conjunction with *k'ung-tsui* (P6) on the pulmonary tract; for abdominal pain and loose bowels, *tsu-san-li* (V36) on the foot yang brightness stomach tract is often used in conjunction with *kung-sun* 公 孙 (LP4) on the foot mature yin splenetic tract.

4.3.3.2.4.   Selection of locus according to the relation of a visceral system to other tissues. For instance, the hepatic system is vented in the eyes (2.1.2.1.3); so for eye disorders *t'ai-ch'ung* (H3) or *hsing-chien* 行 间 (H2) on the hepatic tract, or the "hepatic transmission locus" (*kan-shu* 肝 俞 , VY18) on the urinary bladder tract, may be selected. The renal system is vented in the ears (2.1.5.1.6); so for ear disorders *t'ai-ch'i* 太 溪 (R3) or *shui-ch'üan* 水 泉 (R5) on the renal tract, or the "renal transmission locus" (*shen-shu,* VU23) on the urinary bladder tract, may be selected. The splenetic system controls the flesh; thus for symptoms which involve the flesh such as atrophied, enervated, or pulsating flesh, *t'ai-pai* 太 白 (LP3) or *yin-ling-ch'üan* 阴 陵 泉 (LP9) on the splenetic tract, or the "splenetic transmission locus" (*p'i-shu,* VU20) on the urinary bladder tract, may be selected. The pulmonary system controls the body hair (2.1.4.1.3); thus in cases of nocturnal sweating due to yin depletion in the pulmonary system, *yü chi* (P10) on the pulmonary tract or the "pulmonary transmission locus" (*fei-shu,* VU13) on the urinary bladder tract, may be selected for treatment. For manifestations which involve the Five Sense Organs (wu kuan 五 官 , nose, eyes, lips, tongue, ears) or the Five Somatic Tissues (wu t'i 五 体 , skin, flesh, sinews, blood vessels, bones), choosing for therapy loci associated with the five yin visceral systems or combining them with loci on the corresponding cardinal tracts gives relatively good results. Here we have merely provided examples for the sake of explanation.

4.3.3.3. Special locus selection

This method of selection is mainly based on the special functions of certain loci.[6]

4.3.3.3.1. *Selection of transmission loci.* The dorsal transmission loci (shu hsueh 俞 穴) transmit along the back the circulating ch'i of the visceral systems. The ventral collection loci (mu hsueh 募 穴) are those in which it collects along the thorax and abdomen. Generally speaking, the dorsal loci are mostly used for disorders which involve the yin visceral systems [dorsal = yin], for disorders newly manifested in the yin and yang systems, or for the active phase of diseases. The ventral loci are mostly used for disorders of the yang visceral systems, or for diseases which resist protracted treatment or temporarily constitute a stable condition. The distinction between the dorsal and ventral loci is relative; both regulate the functioning of the visceral systems. Thus in treating disorders of the visceral systems the dorsal and ventral loci are often employed in combination or alternation.

4.3.3.3.2. *Selection of primordial ch'i loci, interstitial loci, and nexic loci.* Each of the twelve cardinal tracts has a primordial ch'i locus (yuan hsueh 原 穴). Distributed on the extremities, these loci are places where the primordial ch'i (yuan ch'i 原 气 [= yuan ch'i 元 气 , 3.1.1]) is retained. When used to treat disorders of the visceral systems they often yield relatively good results. The interstitial loci (hsi hsueh 郄 穴) are mainly distributed in interstices between bones and sinews and are places where the circulating ch'i collects. For acute pain manifestations in general, needling the

---

[6] On this topic see CL59–68 and P335–45.

interstitial loci yields relatively good results. The nexic loci (*lo hsueh* 络 穴 [at the junctions of cardinal and reticular tracts, 4.0]) maintain contact between cardinal tracts that form an inner-outer configuration (2.1.1.3). Thus there is the saying "needle one nexus, treat two tracts."

4.3.3.3.3. Selection of the eight conjunction loci. The eight conjunction loci (*pa hui* 八 会) are:

Locus Corresponding To	Name		Code
yin visceral systems	*chang-men*		H13
yang visceral systems	*chung-kuan*	中 脘	JM12
ch'i	*shan-chung*		JM17
blood	*ko-shu*	膈 俞	VU17
sinews	*yang-ling-ch'üan*		VF34
bones	*ta-chu*	大 杼	VU11
medulla (*sui*)	*hsuan-chung*	悬 钟	VF39
pulsating circulation vessels (*mai*)	*t'ai-yuan*		P9

When the eight conjunction loci are selected to treat chronic disorders, results are often relatively good; for example, *chang-men* for treatment of disorders of the five yin visceral systems (especially those involving the hepatic and splenetic systems); *chung-kuan* for disorders of the six yang systems (especially those of the stomach and large intestine systems); *shan-chung* for respiratory difficulties, asthma, distension and distress in the chest and diaphragm regions, and retching and belching; *ko-shu* for spitting or vomiting blood, nosebleed, excessive or prolonged menses, bloody urine or stool, purpura, and so on; *yang-ling-ch'üan* for hemiplegia, tonic convulsions, palsy, and loss of function in limbs; *ta-chu* for generalized bone and joint pains; *hsuan-chung* for paralysis and loss of function in the lower extremities; and *t'ai yuan* for absence of the pulse and diseases of the cardiac and pulmonary systems.

The dorsal transmission and ventral collection loci, primordial *ch'i* loci, interstitial loci, nexic loci, and conjunction loci described above may be used in combination or singly. In the treatment of chronic illness, effectiveness is often improved when the transmission and collection loci, or primordial *ch'i* and nexic loci, are used in coordination.

4.3.3.4. Experiential locus selection

Selection, based on clinical experience, of loci that have special therapeutic functions for certain disorders is called experiential locus selection (*ching-yen ch'ü hsueh* 经 验 取 穴). Representative of this method is the "Song of the Four General Loci" which served our forebears as a mnemonic summary:

> For the belly *san-li's* for you
> For the back *wei-chung* will do
> Head and neck? Look for *lieh-ch'ueh*
> Face and mouth? You want *ho-ku*.[7]

In clinical situations, if *tsu-san-li* (V36) is chosen for abdominal disorders, *wei-chung* (VU54) for those of the back, *lieh-ch'ueh* (P7) for those of the head and neck, and *ho-ku* (IG4) for those of the face, results are comparatively good. Similarly, *kao-huang* 膏 肓 (VU38), *ta-chui* (TM13), *ming-men* (TM4), *p'i-shu* (VU20), *shen-shu* (VU23), *ho-ku* (IG4), *tsu-san-li* (V36), and *kuan-yuan* (TM4) have a tonic effect in chronic disorders and on constitutionally debilitated patients. *Feng-ch'ih* (VF20) gives comparatively good results if used for profuse watering of the eyes when facing into the wind and for dizziness due to hepatic wind heteropathy (5.1.1.2). *Feng-men* 风 门 (VU12) is often used to treat external wind-cold and wind-hot manifestations (5.1.1.1); *feng-shih* 风 市 (VF31) for Wind-moist Heteropathy Disorder (*feng-shih* 风 湿) and Wind Heteropathy Rash (*feng chen* 风 疹 , 5.1.1.1) of the lower extremities; *feng-lung* 丰 隆 (V40) for mucus manifestations (3.5); *fei-shu* (VU13), *yü-chi* (P10), *ho-ku* (IG4), and *fu-liu* 复 溜 (R7) for nocturnal sweating and perspiration without apparent cause, and so on. All of these are experiential loci [in the sense that these uses are not predicted by theory].

During the Great Proletarian Cultural Revolution, great numbers of revolutionary medical personnel under the guidance of Mao

---

[7] Such jingles were common in introductory textbooks of classical medicine as an aid to memorization.

Tse-tung thought, as a result of needling experiments on themselves and large-scale clinical experience, discovered several new loci and used them to cure a number of recalcitrant disorders. In particular, they accumulated much experience in treating deafmutism, paralysis, eye disorders, and so on. For example, they obtained relatively good results using *t'ing-ling* 听 灵 (lit., "auditory acuity") for deafness, *tseng-yin* 增 音 ("augmented voice") for muteness, *chien-ming* 健 明 ("strengthened light") for blindness, *mai-pu* 迈 步 ("vigorous stride") for palsy, *ting-ch'uan* 定 喘 ("asthma relief") for asthma, and so on; these may be considered when selecting loci.[8]

What we have introduced above are the methods for choosing loci. In clinical applications it is also essential to combine loci in prescriptions (*fang* 方). It is best that not too many loci be used in each prescription. Generally two to three loci are preferable, and local (or adjacent) and distal loci are selected coordinately. One may needle only one side of the body, choose loci on both sides at once, or choose different loci on the two sides, as in insomnia, when *shen-men* 神 门 (C7) on the left side and *nei-kuan* 内 关 (HC6) on the right side may be jointly selected. If the period of therapy is relatively protracted, one should not continue using one locus too long. One should regularly change loci, or needle at set intervals. Otherwise the locus may develop fatigue or adaptation phenomena that will influence its efficacy.

4.4. Introduction to Contemporary Research Materials on the Tract System

Since Liberation [1949], especially since 1958, a great deal of research work has been carried out in China on the tract system and the loci. Important aspects will be introduced briefly below.

---

[8] Academy of Traditional Medicine 1975: 204–16 lists *tseng-yin* as Extra 11 and *ting-ch'uan* as Extra 17; Beijing College of Traditional Chinese Medicine et al. 1980: 291 lists only the latter locus, as no. 6. It is equally clear from publications for internal use that enthusiasm for adding experiential loci has abated alongside the fervor of the Cultural Revolution.

4.4.1. Anatomical studies of the loci

We will be concerned principally with the relations between loci and the nervous and vascular systems. From dissection of cadavers it has been noted that, of the loci on the twelve cardinal tracts, roughly half are distributed along comparatively large nerves or nerve trunks, and that comparatively large nerves or nerve trunks pass through the vicinity of the other half. Under the microscope it has also been observed that the various tissue layers within the loci are rich in nerve endings, plexes, and bundles; but so far no special receptors or other special structures have been seen.[9] Secondly, the distribution of loci and that of cutaneous nerves are intimately related. More than a few loci are located precisely on cutaneous nerve trunks or on the boundaries between contiguous areas of innervation. The ability of moxa and the "plum-blossom needle" [a tool with multiple points with which the skin is struck] to produce therapeutic results by stimulating the skin at the loci is probably related to the association of loci with cutaneous nerves.

In the courses of the circulation tracts along the extremities, the directions of the pulmonary tract (P) and the musculocutaneous nerve; the cardiac tract (C) and the ulnar and medial cutaneous nerves of the forearm; the pericardial tract (HC) and the median nerve; and the urinary bladder (VU) and the sciatic nerve, are basically identical. The places where a reticular tract joins two cardinal tracts are mostly junctions of two nerve branches. For instance, the nexic locus *lieh-ch'ueh* (P7), which connects the pulmonary (P) and large intestine (IG) tracts, is situated precisely at the junction of the musculocutaneous nerve and the superficial ramification of the radial nerve; the nexic locus *kung-sun* (LP4), which connects the splenetic (LP) and stomach (V) tracts, is situated just at the junction of the superficial peroneal nerve branch and the saphenous nerve, and so on.

The distribution of the loci is also closely related to the blood vessels. Loci distributed precisely on vascular trunks are only a minority, but those alongside a vascular trunk are half or more of the total number. On the basis of animal experiments some have concluded that the nervous impulse from needling at a locus is likely to

---

[9] Refer to the discussion of the Bonghan corpuscles, page 146 above.

be transmitted in the medial direction via the nerves in the walls of blood vessels.

4.4.2. Studies of the functions of loci in the human body

4.4.2.1. Digestive system

Needling *t'ien-t'u* 天 突 (JM22), *shan-chung* (JM17), *ho-ku* (IG4), *chü-ch'ueh* 巨 闕 (JM14) or other loci may strengthen esophageal peristalsis, dilating the canal and relieving difficulty in swallowing due to esophageal spasms. Needling *tsu-san-li* (V36), *wei-shu* (VU21), *chung-kuan* (JM12) or other loci may alter peristalsis of the stomach and small intestine, causing an atonic stomach to contract, and may eliminate spasms. Needling *tsu-san-li* (V36), *san-yin-chiao* (LP6), *ta-ch'ang-shu* 大 肠 俞 (VU25), *nei-kuan* (HC6), *t'ien-shu* 天 枢 (V25), *chih-kou* 支 沟 (SC6), or other loci, may alter rectal peristalsis; thus they may be used in constipation to bring about excretion, or in diarrhea to stop it. Needling *tsu-san-li* (V36), *feng-ch'ih* (VF20), *ta-chu* (VU11), and *ssu-feng* 四 鋒, or other loci, may affect the secretion of gastric juice. Needling *yang-ling-ch'üan* (VF34) may cause the gall bladder to contract, promoting excretion of bile.

4.4.2.2. Circulatory system

Needling *jen-ying* 人 迎 (V9), *ch'ü-ch'ih* 曲 池 (IG11), *t'ai-ch'ung* (H3), *feng-ch'ih* (VF20), *tsu-san-li* (V36), or other loci, can reduce blood pressure in hypertensive patients. Applying the needle or moxa to *jen-chung* (TM25), *shih-hsuan* 十 宣 , *ho-ku* (IG4), *tsu-san-li* (V36), *pai-hui* (TM19), and other loci, can also restore the blood pressure of shock patients. Applying the needle or moxa to *nei-kuan* (HC6), *shen-men* (C7), *hsi-men* 郄 门 (HC4), *hsin-shu* 心 俞 (VU15), or other loci, can alter the strength and frequency of heart contractions. Needling *tsu-san-li* (V36) may bring about vasodilatation and reduce vascular permeability. Moxa applied below *shih-ch'i-chui* 十 七 椎 may increase vascular permeability.

4.4.2.3. Respiratory system

Needling *t'ien-t'u* (JM22), *shan-chung* (JM17), *fei-shu* (VU13), *ting-ch'uan*, or other loci, may relieve bronchial spasms, and can cure bronchial asthma.

4.4.2.4. Blood system

Needling or applying moxa to *tsu-san-li* (V36), *yin-ling-ch'üan* (LP9), *ch'ü-ch'ih* (IG11), or *ta-chui* (TM13), may cause the white corpuscles to increase in number and may strengthen their ingesting capacity [i.e., leucocytosis and phagocytosis]. Needling or applying moxa to *tsu-san-li* (V36), *kao-huang* (VU38), or *ssu-feng*, may cause the red corpuscles and hemoglobin to increase.

4.4.2.5. Urogenital system

Needling *shen-shu* (VU23), *fu-liu* (R7), *chao-hai* 照 海 (R6), or other loci has a manifest influence on renal diuresis. Needling or applying moxa to *kuan-yuan* (JM4), *chung-chi* 中 极 (JM3), *ch'ü-ku* 曲 骨 (JM2), *shen-shu* (VU23), *p'ang-kuang-shu* (VU28), *yin-ling-ch'üan* (LP9), *san-yin-chiao* (LP6), or other loci, can alter the motility of the urinary bladder, and thus may be used to treat urine retention or incontinence. Needling *san-yin-chiao* (LP6) or *ho-ku* (IG4) can cause uterine contractions, and thus may induce labor.

4.4.2.6. Endocrine system

Needling *ho-ku* (IG4), *ch'u-ch'ih* (IG11), *t'ien-t'u* (JM22), or other loci, can promote or inhibit thyroid activity, and thus may be used to treat simple goiter and hyperthyroidism. Needling *tsu-san-li* (V36), *kan-shu* (VU18), or *tan-shu* 胆 俞 (VU19), can promote activity of the pituitary-adrenal system, increasing the secretion of cortisone and glucocorticosteroids. Needling *shao-tse* 少 泽 (IT1), *ho-ku* (IG4), or applying moxa to *shan-chung* (JM17) or other loci, serves the function of promoting lactation, probably through promoting secretions of the anterior lobe of the pituitary that produce prolactin (LtH).

4.4.2.7. Nervous system

It has been reported in publications that needling at the loci may affect the reticular formation of the brain stem, causing patients with injuries to this area to return to normal. Needling at the loci may also affect the hypothalamic nuclei and the pituitary-adrenal system, promoting release of ACTH and corticoids, thus under certain conditions strengthening the organism's resistance to disease. It may also improve the balance between excitation and inhibition, as well as adaptability. Needling loci with tonic functions such as *tsu-san-li* (V36), *ho-ku* (IG4), *shao-hai* 少 海 (C3), and so on, may increase the tonus of the sympathetic nervous system. Needling *p'i-shu* (VU20), *t'ai-pai* (LP3), and other loci, may be efficacious in lowering the activity of the sympathetic adrenal system. Because of these manifold functions, it is possible to treat many sorts of nervous system disease by needling at the loci.

On the basis of abundant materials from physiological experimentation, it may be held that the functions of the loci as they affect every aspect of the organism are distinctive, whereas the functions of spots that are not acupuncture loci are by no means marked. The functions of a minority of loci are multiple; *tsu-san-li* (V36) and *ho-ku* (IG4) are of this sort. The locus *su-liao* (TM24), used for first aid, simultaneously stimulates the activity of the respiratory, circulatory, nervous, endocrine, and other systems.

4.4.3. Studies of the material correlates of the tract system

The sensations of soreness, numbness, distension, and electrical shock that signal "striking the *ch'i*" (*te ch'i* 得 气) frequently propagate along the pathways traced by the tract system, showing a "tractwise course" phenomenon.[10] What is the material basis of this? This has not yet been clarified. Preliminary conclusions have been drawn regarding the following three possibilities:

---

[10] "Striking the *ch'i*" refers to feelings of numbness, etc., that follow correct insertion of the needle. See CL192–93 and Academy of Traditional Chinese Medicine 1975: 15–16.

4.4.3.1. The nerves

According to views of this kind, anatomical studies of the loci have revealed that the distribution of loci, especially the courses of the cardinal tracts along the extremities, is closely similar to the distribution of the nerves. From the efficacy of needling at the loci in bringing about changes in the vital functions of the various organs, it is generally believed that this efficacy is inseparable from the functions of the nervous system. Beginning with the reception of the stimulus, every link in its transmission requires involvement of the nerves, including the somatic nerves and those in the walls of the blood vessels, and is closely related to the nerve centers. Experiments have proven that circulation tract phenomena may be suppressed or weakened when surgery or anesthesia blocks nerve pathways. For instance, needling *tsu-san-li* (V36) may strengthen small-intestine peristalsis (in rabbits), but if the sciatic and femoral nerves are both cut the response is suppressed. This shows that there is a close relation between the two nerves and the inward transmission of the stimulus. If the spinal cord in the lumbar or sacral region is completely severed and *tsu-san-li* is then needled, the response is also suppressed. This shows that the spinal cord is also involved in the response. Under spinal anesthesia in the lumbar region, when *tsu-san-li* is needled it is impossible to induce sensations of soreness or numbness until the anesthesia has passed off. If, after the stellate ganglion has been blocked, loci on the face are needled, the response is suppressed. After the cerebral cortex has been anesthetized, the efficacy of *ta-chui* (TM13) in reducing fever is clearly reduced. If the sympathetic and parasympathetic nerves are then blocked, its antipyretic effectiveness is no longer apparent.

In recent research on acupuncture analgesia, it has been observed that *ho-ku* (IG4) can cause the pain threshhold to rise in various parts of the body. If, however, procaine is used to block the superficial and deep levels at the locus, or if only the deeper tissues are blocked off, it is no longer possible to raise the pain threshhold. In addition, the deeper tissues at the *ho-ku* locus are controlled by the ulnar nerve; if a pulsed square-wave electrical stimulus is applied to *ho-ku*, a change in the electrical potential—a complex action potential—may be recorded on the skin surface above the elbow along the route of the ulnar nerve. It has also been observed that when, in cats and monkeys, certain loci corresponding to those on the human body are needled, one can record electrical discharges, induced by the needling, on nerve fibers that control the region of the locus. If the hind extremity of the cat is stimulated with a pulsed square wave at spots that correspond to the loci *san-yin-chiao* (LP6) and *tsu-san-li* (V36), an electrical potential change—an induced potential—may be recorded at the central median nucleus of the thalamus, the central segmental area of the midbrain (mesencephalon), and other sites. According to the above results of clinical observation and animal experimentation, it has been concluded that the material correlate of the tract system is probably the nerves.

4.4.3.2. The general neuro-humoral regulating functions

According to views of this kind, in addition to the nerves serving as pathways for circulation tract phenomena, elements of humoral regulation must be kept in mind, since there is sometimes a relatively long period of latency in the effectiveness of needling, and efficacy is often relatively enduring. Experiments have already proved that in acute appendicitis, needling may increase blood cortisone. Acupuncture and moxibustion can also promote secretion of luteinizing hormone and luteotrophic hormone in the anterior lobe of the pituitary, influencing the discharge of the ovum, and so on.

4.4.3.3. Vegetative electrical phenomena of the organism

Some people as a result of research on skin resistance and skin potentials, have discovered a number of "good conductor points" and "good conductor nexi" (*ryōdōten* 良 导 点 , *ryōdōraku* 络), similar to the acupuncture loci and tracts. They believe this is an objective proof that the tract system exists. The results of research by different individuals show discrepancies, however, so that there is no consensus.[11]

Research materials related to the circulation tract system are rather abundant, and will not be reviewed in detail here. Generally

---

[11] This obviously skeptical paragraph refers to Japanese attempts to make it possible for untrained personnel to locate acupuncture loci using skin resistance meters; see, for instance, CL187–88. Such meters are now manufactured in China, since there is a large market for "electroacupuncture machines" in Europe and the United States.

speaking, these materials show that the tract system has a material basis. In the light of research materials seen to date, it can be held that the relation of the tract system to the nervous system is comparatively close. In the sense that the tracts are responsible for regulating the functions of the entire body, they correspond to the neuro-humoral system. Needling at the loci may also affect the activity of internal secretion. Seen in the light of traditional doctors' descriptions of the tract system, the circulation tracts also include the blood vessels. Thus it is likely that the tract system includes the nervous, endocrine, and vascular systems. The laws that govern the activity of the nervous system are not yet entirely clear; this is probably one reason that the nerve theory cannot entirely explain the theory of the tract system.

The theory of the tract system is one of the fundamental principles of Chinese medicine. It has guiding significance for acupuncture, moxibustion, and every specialty in clinical medicine. Clarifying further its material correlates may not only allow circulation tract theory to better serve the broad masses of workers, peasants, and soldiers, but also is bound to make a comparatively large contribution to the development of medicine.

4.5. Conclusion

The course followed by the circulation tract system is known as a result of countless clinical experiences. It is no fictitious concept, but rather a pathway along which needle response is propagated when acupuncture is applied at the loci. Physiologically speaking, it is a communication net which interconnects every part of the human body; therapeutically speaking, it is the reaction pathways along which responses develop when the body receives a stimulus. Acupuncture and moxibustion therapy proceeds by stimulating the loci, the most sensitive points on the tracts. As a result of the regulative functions of the tracts, the therapeutic goal is reached. What locus to use for what disorder is normally decided according to circulation tract theory. Thus the fact that the theory is able to guide clinical practice shows that this theory definitely makes sense.

The material basis of the tract system remains an unsolved problem. We believe that we must consider not only the aspect of tract theory that guides clinical medicine, but also the aspect that, limited by historical conditions, is insufficiently accurate. We must consider not only what contemporary physiology and anatomy have already accomplished, but also the many questions that they have not yet answered. Thus we must take dialectical materialism as a guide and use the knowledge and methods of modern science in our research. In this way the question of the material correlates of the tract system is certain to be answerable.

5. Causes of Medical Disorders

In etiology Chinese medicine gives the most important role to or-thopathic *ch'i* (3.1.1) in the belief that "when the body's orthopathic *ch'i* is intact, heteropathic *ch'i* cannot interfere," and that "where heteropathy moves in, the *ch'i* is bound to be depleted." That is to say, the main occasion of medical disorders is depletion of this or-thopathic *ch'i*, giving the heteropathic *ch'i* an opening of which to take advantage. If the orthopathic *ch'i* is at an adequate level and the power of resistance strong, one does not readily become ill.[1]

Traditional physicians believe that every medical disorder has its causes. Two thousand years ago the *Inner Canon of the Yellow Lord* [*Huang ti nei ching* 黄 帝 内 经] divided the causes of medical disorders into two categories, "inner causes" (*nei yin* 内 因) and "outer causes" (*wai yin* 外 因). Later there was a theory of three causes, according to which the Six Excesses (*liu yin* 六 淫 , 5.1), bringing on exogenous disorders, were called "outer causes," and the Seven Emotional States (*ch'i ch'ing* 七 情 , 5.4), overexhaustion, and incorrect diet, bringing on disorders due to internal harm, were called "inner causes." Because wounds and in-sect or animal injuries differ from the above, they were called "causes neither inner nor outer" (*pu nei wai yin* 不 内 外 因). This etiological classification was used clinically for a relatively long period.

We do not believe that this sort of classification is reconcilable with the developmental view of dialectical materialism. Climatic changes, external injuries, injuries by insects and animals, mental overstimulation, overexhaustion, unregulated diet: all are external etiological factors, and should belong to the outer causes, whereas

---

[1] This doctrine goes back to the *Inner Canon*. See above, pages 100–1.

only individual mental factors and changes in the organism's power of resistance are inner causes.[2]

The Chinese physician's common saying, "consider the manifestation type and find the cause" means that in the course of determining the manifestation type one deduces the cause of a disorder; this is one aspect of manifestation type determination (7.0). Since causes differ, pathological changes brought about within the body differ. A good grasp of the rules according to which different causes bring about disorders, as well as their clinical characteristics, is important for diagnosis and therapy.

---

[2] On the distinction between outer and inner causes implicit in the *Inner Canon* see, e.g., SW, *23* (77): 496, without parallel in TS. The threefold distinction occurs vaguely in passing in *Chin kuei yao lueh fang lun* 金 匱 要 畧 方 論 (196/200?), *1*: 1b-2a. This seminal work lists only wounds, injuries by insects and animals, and violations of sexual hygiene as causes that are neither internal nor external. The classification was fully developed in the *San yin chi i ping yuan lun ts'ui* 三 因 极 一 病 源 論 粹 (1174 or slightly later), and the categories redefined. To the third category were added, for instance, overeating, fatigue, and spirit possession (*2*: 19). The book emphasizes that many disorders can be due to any of the three types. The *Revised Outline* is thus doubly incorrect in describing overexhaustion and diet as inherently inner causes in this schema.

Why is the account not more accurate? Partly because the threefold division was suspected of idealistic bias, and thus was ideologically unsatisfactory, a matter that has ceased to perturb recent authors. There is another more fundamental reason. Although the three-type etiology was influential, discussions of causation were not very important either in basic or clinical medicine, far less important than accounts of the courses of disorders. This point can be seen in the *Revised Outline*, where the latter is a pervasive theme and the former is little discussed outside this chapter.

5.1. Six Excesses

Wind, cold, heat, moist, dry, and Fire (*feng, han, shu, shih, tsao, huo* 风 寒 暑 湿 燥 火) are manifestations of climatic change in the realm of nature over the four seasons. Under normal conditions they are called the "Six Climatic Configurations" (*liu ch'i* 六 气), but when abnormalities appear these six can become causative factors in medical disorders. In that case they are called the "Six Excesses" (*liu yin*).[3]

When bringing on disorders the Six Excesses generally first invade the outer part of the flesh or enter through the nose or mouth, so they are usually referred to as "external heteropathies" (*wai hsieh* 外 邪). In addition to climatic factors, to some extent they encompass disease-causing microorganisms, although historical conditions prevented the ancients from clearly recognizing this.

Most Six Excesses etiology is seasonal; for instance, in spring there is a preponderance of wind heteropathy disorders, in summer of heat heteropathy disorders, in autumn of dry heteropathy disorders, in winter of cold heteropathy disorders, and at the transition from summer to autumn a preponderance of moist heteropathy disorders. The Six Excesses not only can individually bring on disorders, as in Wind Heteropathy Damage Disorder (*shang feng* 伤 风 [colds, etc.]) and Heat Heteropathy Attack Disorder (*chung shu* 中 暑 [heat stroke, etc.]), but can also do so in combination, as when wind, cold, and moist heteropathies invading the body in concert bring on Localized Pain Disorders (*pi* 痹 [joint pain syndromes, migraine, etc.]).

In addition there are "internal wind heteropathy" and other internal analogues, pathological conditions which appear in the course of disorders resulting from internal causes. Although they are distinct from the exogenous disorders brought on by Six Excesses heteropathies, certain aspects of their clinical manifestations are similar, so they will also be noted here.

---

[3] *Shu* is sometimes referred to as *je* 热 . The first five are sometimes grouped separately, as in 1.2.1. See also CL143 and P62–66. *Liu ch'i* is also used in the *Inner Canon* for the body's six basic vital substances; see TS, *2* (2): 10 = LS, *6* (30): 58–59.

5.1.1. Wind heteropathy

5.1.1.1. External wind heteropathy

The nature of wind is to blow freely, mobile and changeable, readily causing injury to health, bringing on disorders in any season; thus it is said that "wind is the chief over all disorders." Inception is abrupt, and in general abatement is quick. Thus the course of a disorder is not long, as in Wind Heteropathy Rash (*feng chen* 风 疹 , hives) and Wind Heteropathy Damage Disorder (*shang feng* [various mild febrile syndromes]). Such conditions are migratory, as in Wind Heteropathy Localized Pain Disorder (*feng pi* 风 痹 [migratory pains of rheumatoid arthritis, etc.]), which because the painful part does not remain fixed is also called "Migratory Localized Pain Disorder" (*hsing pi* 行 痹). Wind heteropathy often invades the outer part of the flesh, causing an itching sensation, or encroaches upon the defensive *ch'i* of the pulmonary system, in which case there are such symptoms as abnormal sensitivity to wind, hot sensations, perspiration without external cause, itchy throat, coughing, and floating pulse.

The most common heteropathy combinations involving wind factors are wind-cold, wind-hot (for both of these see 9.1), and wind-moist. Wind-moist heteropathy infiltrates the circulation tracts in the peripheral flesh, with symptoms such as headache with sensation of heaviness; pains in all the joints or migratory pains; or in some cases Moist Heteropathy Rash (*shih chen* 湿 疹 [eczema]) or itching sores.

5.1.1.2. Internal wind heteropathy (hepatic wind heteropathy)

Often brought about by pathological changes in the cardiac, hepatic, and renal systems of function, it usually causes abrupt symptomatic attacks, including in light cases dizziness, dullness of vision, or spots before the eyes, moodiness, trembling of the hands and feet, numbness, contortion of the mouth or eye, and in severe cases sudden fainting, unawareness of surroundings (*pu hsing jen shih* 不 省 人 事 [i.e., unresponsiveness, unconsciousness, coma]), muscle spasms, convulsive backward arching of the spine [as in grand mal epileptic seizures], and hemiplegia.

Internal wind heteropathy is often seen in the following circumstances:

Extreme intensity of hot heteropathy giving rise to wind heteropathy: mostly seen in Heat Factor Disorders (9.1.3.5), and especially frequent in infants. Damage by hot heteropathy to dispersed body fluids, constructive *ch'i*, and blood affects the functioning of the cardiac and hepatic systems, causing the appearance of such symptoms as spasmodic Fright Disorders (*ching chueh* 惊 厥) and mental confusion with or without unconsciousness.[4] This predisposing situation is similar to what Western doctors call fever convulsions.

Yin depletion activating wind heteropathy: mainly hepatic wind heteropathy induced when yin depletion in the hepatic or renal system causes the hepatic yang to rise in excess. In light cases there is headache or dizziness, and in severe cases sudden fainting and Wind Attack Disorders [strokes, etc.]. This situation is often seen in high blood pressure disorders (14.2.10), cerebrovascular accident (14.2.17), and so on.

Blood depletion giving rise to wind heteropathy: this situation is generally brought on by blood depletion or depletion of renal yin *ch'i*. Main symptoms include dizziness, spots before the eyes, ringing in the ears, numbness and trembling in the extremities, tetany, and in severe cases convulsions and coma. This situation is often seen in dizziness as a symptom of severe anemia, as well as in connection with low blood sugar, low blood calcium, and so on.

5.1.2. Cold heteropathy

5.1.2.1. External cold heteropathy

Cold heteropathy mostly brings on medical disorders in winter, but can also do so in other seasons as a result of drops in air

---

[4] Fright Disorder (or Fright Syndrome) is an entity recognized by cross-cultural psychiatrists. For descriptions see Topley 1970: 429–34 and Kleinman 1980b: 195–97. Traditional physicians differentiate a number of disorders related to fright and anxiety, discussed in *Cheng chih chun sheng* 證 治 準 繩 (1602), I, 326–34. In modern medicine *ching-chueh* is a general term for convulsions, but a parenthetical comment below (page 422) indicates that the authors of the *Revised Outline* are using it in the traditional sense (which often implies convulsions).

temperature. It readily blocks the yang *ch'i* in the outer part of the defensive circulation (3.1.3), so that such symptoms appear as abnormal sensitivity to cold, hot sensations, inability to perspire, and floating and tense pulse. Cold heteropathy moves from outer aspects to inner,[5] and is readily transformed into hot heteropathy. Generally cold heteropathy, after being transmitted from a mature yang tract and entering a yang brightness tract, can produce hot sensations of great intensity, intense thirst, profuse sweating, and other repletion hot symptoms.

The nature of cold heteropathy is to congeal. After invading the body it often becomes static in the skin and peripheral flesh, the circulation tracts, the bones and sinews, the joints, or the visceral systems, preventing the *ch'i* or blood from flowing freely. The *ch'i* becomes static and the blood coagulates, giving rise to pain manifestations. When cold heteropathy remains in the intestinal systems or stomach system, there are vomiting, stomach pains, and loose bowels.

Cold heteropathy often combines with wind or moist heteropathy to bring about medical disorders. Frequently seen cold heteropathy disorders include the wind cold type (see 9.1.1.5), Wind Attack Disorder—which directly attacks the visceral systems, with cold body and extremities, shivering, pale face and, in serious cases, sudden fainting and coma, pulse sunken and small—and Cold Heteropathy Localized Pain Disorder (*han pi* 寒 痹 , 6.4.1.2.6)—in which cold heteropathy becomes static in the circulation tracts or in the bones and sinews, producing flesh and joint pains that in general do not change location, become more intense when cold, and are relieved by heat.

---

[5] This refers mainly to motion from the periphery of the body toward the visceral systems of function in the abdomen, but its scope is considerably wider than that. "From outer aspects to inner" implies from relatively yang to relatively yin, whether in the body as a whole or in visceral system or circulation tract relationships. The next sentence gives an example of a subtler sense.

5.1.2.2. *Internal cold heteropathy*

This is identical with the inner cold manifestation type (7.2), and is divided into depletion and repletion types (7.3). The depletion type is produced when there is a yin *ch'i* preponderance. Clinical manifestations are abnormal antipathy to cold, lack of warmth in hands and feet, nausea with vomiting of a clear liquid, diminution of appetite with thin stool, abdominal pains with gurgling in the intestine, protracted voiding of clear urine, tongue pale in color with lustrous white coat, pulse sunken and retarded, and so on.

Overeating of raw and cold foods may bring on "submerged cold and accumulated chill factors" (*ch'en han chi leng* 沉 寒 积 冷), which also correspond to internal cold heteropathy. One observes as indicative signs pains in the abdomen, diminution of appetite, constipation, and in serious cases cold sensations and more severe pains in the abdominal region, tongue coat white and thick or white and unctuous, and pulse sunken and retarded but vigorous; this is the cold repletion manifestation type (7.3.2).

5.1.3. Heat heteropathy

Heat heteropathy (*shu* 暑 [also called "hot heteropathy," *je* 热]) brings on medical disorders in summer. Summer heat heteropathy disorders [i.e., acute febrile diseases with onset in summer, 9.1.1.2] are called "Heat Heteropathy Damage Disorders" (*shang shu* 伤 暑) or "Heat Heteropathy Stimulus Disorders" (*kan shu* 感 暑). The disorders that result from prolonged activity under a hot sun are called "Heat Heteropathy Attack Disorders" (*chung shu* 中 暑). In heat heteropathy disorders one generally observes such typical signs of the hot manifestation type (7.2.2) as high fever, intense thirst, and profuse sweating. They readily bring about *ch'i* debilitation and damage to the yang body fluids (*chin*; 3.4); symptoms include general languor and lack of vigor, mouth and tongue dry, and constipation and scanty urine. Heat heteropathy disorders also mostly entail moist heteropathy complications, partly because of summer humidity and partly because in summer people tend to eat raw and cold foods, which can easily damage the splenetic and stomach systems and give rise to internal moist heteropathy. Thus heat heteropathy disorders are often attended by such symptoms as feelings of distress in the chest, nausea, and poor appetite.

Commonly seen heat heteropathy disorders include the following.

5.1.3.1. Heat Heteropathy Damage Disorders

When the stimulus from heat heteropathy is relatively weak, manifestations include hot sensations, intense thirst, perspiration, headache, nausea and vomiting, loose bowels, rapid breathing, lack of strength in the extremities, and pulse swollen and accelerated.

5.1.3.2. Heat Heteropathy Attack Disorders

This is mainly a result of over-stimulation by heat after protracted labor under a hot sun or in a high-temperature environment. Its manifestations include such symptoms as sudden fainting, confused state of mind, hot sensations of great intensity, inability to sweat or cold perspiration, breathing rough and face flushed, tongue red and lips scarlet, and pulse swollen and large but debilitated.

5.1.4. Moist heteropathy

5.1.4.1. External moist heteropathy

Medical disorders brought on by external moist heteropathy are mostly related to climate and environment. Whether due to protracted rainy weather, a long sojourn in a misty, humid place, wading through water or soaking by rain over a long period, if prevention is not thorough or physical conditioning has been neglected, moist heteropathy disorders can easily occur. People with long-established weakness in the splenetic and stomach systems also readily respond to external moist heteropathy.

This agent usually enters by way of the peripheral flesh and skin. In light cases it invades the skin, sinews, circulation vessels, or joints; in serious cases the damage extends to the visceral systems. After penetrating the body the heteropathy may turn cold or hot. This transformation is usually related to the state of functioning of the patient's visceral systems as well as to the appropriateness of medical treatment. For instance, in patients with chronic yang depletion in the splenetic system, moist heteropathy readily turns cold; in patients with a hot heteropathy [i.e., yang repletion] in the stomach system, it readily turns hot. When an excess of chilling or cooling drugs has been taken, it readily turns cold; and when warming or heating medicines have been used without good reason, it readily turns hot.

The special features of medical disorders brought on by moist heteropathy are as follows.

1. Since it is characteristic of moisture to weigh heavily, one often sees the head heavy as if bound up, the body weighed down, and the extremities lacking in strength. Most moist heteropathy disorders begin in the lower part of the body, so one often observes sluggishness in the lower extremities and swollen ankles.

2. Since the character of moisture is yin, cold, and congealing, it can impede the mobility of the body's energies, so that one often notes feelings of distress in the chest, distension and fullness in the stomach cavity, and other symptoms of *ch'i* stasis.

3. Since it is characteristic of moisture to be contaminated, such symptoms belong to it as White Band Disorder (*pai tai* 白 带 [light-colored vaginal disorders, abnormal leukorrhea]), Urinary Discomfort Disorders (*lin* 淋 [involving inability to urinate or difficult urination, 6.1.4]), and Urethral Turbidity Disorders (*cho* 浊 [turbid urine or discharge]), and diarrhea (*hsia li* 下 利), Moist Heteropathy Rash, and running sores.

4. Since it is characteristic of moisture to be persistent, a number of moist heteropathy disorders cannot be cured quickly.

5. White and smooth or unctuous tongue coating ["bald" tongue?] and moderate or soft pulse are often observed.

Moist heteropathy often combines with wind or cold heteropathy to bring about disorders. Common moist heteropathy disorders include:

5.1.4.1.1.   Moist Heteropathy Damage Disorders. This refers to damage to the outer aspect (7.1.1) by moist heteropathy, and is also called "Outer Aspect Moist Heteropathy Disorders" (*piao shih* 表 濕). Its manifestations are aversion to cold, hot sensations without great intensity, distended and heavy feeling of the head, heavy feeling in the body with languid limbs, feelings of distress in the chest, lack of thirst, white and smooth tongue coating, and floating or moderate pulse. It is often seen in the early stages of exogenous disorders during rainy seasons.

5.1.4.1.2.   Moist Heteropathy Rheumatic Disorders. Also called "Lodged Localized Pain Disorders," (*cho pi* 著 痹). When moist heteropathy encroaches on the circulation tracts it brings on pains all over the body. The most serious are joint pains. They are fixed in location, with skin numbness and difficulty in locomotion.

5.1.4.1.3.   Moist-hot Disorders. Generally with hot sensations, but not of great intensity; thirst and perspiration without external cause; worry and mental upset with sensations of fullness in the chest; urination brief, urine tinged scarlet; tongue coating yellow and unctuous; and pulse smooth and accelerated or soft and accelerated. If the heteropathy becomes pent up in the splenetic or stomach system, Yellow Jaundice Disorders (*huang tan* 黃 疸) may be the outcome.[6] If it is locked in struggle [with the body's normal *ch'i*] in the large intestine system one may observe purulent or bloody diarrhea.

If the moist-hot heteropathy runs down into the urinary bladder one may observe painful, frequent, or bloody urination, excessive urge to urinate, Urinary Discomfort Disorders, or White Band Disorder. If moist-hot heteropathy becomes blocked up in the skin, one may observe its toxicity manifested in sores, abscesses, and swellings, as well as Moist Heteropathy Rash.

5.1.4.1.4.   Internal moist heteropathy. Generally when lack of moderation in eating and drinking damages the splenetic or stomach system, bringing about inability of the splenetic yang *ch'i* to exert itself, and consequent abnormalities in the transmission and as-

---

[6] On jaundice as a symptom and a group of disorders see the introductory study, pages 301-2.

similation functions, moist heteropathy is produced from within and becomes a source of trouble as it accumulates. Clinical manifestations may include loose bowels, dropsy, or excretory mucus. The saying that "moist heteropathy swellings all belong to the splenetic system" comes from this.

5.1.5. Dry heteropathy

5.1.5.1. External dry heteropathy (autumnal dry heteropathy)

In autumn, when the weather is dry, one readily contracts dry heteropathy disorders. When the weather turns cool and dry, cool-dry manifestations readily arise; when dry heteropathy is transformed by hot heteropathy the result is warm-dry manifestations.

The special features of medical disorders brought on by dry heteropathy are:

1. Likelihood of harm to the pulmonary system, involving dry cough, or in some cases excretion of blood mucus, dry nasal passages, pains in the chest, or hot sensations.

2. Likelihood of damage to the body's yin *ch'i* and dispersed body fluids. Thus one often observes dryness of the mouth, tongue, lips, and skin, thirst temporarily relieved by drinking, hot sensations without perspiration, dry stool, small and rough pulse, and similar symptoms.

In the cool types of external dry heteropathy, abnormal sensitivity to cold is more noticeable than hot sensations, the tongue coating is white, and the pulse is floating. In the warm type, hot sensations are more noticeable than aversion to cold; there is thirst, and in some cases inflamed eyes, pain in the esophagus, coughing up of mucus streaked with threads of blood, urination brief with a scarlet tinge, redness on the sides and tip of the tongue, and floating and accelerated pulse.

5.1.5.2. Internal dry heteropathy

On the whole there are three types of causes that produce internal dry heteropathy:

1. excessive vomiting, diarrhea, sweating, or loss of blood [all of which involve body fluid loss];

2. drawn-out heat factor disorders [chapter 9] that damage the dispersed body fluids, or wasting diseases that diminish the yin dispersed fluids;

3. excessive use of diaphoretics, purgatives, or warming or drying drugs.

External clinical manifestations of internal dry heteropathy include skin and body hair dry, worn-looking, and lacking in luster; throat parched and lips cracked; a rough sensation in the eyes, and a hot sensation in the nostrils. Internal symptoms include intermittent hot sensations or nocturnal sweating, insomnia from worry and mental upset, large liquid intake accompanied by hunger (*k'o yin shan chi* 渴 饮 善 饥),[7] dry and hardened stool, and scanty urination. The tongue is red and saliva scanty, the coating thin or absent, and the pulse small and accelerated or in some instances rough.

5.1.6. Fire heteropathy

The difference between Fire and hot heteropathy is only a matter of degree. When hot heteropathy reaches extreme intensity it may transform into Fire, as may wind, cold, heat, moist, and dry heteropathies as they move inward. In addition, imbalances in the functioning of the visceral systems, and mental stimuli, etc., may also be so transformed. Thus it may be said that Fire manifestations mostly belong to the inner manifestation type (7.1.2), and

---

[7] Literally, "thirst [relieved by] drinking but with a tendency to be hungry," which suggests considerable loss of nutrients. I am grateful to Lu Gwei-djen for a conversation about this term.

clinically may be divided into repletion Fire and depletion Fire [which correspond generally to external and internal etiology].

5.1.6.1. Repletion Fire

This form mostly develops when exogenous heteopathy is transformed. Its clinical characteristics are as follows.

1. It has an abrupt onset and rapid changes.

2. Because Fire and hot heteropathies are particularly injurious to dispersed body fluids, one generally observes hot sensations of great intensity, aversion to heat, sensations of dryness and thirst with a preference for drinking cold liquids, copious perspiration, red face and inflamed eyes, mouth and lips parched, stool dry and hardened, urination brief with scarlet tinge, tongue reddened and coating yellow, and similar symptoms.

3. It is characteristic of Fire to flame upward, with symptoms that differ according to visceral system. If the Fire of the cardiac system flames upward (*hsin huo shang yen* 心 火 上 炎) one may observe insomnia from worry and mental upset, and in serious cases, confused state of mind, raving, and manic agitation. If the Fire of the stomach system flames upward one may observe swollen and painful gums, vomiting of blood, nosebleed, headache, and so on. If the Fire of the hepatic system flames upward one observes irritability, inflamed, swollen, and painful eyes, headache, and other symptoms.

4. Fire is the relatively yang type of hot heteropathy. It can force the blood into uncontrolled motion (*hsueh wang hsing* 血 妄 行), often bringing on vomiting of blood, nosebleed, skin rash, and other hemorrhagic symptoms.

5. In most Fire manifestations one observes the tongue red or crimson, the coating yellow and dry with scanty saliva, and the pulse swollen and accelerated.

5.1.6.2. Depletion Fire

Mostly brought about by internal dysfunctions, as when the functioning of the visceral systems (pulmonary, renal, hepatic) is unbalanced, or the *ch'i* and blood do not flow freely, or as a result of incorrect care for a drawn-out disorder, overconsumption of vital energy (*ching-ch'i* 精 气), emotional tension, and so on.

The special clinical features of depletion Fire heteropathy are gradual onset and comparatively long course. Main symptoms are intermittent fever and nocturnal sweating, sensitivity to heat in the Five Hearts [i.e., heart, palms of the hands, and soles of the feet], reddening about the cheekbones in the second half of the day, insomnia as in Depletion Agitation Disorder (*hsu fan* 虚 烦 [agitation, wakefulness, and related symptoms of the depletion hot manifestation type]), dry mouth and throat, dry cough without phlegm or in some cases with bloody phlegm, ringing in the ears, forgetfulness, aching loins, involuntary loss of semen, tongue red with scanty saliva and peeling coating or no coating, pulse small and accelerated, and so on.

5.2. Pestilential *Ch'i*

Extremely communicable acute infectious disorders are called "Epidemic Disorders" (*i li* 疫 疬). Such disorders are brought on by certain pestilential *ch'i* (*li ch'i* 疬 气), or epidemic heteropathies (*i hsieh* 疫 邪), distinct from the Six Excesses and communicable. The clinical manifestations of each epidemic disorder are on the whole constant. As has been said, "when the various epidemic disorders (*wu i* 五 疫) appear they spread easily. No matter how big or small [the patient?], the symptoms are similar."[8] The danger of epidemics to human health is very great. Their production and spread are often related to such factors as serious climatic abnormalities and deficiencies in sanitary conditions.

---

[8] The quotation originates in what claims to be a "lost" chapter of the *Huang ti nei ching su wen*; Ch'eng Shih-te 程 士 德 ed. 1982: II, 522.

5.3. Wounds and Injuries from Animals and Insects

[Text omitted from the original book.]

5.4. Seven Emotions

Joy (hsi 喜), anger (nu 怒), sorrow (yu 憂), ratiocination (ssu 思),[9] grief (pei 悲), apprehension (k'ung 恐), and fear (ching 驚), seven kinds of emotional activity, are called the Seven Emotions (ch'i ch'ing 七 情). Emotional activity is basically a biological response of the body to the external environment. Within normal limits it does not bring on medical disorders, but when excessive can lead to unbalance of yin and yang [function], disharmony of ch'i and blood, blockage of the circulation tracts, and unbalance of the visceral systems of function, providing the conditions for development of disease. Not only can emotional disharmony lead to depletion and debilitation of the orthopathic ch'i (3.1.1) and a tendency to be affected by external heteropathy, but emotional changes themselves can bring on medical disorders. In particular they can lead to visceral system and ch'i symptoms. For instance, excessive ratiocination injures the splenetic system, with such symptoms of splenetic and stomach system unbalance as distension and pain in the stomach cavity and poor appetite. As another instance, great anger injures the hepatic system, so that the hepatic ch'i is congealed or backs upward. It may transform into Fire, in which case such symptoms appear as headache, dizziness, inflamed eyes, ringing in the ears, deafness, agitated disposition, bitter taste in the mouth, and pain in the flanks.

---

[9] Ssu is a general word for thought, but its meaning also includes a range of emotions, among them worry, longing, and preoccupation (if that is an emotion). A famous passage in the Inner Canon that relates various terms for thought and emotion makes a single translation for ssu even less feasible: "what the mind recalls is called thought (i 意). What thought retains is called intent (chih 志). Change of what is retained, in accord with intent, is called ssu. Yearning for something distant in accordance with ssu is called concern (lü 慮). Making decisions with regard to things on the basis of concern is called wisdom (chih 智)" (TS, 6 (1): 71 = LS, 2 (8): 20, tentative translation).

5.5. Lack of Moderation in Eating and Drinking

Lack of moderation in eating and drinking is often a factor in medical disorders. Gluttony, eating too much of cold or raw foods or of fat, sweet, or richly flavored dishes, or mistakenly eating unclean or poisonous substances, can all lead to illness.

1. Eating too much of cold or raw foods can injure the yang *ch'i* of the splenetic and stomach systems, creating a depletion cold condition (8.3.1) with vomiting of colorless fluid, abdominal pains diminished by pressure, an urge for hot liquid satisfied by small amounts, poor digestion, tongue pale with white coating, retarded pulse, and similar symptoms.

2. Eating too much of fat, sweet, or richly flavored dishes can give rise to hot or moist heteropathy or to mucus, and these become the causes of many sorts of visceral system disorder manifestations.

3. Overeating gives rise to Alimentary Stasis Disorders (*shih chih* 食 滯). Symptoms are lack of interest in eating, malodorous belching and regurgitation of gastric acid, nausea and vomiting, abdominal pains aggravated by pressures, foul-smelling excrement, smooth pulse, and so on.

5.6. Overexhaustion

Overexhaustion can bring on disharmony of *ch'i* and blood and lower the powers of resistance, inducing certain illnesses.

5.7. Conclusion

Chinese medicine's theories of the causes and beginnings of illness were developed out of thousands of years of therapeutic practice by the workers of our country, and are products of the struggle against religious superstition and idealism. When studying these theories we must be aware not only of their acceptable dialectical viewpoints but also of their historical limitations.

The occurrence of every illness has its definite causes. As noted earlier (5.0), the threefold classification of causes formerly prevalent is inadequate, since most of the causes of medical disorders that it encompassed would now be classified as exogenous. The Seven Emotions, as mental activities of the human body itself, might be considered internal causes, but the stimuli which lead to changes in the emotions must be considered to come from outside the body. Analogously, overexhaustion as an etiological agent would be an external cause, but the lowering of the organism's power of resistance which results from it also falls within the scope of internal causes.

The theory of the onset of disorders emphasizes internal causes. The Chinese doctor believes that illness is a process of struggle between orthopathy and heteropathy, and at the same time is the reaction of orthopathic *ch'i* to heteropathic *ch'i*. One must pay attention not only to the external heteropathy, but even more to depletion of the orthopathic *ch'i*. As the *Inner Canon of the Yellow Lord* puts it, "where heteropathy gains admission the [orthopathic] *ch'i* is bound to be depleted," and "if the orthopathic *ch'i* is intact within, external heteropathy cannot cause trouble."[10] This emphasizes the point that only when changes take place in the orthopathic *ch'i* of the body itself is external heteropathy able to take advantage of the depletion and enter. This source also recognizes that the inborn constitition, mental activity, conditions of life, natural environment, and other factors can influence the orthopathic *ch'i*, providing the conditions for occurence of illness. With these ideas in mind, in the course of prevention and treatment of medical disorders, traditional physicians pay full heed to the operation of internal causes. Citing the viewpoint that "if the orthopathic *ch'i* is preponderant, the heteropathic *ch'i* is likely to depart; if the heteropathic *ch'i* departs, the orthopathic *ch'i* is likely to return to normal," in clinical therapy they are unremittingly attentive to the changing comparative strength of orthopathy and heteropathy, tightly grasping the link between "reinforcing the orthopathic *ch'i*" (*fu cheng* 扶 正) and "expelling the heteropathic *ch'i*" (*ch'ü hsieh* 祛 邪). Thus they do away with conditions detrimental to the or-

---

[10] The first quotation is from TS, *29* (5): 558 = SW, *9* (33): 176. The second turns out to be, not from the original *Inner Canon*, but from the questionable "lost chapter" cited in note 8 above.

ganism and normalize factors beneficial to it, thereby attaining their goal, the restoration of health.

6. The Four Methods of Examination

Examination in Chinese medicine consists of four methods: interrogation (*wen* 问), visual inspection (*wang* 望), auditory and olfactory examination (*wen* 闻), and palpation (*ch'ieh* 切).[1]

6.1. Interrogation

Through detailed interrogation it is often possible to find a clue to correct diagnosis. The subject matter of interrogation is on the whole the same as in Western medicine. The aim is to understand the location of the patient's major discomfort, the time of onset of the illness, its causes, its course, previous treatment (including drug reactions), previous history, as well as the patient's living habits, preferences in food or drink, mental condition, and family history.

Interrogation in Chinese medicine has its own distinctive features. Its main points were once summed up in a mnemonic on the "Ten Inquiries," which is still worth referring to:

First ask about chills and fevers, second ask about sweat
Third, about diet, fourth, about elimination
Fifth, about head and body, sixth, about chest and abdomen
Seventh, deafness, eighth, thirst, must be made clear
Ninth, ask about old illnesses, tenth, about causes
Again, about drugs taken, then about changes in vitality

---

[1] The second *wen* used as a verb means only "to smell" in modern vernacular, but in the Chinese classics it may mean either "to smell" or "to hear."

For women, ask about menstruation, discharges, childbirth
For infants, ask about poxes and rashes.[2]

Now let us outline the subject matter of interrogation.

6.1.1. Chills, fever, and sweat

One should ask whether there is fever or aversion to cold; how severe the alternating fever and chills are; what the special characteristics of the fever are; whether there is sweating; when the sweating takes place; and what its character and quantity are.

6.1.1.1. In the case of a new illness, if there is fever with sensitivity to cold it is an outer manifestation type of external origin [on manifestation types see chapter 7]. If the fever is mild, the sensitivity to cold strong, and there is no sweating, it is a wind-cold outer repletion manifestation type of external origin. If the fever is serious, the sensitivity to cold mild, and there is perspiration, it is a wind-hot outer depletion manifestation type of external origin.

6.1.1.2. A bout of chills succeeded by a bout of fever is called "hot-cold alternation" (*han-je wang-lai* 寒 热 往 来). If the period is comparatively short, and there are also a bitter taste in the mouth, dry throat, dizziness accompanied by disturbances of vision, and fullness and distress in the chest and flanks, it is a semi-outer, semi-inner manifestation type.

6.1.1.3. If there is fever without sensitivity to cold, but with sweating, thirst, and constipation, it is an inner repletion hot manifestation type.

6.1.1.4. A chronic disorder with mild hectic fever, mental upset accompanied by hot sensations in the chest, palms of the hands, and

---

[2] This rhymed jingle for beginners is originally from *Ching-yueh ch'üan shu* 景 岳 全 書 (1624), *1*: 29a ("Ch'uan chung lu 傳 忠 録 ," chapter 1). The *Revised Outline* quotes (with some modifications) the rewritten version in *I hsueh shih-tsai i* 醫 學 實 在 易 (1808), *1*: 31–32, which is annotated.

soles of the feet (the Five Hearts, *wu hsin*), reddening about the cheekbones and dry lips, and nocturnal sweating, is "yin depletion hot sensations." Constant sensitivity to cold, shortness of breath and lack of vigor, and perspiration without external cause mean yang depletion.

6.1.2. Head, body in general, chest, and abdomen

It is important to determine clearly the location, character, and time of discomfort.

6.1.2.1. Headache and dizziness

Headaches without remission, with pain located at the two mature yang acupuncture loci (*t'ai-yang hsueh* 太 阳 穴 [*t'ung-tzu-liao* 瞳 子 髎 is the official name, VF1, slightly outside the outer corners of the two eyes]), accompanied by fever and sensitivity to cold, are mostly of external origin. Headache pain disappearing and recurring, often accompanied by faintness or dizziness, but without fever or chills, is usually of inner manifestation type and internal origin. Pain on one side only [migraine, etc.] mostly belongs to internal wind heteropathy or blood depletion. Headache during the day, increasing in severity with fatigue, is mostly yang depletion. Afternoon headache mostly belongs to blood depletion. Headache at night mostly belongs to yin depletion. Headaches with faintness or dizziness, inflamed eyes and bitter taste in the mouth are mostly preponderance of Fire heteropathy in the hepatic or gall bladder system. Dizziness with regular throbbing of the heart, shortness of breath and lack of vigor mostly means depletion and debility of the *ch'i* and blood. Sudden dizziness is mostly repletion type; persistent dizziness, mostly depletion type. Feelings of distress, pain, heaviness, and distension in the head, as though it were wrapped in cloth, are mostly the heavy sensation associated with moist heteropathy in the upper part of the body (*shih chung* 湿 重).

6.1.2.2. Body pains

Soreness and pains over the whole body with fever and sensitivity to cold are mostly of external origin. Drawn-out disorders with body pains are mostly *ch'i* and blood insufficiencies. Aches and pains in the loins are mostly renal system depletion. Aches, pains, and numbness in the joints of the extremities, the flesh, and the sinews—or swellings in the joints, with pain either migratory or fixed—are mostly wind, cold, or moist heteropathy Localized Pain Disorders.

6.1.2.3. Chest pains

Chest pains with fever and coughing or spitting of pus or blood are mostly Pulmonary System Abscess Disorders (*fei yung* 肺 痈). Chest pains with hectic or intermittent fever, and dry cough with scanty mucus or bloody mucus, are mostly Pulmonary Consumption Disorder (*fei lao* 肺 痨 , pulmonary tuberculosis).[3] Chest pains radiating toward the shoulders or back, severe pains in back of the breastbone, or a sensation of pressure in the vicinity of the heart is chest Localized Pain Disorder (but note whether it is actually angina pectoris).[4] Pains in the rib region are usually impeded flow of hepatic *ch'i*.

---

[3] These classes of disorders are of different extent than the lung abscess and pulmonary tuberculosis of modern medicine, as one would expect from the lack of access in premodern medicine to pathology and laboratory reports. According to *Chu ping yuan hou lun* 諸 病 源 候 論 (610), the most authoritative source on semeiology, the main symptoms of Pulmonary System Abscess Disorders are cough, congestion, and in many instances trembling. Cases in which the cough is productive of purulent or bloody sputum were generally considered untreatable (*33*: 177b-78a). *Fei lao* (roughly synonymous with *hsu lao* 虚 勞 or *lao chai* 勞 瘵 in various sources) was only one of several groups of disorders characterized by chronic spitting of blood and feelings of consumption or "bone-steaming" (*ku cheng* 骨 蒸 ; ibid., *3*: 17a-4: 27b). From the modern viewpoint each of these groups includes pulmonary tuberculosis, various anemic and neurasthenic syndromes, and assorted diseases in which hemotypsis is a symptom. See also note 3, page 408.

[4] This statement is puzzling. The first symptoms would generally indicate angina pectoris (a modern category), of which the radiating pains are characteristic, if they do not indicate something

6.1.2.4. Abdominal pains

Pains in the upper abdomen accompanied by dry retching or spitting of clear saliva, becoming more severe on exposure to cold, are mostly the stomach system cold manifestation type. Distension and pain in the upper abdomen accompanied by malodorous belching and regurgitation of gastric acid is mostly Alimentary Stasis Disorders (5.5). Recurring pains around the navel, with a local mass appearing during painful periods, are mostly from roundworms [ascariasis]. Abdominal pains with fever; diarrhea with or without pus or blood in the stool; and tenesmus are mostly the moist hot repletion manifestation type (8.4.7).[5] Lingering abdominal pains with thin, decomposed stool, sensitivity to cold, and chilly extremities are mostly depletion manifestations of Cold Moist Disorder (*han shih* 寒 濕 [yang depletion and fluid stasis due to moist heteropathy in the stomach and associated visceral systems]).

Generally speaking, sudden pains are mostly the repletion manifestation type, and persistent pains mostly the depletion type. Distension and pain after eating is repletion, and lessening of pain after eating is depletion. Excruciating pains fixed in location, and increased pain or resistance to pressure when the place is pressed, is repletion; steady diffuse pain, lessening or temporarily relieved when the site is pressed, is depletion.

---

more serious. The text provides no guidance about differential diagnosis between traditional and modern entities. Presumably the reader is left to diagnose angina pectoris, with Localized Pain Disorder determined by a negative finding. That is not, to say the least, a traditional procedure. It is also incorrect by classical standards, since often chest Localized Pain Disorder and angina pectoris coincide in point of symptoms!

[5] The Chinese syndrome corresponding to tenesmus is *li chi hou chung* 里 急 後 重 , literally, "urgency within and heaviness in back." It combines rectal urgency, pain, ineffectual straining, and heavy sensation at the anal opening.

6.1.3. Diet

It is important to determine clearly the patient's appetite, food intake, dietary preferences, reactions after eating, and conditions in which the patient is thirsty.

6.1.3.1. Normal diet during illness shows that the *ch'i* of the stomach system has not been injured. Lack of desire to eat or drink combined with repeated belching means a stasis due to an Accumulation Disorder (*chi chih* 积 滞) in the stomach system. Increase in the amount eaten combined with a tendency toward hunger mostly indicates repletion Fire in the stomach system (note whether it is actually a manifestation of Wasting Thirst Disorders (*hsiao k'o* 消 渴 [diabetes mellitus, diabetes insipidus, and diseases with similar symptoms]).

6.1.3.2. Thirst with preference for cold drinks generally means that hot heteropathies in the stomach system have injured its yin *ch'i*. Thirst with preference for hot drinks generally means stomach system yang insufficiency. An insipid taste in the mouth unaccompanied by thirst may mean that an outer manifestation type has not yet passed to the inner aspect, or may indicate an inner manifestation type with yang depletion and preponderance of cold heteropathy. Dry mouth without desire to drink means splenetic system depletion with preponderance of moist heteropathy.

6.1.3.3. A bitter taste in the mouth indicates that there is a hot heteropathy in the hepatic or gall bladder system; an acid taste indicates a stasis due to an Accumulation Disorder in the stomach or intestine systems; a sweet taste developing in the mouth generally indicates that there is a Moist-hot Heteropathy Disorder (5.1.4.1.3) in the splenetic system; an insipid taste [with loss of taste sensation and appetite, *k'ou tan* 口 淡] mostly indicates the depletion manifestation type.

6.1.4. Elimination

It is important to determine clearly frequency and character of elimination, whether there is hemorrhaging, and so on.

6.1.4.1. Constipation or stool dry and difficult to pass, accompanied by fever, mostly belongs to the hot or repletion manifestation type. The constipation which accompanies persistent disorders, or which occurs in the period shortly after childbirth or in old age, mostly indicates *ch'i* depletion or dispersed body fluid loss.

6.1.4.2. Thin, decomposed stool not preceded by abdominal pains is mostly the depletion cold manifestation type in the splenetic or stomach system. Pre-dawn abdominal pains and loose bowels (called "fifth night-watch diarrhea," *wu ching hsieh* 五 更 泄) mostly indicate renal system yang depletion. Watery stool excreted in a gushing manner, accompanied by a burning sensation at the anal opening, means that there is a hot heteropathy in the stomach or intestinal systems. Sour, malodorous, thin, frothy stool, abdominal pains and diarrhea, with the pain abating after defecation, means alimentary stasis (5.5).

6.1.4.3. Pus or blood in the stool, tenesmus, abdominal pains and hot sensations is moist hot heteropathy diarrhea. Stool reddish-black, resembling dried glue or varnish, is mostly "distant blood" (*yuan hsueh* 远 血 [voiding blood after stool, so-called because the origin of the blood is distant from the anus]); blood of fresh red color in the stool is generally "proximate blood" (*chin hsueh* 近 血 [voiding blood before stool]). The location and cause of hemorrhage should be further clarified in either case.

6.1.4.4. Urine copious and clear mostly belongs to the depletion cold manifestation type. Clear urine frequently voided, even to the point of incontinence, is *ch'i* depletion. Urination brief and urine yellow belong to the hot manifestation type. If at the same time the urine is turbid, is voided painfully and is not excreted freely, it generally means Moist-hot Heteropathy Disorders.

6.1.4.5. Copious urination at night or bedwetting indicates renal system depletion. Repeated urination, excessive urge to urinate [urgent dysuria], and painful or difficult expulsion of urine, in some cases accompanied by blood or fine stones, are manifestations of Urinary Discomfort Disorders (*lin* 淋). Thirst, copious drinking and urination, and rapid emaciation are manifestations of Wasting Thirst Disorders. Sudden retention of urine, or inability to void except in drops, accompanied by extremely unpleasant odor of the urine, intense pain in the urinary bladder system, and hot sensations, is the repletion manifestation type. Gradual diminution in the quantity of urine even to the point of disappearance, with face pale and loins, thighs, hands and feet chilly, is the depletion manifestation type.

6.1.5. Sleep

6.1.5.1. Insomnia

It is necessary to understand whether it is a matter of difficulty in going to sleep or a tendency to be easily awakened, and also whether there is much dreaming, and so on. Difficulty in going to sleep at night, lessening of the appetite, fatigue and lack of vigor, regular throbbing of the heart, forgetfulness, and mental vagueness are associated with simultaneous depletion in the cardiac and splenetic systems, mostly brought on by excessive ratiocination. Depletion Agitation Disorder (5.1.6.2) accompanied by inability to sleep, intermittent hot sensations with nocturnal sweating, tongue red and saliva scanty, and pulse small and accelerated, mostly mean yin depletion. Simultaneous depletion of *ch'i* and blood after a major illness or in old people often leads to diminished sleep. Inability to sleep soundly at night, diminished sleep with a tendency to awaken, worry and mental upset, sores in the mouth and on the tongue, and reddening of the tip of the tongue mean cardiac Fire rising in excess (8.1.6). Insomnia and a tendency to dream, headache with a bitter taste in the mouth, and an agitated and irritable disposition are mostly hepatic Fire excess (8.2.2). Crying out in fright while dreaming mostly indicates gall bladder system *ch'i* depletion or stomach system hot heteropathy.

6.1.5.2. Excessive sleep

Fatigue of the mental faculties and extremities along with excessive sleep is *ch'i* depletion. Lassitude and sleepiness after meals is mostly splenetic system *ch'i* insufficiency. Excessive desire to sleep after illnesses indicates that the orthopathic *ch'i* has not yet recovered. Overweight, moderate pulse, and excessive sleep indicate preponderance of moist heteropathy.

6.1.6. Deafness and ringing in the ears

The relation between the renal, hepatic, and gall bladder systems and the ears is intimate. Sudden deafness mostly indicates repletion manifestation type with intense Fire in the hepatic or gall bladder system; persistent deafness is mostly renal depletion or *ch'i* depletion. The appearance of deafness in heat factor disorders is an indicative sign of injury to the yin aspect by hot heteropathy (9.2.2).

Ringing in the ears if accompanied by regular throbbing of the heart and dizziness mostly belongs to the depletion manifestation type; if accompanied by feelings of distress in the chest, pains in the rib region, bitter taste in the mouth, dry and hardened stool, and vomiting, it indicates the repletion manifestation type.

6.1.7. Women and children: special characteristics

For women and small children, in addition to the above inquiries the following subjects should be asked about:

6.1.7.1. It is necessary to determine clearly from female patients whether or not they have married, whether they have menstruated (including age of onset, period, character and amount of bleeding, whether the menses are painful, aroma and color of vaginal discharges, and so on), and circumstances of childbirth (number of pregnancies, whether there have been any difficult deliveries or miscarriages, and so on).

Early menses. Copious menses, thick and dark red, dry mouth, and reddened lips indicate hot heteropathy in the blood. Menses purple or blackish with clots mostly indicate the repletion hot manifestation type.

Delayed menses. Scanty menses, pink and thin, with faded yellow facial color, indicate blood depletion; if the extremities are chilly and the face white, the depletion cold manifestation type is indicated. If the menses are purplish, dark, and clotted, and if the lower abdomen is painful and the pain is aggravated by pressure, perhaps also with areas of swelling, it is *ch'i* stasis with blood coagulation.

Foul-smelling menses indicate the hot manifestation type; a rank smell indicates the cold manifestation type. White Band Disorder (*pai tai* 白帶) discharges [syndromes involving leukorrhea] that are clear, thin, and rank are depletion cold manifestation type.

Those yellow, thick, and foul-smelling are moist hot manifestations. Protracted bloody discharges after childbirth, accompanied by pain in the abdomen worsened by pressure, indicate blood coagulation [which prevents the termination of such discharges within a normal period of about three weeks].

6.1.7.2. It is necessary to determine clearly with respect to children the history of development and of previous illnesses; for instance how early the fontanelle closed, how early the patient walked and talked, whether preventative inoculations have been given, whether the patient has had measles and chickenpox, circumstances of breast feeding, and so on.

6.2. Visual Inspection

Through the visual inspection phase of physical examination one arrives, by way of scrutinizing general vitality (*shen* 神), facial appearance (*se* 色), body form (*hsing* 形), and body state (*t'ai* 態), at an understanding of the general situation. By looking at changes in the tongue one is further aided in determining the character of the disorder. For children aged under three *sui* [or about two years by Western reckoning] examination of finger veins (*chih wen* 指 紋) can provide supplementary information for diagnosis (6.2.3).

6.2.1. General situation

6.2.1.1. Animation, facial appearance

Listlessness, dull look in the eyes, dull facial expression, and complexion dark and dull indicate that there has been injury to the orthopathic *ch'i*. Face pale and dried-out or withered-looking with pale lips is generally blood depletion. Faded yellow complexion is mostly splenetic system depletion. Dark complexion accompanying long illness is mostly renal depletion. Recurrent flushes about the cheekbones and hot sensations in the afternoon are generally yin depletion and internal hot heteropathy. In small children, a greyish or bluish color developing in the face and about the lips is mostly hepatic wind heteropathy (5.1.1.2). In every sort of complexion modified by illness, the disorder is less serious if the complexion is light and lustrous, and more severe if it is dark and dull.

In Heat Factor Disorders and childhood Fright Wind Disorders (*ching feng* 惊 风 [convulsions or withdrawal as complications of certain acute or chronic illnesses]), unresponsive eye movement and occasional fixed gaze—whether fixed upward, straight ahead, or sideways—is usually due to internally stimulated hepatic wind heteropathy or to obstruction of circulation by mucus or hot heteropathy; this is one of the symptoms of Fright Wind Disorders. In childhood illnesses, crying without tears and dry nostrils that are without mucus are generally serious manifestations. A pale nose indicates *ch'i* and blood depletion and debilitation.

6.2.1.2. Body state, skin condition

Emaciated body, languid extremities, and skin dried out or withered-looking indicate *ch'i* and blood depletion and debilitation. Obesity of the depletion manifestation type with low food intake [i.e., mainly due to fluid retention] indicates depletion and debilitation of the medial *ch'i* (3.1.2); emaciation with large food intake means Fire heteropathy in the medial *chiao* (2.1.6).

Yellowing of the skin over the whole body as well as of the sclerae of the eyes is Yellow Jaundice Disorder (*huang tan* 黄 疸 [symptomatic jaundice]). A deep and vivid coloration like that of orange peel, accompanied by hot sensations, is Yang Jaundice Disorder (*yang huang* 阳 黄 , generally acute). Pale or dull yellow color as if smoked, with slight or no hot sensations, is Yin Jaundice Disorder (*yin huang* 阴 黄 , generally chronic).

Edema over the whole body: rapid onset, extremities and joints aching and heavy, sometimes accompanied by abnormal sensitivity to cold or aversion to wind, indicate occlusion of liquid *ch'i* (*shui ch'i* 水 气 [which forms edema]) within and invasion of wind heteropathy from without. Heavy feeling in the body accompanied by an exceptional degree of mental fatigue is the heavy sensation characteristic of moist heteropathy in the upper part of the body (*shih chung*, 6.1.2.1). Aching loins and cold extremities with greyish, dull complexion is renal system yang *ch'i* depletion. Edematous lower extremities, faded yellow complexion, poor appetite, distended abdomen, and thin, decomposed stool indicate splenetic system yang *ch'i* depletion.

Skin rashes mostly mean internal hot heteropathy, and in Heat Factor disorders are an important sign of hot heteropathy entering the blood sector (9.1.4). Rash of vivid red, lustrous color means a relatively mild condition; dark, dull color means a more serious condition.

6.2.1.3. Appendix: Inspection diagnosis of intestinal worms

There are ancient records of diagnosing intestinal worms by visual inspection. Not long ago there was a survey of over a thousand child victims of intestinal worm infection, which proved that this technique has a definite significance. The children often presented the following symptoms:

1. large red spots on the tongue, of even, round outline, protruding above the surface of the tongue like nipples, and varying in location and number;

2. granules in the mucous membrane of the lower lip, mainly ashen white, small convex spots as big as the head of a needle, from a few to a dozen or so;

3. blue spots in the sclerae of the eyes, triangular, round, or semicircular in shape, distributed among the tips of the capillary reticulations [which lead out of the arterioles to supply the cornea] but not protruding;

4. large white spots appearing on the face, generally round and comparatively even in outline with pale whitish centers, not protruding above the skin.

These four positive signs may appear singly or in combination; the spots on the tongue are most common. The number of signs is generally in direct proportion to the number of parasites in the belly. According to the survey statistics, the proportion of positive findings from inspection was higher than that from microscopic examination of feces (including the egg-collecting technique). The above method, which requires no equipment and is simple and convenient, is worth using.[6]

---

[6] Some of the symptoms noted suggest tissue reactions to dead encysted larvae of the pork tapeworm, *Taenia solium*. The wide utility claimed and the range of signs still await explanation.

6.2.2. Tongue inspection

Observation of the tongue is particularly detailed in Chinese medicine, since from it one can learn whether there is depletion or repletion of the visceral systems, preponderance or deficiency of the *ch'i* or blood, abundance or deficit of dispersed body fluids, and can also find out the character of external heteropathies. Thus to a certain extent it is helpful in determining the character, seriousness, and prognosis of the disorder. Whether the disorder is of the hot or cold manifestation type, and of the yin or yang depletion manifestation type, is relatively clearly reflected in tongue phenomena (including changes in the tongue tissue and tongue coating). On the basis of contemporary large-scale clinical experience, it has been observed that in the course of disorders changes in the tongue are rapid and clear, reflecting at an early stage and in a relatively objective way the character, seriousness, and changing trend of an illness.

6.2.2.1. Tongue tissues

"Tongue tissues" refers to the body of the tongue, which is closely associated, part by part, with the visceral systems. The tip of the tongue mainly reflects pathological changes in the cardiac and pulmonary systems; for instance, reddening of the tongue means flaming up of the cardiac Fire (5.1.6.1, 8.1.6). The sides mainly reflect pathological changes in the hepatic and gall bladder systems, as when large purplish spots indicate a stasis of the hepatic system (clinically one often observes certain liver disease patients with large virid or purplish spots on the sides of the tongue or engorged veins on its underside). The medical portion mainly reflects pathological changes in the splenetic and stomach systems, and the dorsal part those in the renal system.

The color, degree of moistening, form and state of the tongue are used to analyze its alterations.

1. Color and degree of moistening of the tongue

The normal tongue is pink and moist.

Stool examination allows identification of only 50 to 75 percent of infections. Hoeppli 1959 provides a trove of information on parasitic diseases in classical Chinese medicine.

A color paler than normal indicates blood depletion, yang depletion, or cold manifestation type. Pale color without a coating is mostly simultaneous *ch'i* and blood depletion. Pale color and good lubrication indicate cold heteropathy. This tongue coloration is also called "whitish tongue," which is to say that white is preponderant over red. It can be observed in nutritional deficiencies, anemia, and certain endocrine disorders such as myxedema.

Dry tongue of a vivid red color means yin depletion. Vivid red color without coating indicates yin depletion with intense Fire heteropathy. In the last stages of Warm Factor Disorder [chapter 9], pulmonary tuberculosis, hyperthyroidism, diabetes mellitus, and so on, yin depletion tongue can be observed. A crimson or deeper red color belongs to the repletion manifestation type; in general, the deeper the red the stronger the hot heteropathy. In relatively serious acute infectious illnesses or toxemic symptoms brought on by infections, red or deep red tongue may be observed.

A crimson tongue is an important sign that Heat Factor Disorders have been transmitted from the active *ch'i* sector to the constructive *ch'i* sector (9.1.3). When the deep red color is accompanied by a spiky growth [i.e., elongation of filiform papillae, "hairy" tongue], preponderance of hot heteropathy in the constructive *ch'i* sector is indicated. Crimson of a fresh hue indicates that hot heteropathy has injured the pericardial system. Crimson tongue may be observed among septic symptoms and in serious acute infections. If at the same time the tongue is bald, disappearance of stomach system yin *ch'i* is indicated—a serious condition.

Alteration of tongue color from crimson to purplish red, with the tongue dry, is an important sign that a Heat Factor Disorder has developed as far as the blood sector (9.1.4). When serious infections have developed to the point of respiratory and circulatory collapse, purple tongue may be observed. A purplish dull coloration is usually blood coagulation. Light purple, moist tongue mostly indicates cold manifestation type.

Blue tongue is a grave symptom of simultaneous *ch'i* and blood deficit. If at the same time the tongue is bald, the prognosis is not favorable. In respiratory and circulatory collapse, serious hypoxia may give rise to [cyanotic] blue tongue.

2. Physical form and state of the tongue

Mainly to be observed are whether the tongue is fat or thin, hard or soft, and dry or moist, as well as fissures and state of activity.

If the tongue is fat, soft, and pink, with impressions of the teeth in its sides, general depletion or cold manifestation type is indicated. Enlarged tongue may be seen in hypothyroidism, acromegaly, and so on. Tongue enlarged and deep red mostly indicates hot heteropathy in the cardiac or splenetic system. Emaciated, thin tongue crimson in color indicates that the dispersed body fluids have already been injured. Compact, coarse tongue usually is associated with the repletion or hot manifestation type. Spikes growing on the tongue indicate internal stasis due to congelation of hot heteropathy. The greater the size or number of the spikes, the greater the extent of congelation. In high fever, scarlet fever, and serious pheumonia symptoms, spiky tongue growths may be observed.

Fissures in the tongue mostly mean yin depletion or poor nutrition, but they are also seen accompanying high fever and dehydration. Certain fissues are congenital.

Pink tongue tremulous when protruded and withdrawn indicates *ch'i* insufficiency. This manifestation may be observed in neurasthenia and in general depletion during convalescence. Tremor with vivid red color is mostly yin depletion, and can be observed in "hepatic Wind stirring within" (*kan feng nei tung* 肝 风 内 动 [wind heteropathy disorders of internal origin, 8.2.2]), Wind Attack Disorders (3.5), hyperthyroidism, and so on.

Tongue deviating to one side when protruded is often seen in Wind Attack Disorders.

Stiff tongue, lacking flexibility and unresponsive in movement, causing unclear speech, is brought about by "hepatic Wind stirring within." It often occurs as a precursor, and sometimes as a sequela, of Wind Attack Disorders.

Flaccid, wasted tongue lacking strength can develop in a variety of circumstances. In a new illness, dry, red, and wasted tongue indicates that hot heteropathy preponderance has injured the yin aspect. In a drawn-out illness, whitish, wasted tongue means simultaneous *ch'i* and blood depletion. Crimson, wasted tongue indicates that the yin deficit is already extreme.

6.2.2.2. Tongue coating

The normal tongue coating is formed by the *ch'i* of the stomach system; it is thin, whitish, lustrous, and moist. In illness it may undergo all sorts of alteration. For diagnosis the most important observations have to do with color, fluids, thickness, and so on. One must take care to reject specious phenomena, since a number of foods and medicinal substances may change the color of the tongue coating, e.g., blackening of the tongue's surface from eating Chinese olives (*kan-lan* 橄 欖 [Carnarium album]) or smoked, dried plums (*wu mei* 烏 梅).

1. Whitish coating

Mostly belongs to cold or depletion manifestation type (although sometimes the type is hot or repletion). Thin, white and smooth coating means wind or cold heteropathy of external origin. A soft, white, smooth coating which can be scraped clean indicates inner depletion cold manifestation type. White, smooth, and unctuous means phlegm associated with stasis of moisture (*t'an shih* 痰 濕).[7] White like a thick layer of flour indicates a Warm Factor Epidemic Disorder (*wen i* 瘟 疫, 5.2, 9.1). If in hot heteropathy disorders yellow is intermixed with the white of the tongue coating, the heteropathy has changed to hot and has passed from the outer to the inner aspect; this indicates the development of the condition.

2. Yellow [including brownish] coating

Belongs to the hot manifestation type, the strength of which increases with the depth of the yellow coloration. A slightly yellowish, thin coating means wind-hot heteropathy of external origin. The yellow coating thick and dry means stomach system hot heteropathy has injured the dispersed body fluids. Thick and unctuous coating indicates splenetic or stomach system moist-hot heteropathy, or clogging in the stomach or intestine systems. Yellow coloration pale and moist, sometimes also thick, is "dirty coating" (*cho t'ai* 濁 苔) mainly brought about by moist heteropathy stasis.

3. Black coating

Mostly belongs to the inner manifestation type, and generally indicates that a condition is serious. Hot and cold types are distinguished. Black, smooth coating on a vivid red tongue indicates that Fire or hot heteropathy has damaged the yin aspect. Parched black tongue coating indicates preponderance of Fire with drying up of the dispersed body fluids. Parched, cracked black coating with protrud-

---

[7] "T'an shih" is also written "shih t'an," and is equivalent to the self-explanatory "t'an-yin shih cho nei t'ing 痰 飲 濕 濁 內 停" in table 6.1, item 6. On *t'an-yin*, excretory mucus or phlegm, see section 3.5.

ing spiky growths indicates near-exhaustion of the renal Water (2.1.5.1.4), a critical condition.

4. Disappearance of a thick coating, with the surface of the tongue becoming smooth as a mirror or with a portion of the coating peeled off, means deficit of dispersed body fluids, with yin depletion and Water dried up; these are indications of a serious condition. In case of the white or slightly yellowish thin coating observed in pernicious anemia patients and in stomach and intestine system moist-hot heteropathy or parasites in children, a portion may peel off. The cause of this peeling is local atrophy of mucous membrane proceeding to the point of destruction.

Generally speaking, a whitish coating turning yellow and the yellow fur receding with the growth of a new thin, whitish coating is a manifestation of a normal course (*shun cheng* 顺 证). A whitish coating turning ashen gray and then black is a manifestation of an abnormal course (*ni cheng* 逆 证). Sudden recession or dissolution of a tongue coating is also a sign of deteriorating condition.

6.2.2.3. Conclusions

This separate discussion of tongue tissue phenomena and coating phenomena is merely an expedient. Body and coating must be observed in conjunction, since their alterations are related in complicated ways. Combining tongue tissue and coating changes, generally their relation to manifestation type is:

Hot: tongue always red, coating always yellow and dry.
Cold: tongue always pale, coating always well supplied with saliva and smooth.
Repletion: tongue always hard.
Depletion: tongue always enlarged and soft.
Outer: coating usually thin, whitish, not dried out.
Hot heteropathy transmitted from outer aspect to inner: coating turning from whitish to yellow, thin to thick, moist to dry.

Considering separately the significance of tongue and coating, generally when investigating the energetic state—depletion or repletion—of the visceral systems, the center of attention is the tongue tissues. When investigating the depth of the heteropathy and determining the presence or absence of *ch'i* needed for digestion (*wei ch'i*

胃 气) the center of attention is the tongue coating. *Ch'i* disorders are mainly manifested in coating alterations, and blood disorders mainly in tongue tissue changes.

For the reader's convenience in mastering tongue examination, in table 6.1 common tongue and coating changes are combined for the purpose of manifestation type determination.

6.2.2.4. Appendix: Some modern studies of tongue diagnosis

[Omitted from translation.][8]

6.2.3. Finger veins of small children

"Finger veins" are the small superficial veins on the palmar radial side of the index fingers. The skin of an infant is soft and thin, and the veins are likely to be exposed, so that the finger veins are comparatively easy to see. With age, as the skin thickens, they gradually become indistinct. These veins to a certain extent reflect the character and severity of pathological changes. Because in small children the blood vessels are short and small in diameter [which makes palpation difficult] and because the frequent crying of children during physical examinations can affect the veracity of pulse phenomena, in pediatric practice with children under three *sui* [about two years], visual inspection of finger veins is often used to supplement palpation.

---

[8] This section is neither up to date nor informative. Generally speaking, except for a few well-known changes in color and furring of the tongue connected with particular disorders such as the "magenta cobblestone tongue" of riboflavin deficiency, examination of the tongue's surface no longer plays an important part in modern diagnosis. For accounts comparable with that given in this section the reader is referred to the major symptomatically oriented handbooks of clinical medicine of the late nineteenth and early twentieth century (for instance, Savill's *A System of Clinical Medicine*, *s.v.* through many editions) or the substantial discussion in De Gowin and De Gowin's recent but old-fashioned *Bedside Diagnostic Examination* (first published 1965; 1981: 156–66).

Table 6.1
Determination of Manifestation Types from Commonly Observed Tongue Phenomena

Tongue Body	Tongue Coating	Manifestation Type
Whitish (i.e., white pre-ponderant over pink)	White, very thin	*Ch'i* and blood depletion and debilitation
Whitish, thick, soft, tooth marks in sides	Thin, white	Yang depletion
Whitish, thick, soft	Gray or black, moist, smooth and lustrous	Yang deficiency with cold heteropathy in visceral systems; phlegm associated with moisture stasis
Pink, tender, fissured	None	*Ch'i* depletion, yin deficit
Pink	White, thin, moist	Wind-cold heteropathy of external origin
Pink	White, thick, unctuous	Phlegm and moist heteropathy stopped up, or food not assimilated
Pink	White, thick, floury	Warm Factor Epidemic Disorder or internal abscess
Pink	White with faint yellow	Heteropathy about to transfer from outer to inner aspect
Pink	Medial and dorsal yellow, thick; sides thin, white, moist	Outer heteropathy transferred to inner aspect, accumulated hot heteropathy in stomach and intestine systems
Vivid red	White, extremely thin	Yin depletion, Fire intense
Red, fissures plentiful and deep	Hardly any coating	Water not reinforcing Fire (1.2.2) or deficit of true yin *ch'i* (3.1.1)
Red	Yellow, thin	Hot heteropathy preponderant in active *ch'i* sector (9.1.2) or established in stomach or intestine system
Red	Yellow, unctuous	Moist-hot heteropathy passed into active *ch'i* sector
Red	Yellow, thick, dry	Hot heteropathy penetrated deeply, con-gealed in inner aspect
Red	Black, dry	Injury to yin from Fire or hot heteropathy
Orange-red	Scorched yellow	Hot heteropathy passed from active *ch'i* sec-tor into constructive *ch'i* sector
Orange-red, purple	Deep yellow or yellowish white, dry, little or no coating	Hot heteropathy passed into blood sector
Greyish, purple	White, moist	Internal cold heteropathy extremely serious, *ch'i* and blood congealed

The main points in examination are the color and fullness of the vein. The child's fingers are made to face the light, and the doctor holds the tip of the child's index finger between his or her own left thumb and index finger. With the thumb of his right hand he very lightly presses longitudinally from the fingertip to the metacarpophalangeal joint [i.e., toward the hand] several times to make the vein more apparent, and then observes it.

The index finger is divided into three "passes"; the first joint [i.e., proximal phalanx] is called the "Wind Pass" (feng kuan 风 关), the second the "Ch'i Pass" (ch'i kuan 气 关), and the third the "Life Pass" (ming kuan 命 关; cf. 6.4.1; figure 4).

The normal finger vein is a pale but vivid purple, and generally does not extend beyond the Wind Pass. In medical disorders, changes occur in both the fullness and color of the finger veins. Cases in which the vein is exceptionally apparent mostly belong to the outer manifestation type; those in which it is submerged, to the inner. Pale color is mostly depletion or cold manifestation type; purple or red, hot manifestation type. Virid color is mostly Wind-cold Heteropathy Disorders or Fright Wind Disorders, or sometimes a manifestation of pain, Dietary Damage Disorders (shang shih 伤 食 [including stomach catarrh, symptoms from overeating, and so on]), or backflow of mucus and ch'i (t'an ch'i shang ni 痰 气 上 逆). Black color is mostly blood coagulation. A stagnation in the finger vein, in which when it is pushed longitudinally the blood does not flow freely, is usually phlegm associated with stasis of moisture, Alimentary Stasis Disorders (5.5), static congelation of heteropathic hot factors, or some other repletion manifestation type.

From the point of view of location, when the vein is visible in the Wind Pass, the condition is comparatively mild and superficial. If the vein extends through the Ch'i Pass the condition is more serious. Extension through the Life Pass to the fingertip is called "penetrating the pass and piercing the armor."[9] The condition is usually critical.

To simplify, the main points in manifestation type determination by vein inspection are: floating or submerged to distinguish outer from inner; red and purple to distinguish cold from hot; thin or thick [blood] to determine depletion or repletion; and the Three Passes to measure seriousness of the disorder.

---

[9] This is a pun; "chia 甲 " means both "fingernail" and "armor."

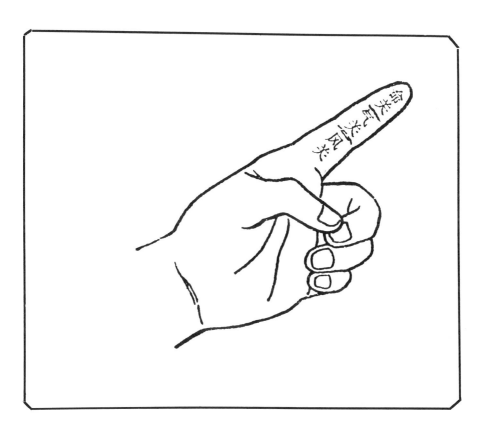

Figure 4

Locations of the Three Passes in the
Finger Veins of Small Children.

The Life Pass is nearest the fingertip.

6.2.3.1. Appendix: Some modern studies of the finger veins

The general belief is that changes in the fullness of the finger vein are chiefly related to alterations in venous blood pressure. In most cases of children with heart failure or pneumonia one can see the finger vein extended toward the Life Pass; this is brought about by a rise in venous blood pressure. The greater the venous pressure, the greater the fullness of the finger vein and the greater its extension in the direction of the fingertip. To a certain extent the color of the finger vein can reflect the extent of hypoxia; the more serious the hypoxia, the greater the amount of reduced hemoglobin in the blood, and the more apparent a virid or purple coloration of the finger vein. For this reason, most children suffering from pneumonia and heart failure present virid-purple or purple finger veins. In anemic patients, because of the decrease in red corpuscles and hemoglobin, the finger vein turns pale.

6.3. Auditory and Olfactory Examination

6.3.1. Auditory Examination

This includes listening to the patient's speech, breathing, coughing, hiccupping, and so on. Weak or jerky voice and shortness of breath shown in drawling or slurring speech generally belong to the depletion or cold manifestation type, and loud and powerful voice or agitated talkativeness, to the repletion or hot manifestation type. Sudden hoarseness usually means the repletion manifestation type, and is brought on by wind-cold heteropathy or phlegm; gradual hoarseness is usually the depletion manifestation type, reflecting loss of function of the pulmonary system and drying up of its fluid (*chin* 津).

Short, hurried, and weak breaths with a feeling of relief after inhalation is mostly the depletion manifestation type; coarse breathing with a feeling of relief after exhalation is mostly the repletion or hot manifestation type. The jerky coarse breathing seen in the last stages of chronic pulmonary or renal system disorders is not repletion but depletion manifestation type; the weak respiration observed when hot heteropathy has entered the Cardiac Envelope Junction system (2.1.1.1.5) and the mind is beclouded is not depletion but repletion manifestation type.

If the sound of coughing lacks strength, it is depletion of the pulmonary system's *ch'i*. If it is heavy and mucous and the excretory phlegm is white, it generally is associated with wind-cold heteropathy of external origin. If the sound is clear and resonant and the phlegm is difficult to expel, it is usually pulmonary hot heteropathy. If the coughing occurs in spasms and is vigorous, it is generally the pulmonary repletion manifestation type.

If the sound of hiccupping is strong and vigorous and the pulse smooth and full, it is mostly "repletion hiccup" (*shih o* 实 呃). If loud, short, labored, and accompanied by thirst, and the pulse is accelerated, it is usually "hot heteropathy hiccup" (*je o* 热 呃). If the sound is weak and the pulse lacks vigor, and symptoms of the depletion manifestation type are observed, it is "depletion hiccup" (*hsu o* 虚 呃). In serious or chronic disorders, sudden appearance of hiccupping is a grave sign.

6.3.2. Olfactory examination

Involves examining the odors of the body, oral cavity, and various excretions.

Body odor. In certain illnesses the patient has a special smell. For instance, ulcerating body sores give out a putrid odor. In the critical stage of Warm Factor Epidemic Disorders and pulmonary or renal system disorders there is often a peculiar odor.

Mouth odor. A foul smell usually is associated with hot heteropathy in the pulmonary or stomach system; a sour stench is generally Overnight Food Accumulation Disorder (*su shih* 宿 食 [stasis of alimentary matter, indigestion, etc.]) in the stomach system. Rank-smelling phlegm means pulmonary system hot heteropathy; strong odor and purulent appearance indicate Pulmonary System Abscess Disorders (6.1.2.3).

Excreta and menses have been remarked upon in section 6.1.1; further discussion is omitted here.

6.4. Palpation

Palpation includes the reading of the pulse and tactile examination of the extremities and trunk.

6.4.1. Pulse palpation

The Chinese physician's discrimination of pulse phenomena is extraordinarily detailed; generally twenty-eight types are noted. These form an important aspect of clinical examination.

6.4.1.1. Method of pulse palpation

Pulse palpation is usually performed at the place where the radial artery pulse beats on the palmar side of the wrist joint, called the "Inch-mouth vessel" (ts'un k'ou mai 寸 口 脈). This segment is further divided into three sections, called the "Inch Section" (ts'un pu 寸 部), "Pass Section" (kuan pu 关 部), and "Foot Section" (ch'ih pu 尺 部). The Pass Section corresponds to the level of the styloid process of the radius, with the Foot and Inch Sections above and below (figure 5). Before palpation the patient's body should be in a comfortable position, and his mind at rest. If the patient has just performed any strenuous activity, he should rest briefly before palpation. His lower arm should be stretched horizontally, with the palm at rest facing upward. The doctor first places the tip of his middle finger on the Pass Section, and then the index finger on the Inch Section and the ring finger on the Foot Section. Generally the three fingers remain together, although if the patient is unusually tall they may be separated.

In children the Inch-mouth Tract is so short that the three sections must be examined with one finger. When examining children under eight sui [about seven years], the thumb may be placed on the Pass Section and rolled to the right and left to read the Inch and Foot Sections. For children over eight sui the thumb may be shifted to read the three sections.

Readings must be taken at different finger pressures. Light contact is called the "floating reading" (fu ch'ü 浮 取 , or "lifting," chü 举); a small amount of pressure is called "median reading" (chung ch'ü 中 取); and firm pressure is called the "sunken reading" (ch'en ch'ü 沉 取 , or "pressing," an 按). Sometimes in order to feel the pulse clearly it is also necessary to search by shifting the finger (called "searching," hsun 寻).

The three sections of the pulse can give separate determinations of symptoms in the various visceral systems; in this respect there are differences between the pulses on the left and right wrists. On the left wrist the Inch Section is examined for cardiac system in-

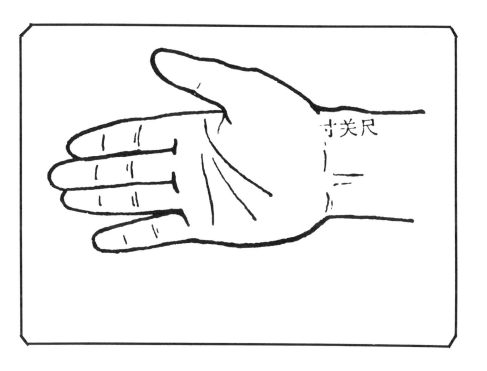

Figure 5

Locations of the Three Sections of the Radial Pulse.
The Inch Section is nearest the hand.

dications, the Pass Section for the hepatic system, and the Foot Section for the renal system. On the right side the Inch Section is read for the pulmonary system, the Pass Section for the splenetic system, and the Foot Section for the renal Gate of Life (the division between renal system and Gate of Life is used only in pulse examination; 2.1.5.1.4).

6.4.1.2. Special features of pulse phenomena and disorders determined by them; moderate pulse

The pulse phenomena observed with relative frequency in Chinese medicine are introduced below [cf. P30]. They vary as to depth of the pulse and rate, rhythm, strength, amplitude, and configuration of the beat. The normal pulse beats on the average four to five times per respiration (corresponding generally to 72–80 beats per minute), and is neither floating or sunken nor large or small, but rather is equable; it is called the "moderate pulse" (huan mai 缓 脉). This pulse is also observed when the ch'i and blood are constrained by moist heteropathy. It is also believed by some that a moderate pulse as a combination of floating, sunken, large, and small pulses may be an abnormal pulse.

6.4.1.2.1. Floating and sunken pulses. Special features: The floating (fu 浮) and sunken (ch'en 沉) pulses are opposites with respect to depth. The location of the floating pulse is high; on light contact the sensation is clear, but the beat is felt more weakly under slightly greater pressure. The sunken pulse is lower; on light contact the pulse is imperceptible. With light pressure it remains indistinct. Heavy pressure is required to feel it clearly (figure 6).[10]

Disorders determined by the floating pulse. Outer manifestation type. Vigorous and floating pulse is outer repletion type; floating pulse without strength is outer depletion type. If the pulse is floating and tense in a disorder of external origin, accompanied by hot sensations and aversion to cold but without perspiration, the manifestation type is outer cold repletion. If the disorder is of ex-

---

[10] The method by which these sphygmograms was obtained is not explained. I do not believe most highly qualified traditional physicians would agree that all the canonical pulses can be identified from mechanical traces.

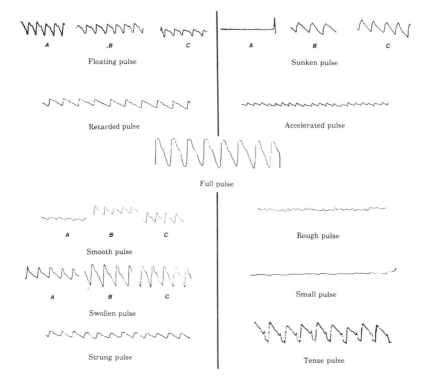

Figure 6
Sphygmograms Showing Pulse Characteristics

A = floating reading; *B* = median reading; *C* = sunken reading.

ternal origin with hot sensations and perspiration, aversion to wind, and floating and weak pulse, the manifestation type is outer cold depletion. But in patients with debilitated constitutions, when the disorder is of external origin the pulse is not ordinarily floating. In the first stages of acute infectious disorders the floating pulse is often observed.

Disorders determined by the sunken pulse. Inner manifestation type. Vigorous sunken pulse is inner repletion manifestation type; sunken pulse without strength is inner depletion type. Coughing without strength, excretory mucus thin and white, breath short, face white, appetite small, fatigue, and pulse sunken and weak indicate pulmonary system *ch'i* depletion, which belongs to the inner depletion manifestation type.

6.4.1.2.2. Retarded and accelerated pulses. Special features: The retarded (*ch'ih* 迟) and accelerated (*shuo* 数) pulses are opposites with respect to rate. The retarded pulse beats three times per respiration (corresponding to sixty or fewer beats per minute); the accelerated pulse, five times or more (corresponding to ninety or more beats per minute).[11]

---

[11] In the early classics pulse types and pulse rates—the latter counted against the physician's respirations—were on the whole independent, and probably originally represented different traditions of diagnosis. They were first combined mainly for prognosis, not for diagnosis, as in the *Mai ching* 脉 经 (ca. 280), *4* (5): 14a, *4* (6): 20a, *5* (3): 4b-5a (IV, 2629–43, 2666–67), *et passim*. They were combined for diagnosis in many latter works, including the most widely used source from the Ch'ing period on, *Pin-hu mai hsueh* 瀕 湖 脉 學 (1564). Li differs fundamentally in some respects from the *Mai ching* and from the other late classical authority on the pulse, *Ching-yueh ch'uan shu*, *5*: 88a-88b. Nan-ching Chung-i hsueh-yuan 南京中医学院 ed. 1958: 185, the first of the great textbooks for schools of traditional medicine, followed Li's book, pages 2–3, in defining the retarded pulse as three beats and the accelerated pulse as six beats per respiration.

The *Revised Outline* here departs from this standard, as do other textbooks after 1972. See, for instance, Nan-ching Chung-i hsueh-yuan ed. 1983: 56. The wording of the definition varies from one book to another. The latter characterizes the *shuo* pulse

Disorders determined by the retarded pulse. Cold manifestation type. Floating and retarded pulse is outer cold type; sunken and retarded pulse is inner cold type. Retarded and vigorous pulse is the repletion type with accumulated cold heteropathy; without strength it is the depletion cold type. For instance, aching loins and weak legs; predawn abdominal pain and loose bowels; tongue pale and moist; and pulse sunken, retarded and without strength indicate renal system yang depletion, which belongs to the inner depletion manifestation type.

Disorders determined by the accelerated pulse. Hot manifestation type. Accelerated and vigorous pulse means yang preponderance; accelerated and small or weak pulse means yin depletion with internal hot heteropathy. Flushed face, dry throat, mental upset accompanied by hot sensations in the heart [region], and pulse accelerated and vigorous indicate intense Fire heteropathy in the cardiac system, a condition that belongs to the yang preponderance manifestation type. Erosions in the mouth, swollen gums, and indigestion, with pulse small and accelerated, indicate stomach system yin depletion or "depletion Fire flaming up" (*hsu huo shang yen* 虚 火 上 炎), and belong to the depletion hot manifestation type.

6.4.1.2.3.   Empty and full pulses. Special features: The empty (*hsu* 虚) and full (*shih* 实) pulses are opposites with respect to the strength of the pulse beat.[12] In the empty pulse there is no strength in either the floating, median, or sunken reading, only an empty and flaccid response to pressure. The full pulse is vigorous on all three readings.

Disorders determined by the empty pulse. Simultaneous depletion of ch'i and blood. Floating and empty pulse indicates Heat Heteropathy Damage Disorders (5.1.3).

---

as "pulse rate accelerated, five times or more per respiration (more than ninety times per minute)." Only the latter clause does not vary. The obvious conclusion is that from the *Revised Outline* on, the standard shifted from the doctor's breathing to his watch.

[12] "Hsu" and "shih" are used for *ch'i* and blood "depletion" and "repletion" in section 7.3 and elsewhere. Here the translation must differ since the terms refer to the sensation directly felt by the diagnostician.

Disorders determined by the full pulse. Repletion manifestation type. Hot sensations of great intensity, manic agitation, constipation, and so on can bring on the full pulse. Full, smooth pulse indicates congelation of persistent phlegm; full, taut pulse means static congelation of the hepatic *ch'i.*

6.4.1.2.4.   Smooth and rough pulses. Special features: The smooth (*hua* 滑) and rough (*se* 澀) pulses are opposites with respect to configuration of flow. The travel of the smooth pulse is fluid, with a smooth sensation under the finger. The travel of the rough pulse is harsh, not following through either in coming or going. Electrocardiograms in cases of rough pulse show bundle branch block, and pulse diagrams also have a characteristic unevenness of wave amplitude.[13]

Disorders determined by the smooth pulse. Phlegmatic moist heteropathy, Overnight Food Disorder. Heavy and mucous cough; phlegm excessive, white, and easily expectorated; feelings of distress in the chest and diminished appetite; tongue coating white and unctuous; and smooth pulse are phlegmatic moist heteropathy cough. In pregnancy the smooth pulse is also often observed.

Disorders determined by the rough pulse. Decrease of blood, *ch'i* stasis, blood coagulation, and so on. For example, anemia, Wind Attack Disorders, hemiplegia, or coronary heart disease may manifest the rough pulse.

6.4.1.2.5.   Swollen and small pulses. Special features: The swollen (*hung* 洪) and small (*hsi* 細) pulses are opposites with respect to both amplitude and configuration. The form of the swollen pulse is large and its onset full, like the onrush of a flood; it is clearly felt in the floating reading. The small pulse is fine as a thread and its onset is not full. It is clearly felt under the finger when heavy pressure is applied.

Disorders determined by the swollen pulse. Hot heteropathy preponderance. For instance, preponderance of hot heteropathy in the active *ch'i* sector in Heat Factor Disorders (9.1.2) produces intense hot sensations, intense thirst, copious perspiration, swollen [or?] large pulse, and other symptoms. In cases of injury to the yin aspect by preponderance of hot heteropathy, with yin depletion bringing on rising yang *ch'i* (*yin hsu yü nei, yang fu yü wai* 阴 虚

---

[13] Note in figure 6 how the smooth pulse varies with pressure.

于 内 阳 浮 于 外　　　[indicated by headache, intermittently flushed cheeks, toothache, and other symptoms concentrated in the head]), the swollen pulse may also be observed. There is often a swollen pulse in the most critical period of infectious diseases.

Disorders determined by the small pulse. Mainly depletion manifestation type. In every variety of Depletion and Wasting Disorder (*hsu lao* 虚 劳 or *hsu sun* 虚 损), the small pulse may be observed.[14] It may also be seen when moist *ch'i* pours downward and moist heteropathy deters the flow in the circulation tracts (5.1.4); but that is repletion, not depletion, manifestation type. For example, pale complexion, whitish lips and tongue, dizziness accompanied by disturbances of vision, regular throbbing of the heart accompanied by languor, and small pulse are blood depletion. Feces of purulent appearance; mental exhaustion; diminished diet; abdominal distension; lack of warmth in the extremities; and mainly taut, small, and moderate pulse is cold-moist heteropathy dysentery (*han shih li chi* 寒 湿 痢 疾), which belongs to the repletion manifestation type.[15]

6.4.1.2.6. Strung and tense pulses. Special features: It is a common characteristic of the strung (*hsuan* 弦) and tense (*chin* 紧) pulses that the pulse waves for the Inch, Pass, and Foot Sections form a single impulse, so that the sensation under the three fingers is like that of a stretched cord. They differ in that the strung pulse feels like pressing on a zither (*ch'in* 琴) string, while the tense pulse feels like pressing on a taut rope, which vigorously resists the fingers. The strung pulse lacks this tightly stretched character, and its wave form is smaller.

Disorders determined by the strung pulse. Pain manifestations, wind manifestations, malaria, excretory mucus. In yin depletion and yang excess the strung pulse is often observed. For instance, in the hepatic system yang excess type of high blood pressure the pulse is mostly strung and vigorous; in the hepatic system yin in-

---

[14] This is a very broad group of disorders. *Chu ping yuan hou lun,* chapters 3–4, gives 75 varieties listed under *hsu lao.*

[15] "*Han shih li chi*" appears to be half a traditional term and half modern (see the next note). The classical *li* is not precisely dysentery, defined by inflammation of the intestinal membrane, but a group of symptoms corresponding to diarrhea with passage of foreign matter, not restricted to mucus and blood.

sufficiency type the pulse is generally strung and small.[16] In hepatic and stomach system disharmony (the manifestations of which are stomach pain extending to the rib region, belching, and irritability) the pulse is mostly strung. In hepatic system disorders, duodenal ulcer, gall bladder inflammations, irregular menstruation, uterine cervical cancers, renal system complaints, and so on, the strung pulse is commonly observed.

Disorders determined by the tense pulse. Cold and pain manifestations. In cases of wind-cold heteropathy of external origin the pulse is floating and tense; in inner cold manifestation type it is sunken and tense. An example [of the latter] is Cold Heteropathy Localized Pain Disorder (5.1.2.1), in which intense pain is felt in the joints of the extremities, the site of the pain does not shift, and the pain diminishes upon application of heat; the pulse is mostly strung or tense. In hardening of the arteries the tense pulse may also be observed.

6.4.1.2.7. Other pulse phenomena. The twelve pulse phenomena described above are often clinically observed. Several types sometimes seen in clinical practice are introduced below (others seldom observed are omitted).

1. Hurried, hesitant, and intermittent pulses.

These three pulse phenomena are all manifested as uneven rhythms with pauses.

Hurried (*ts'u* 促) pulse: pulse accelerated with irregular pauses. Determines repletion hot manifestation type, *ch'i* stasis, and blood coagulation.

Hesitant (*chieh* 結) pulse: pulse moderate with irregular pauses. Determines yin preponderance with *ch'i* congelation, and cold heteropathy mucus with coagulated blood.

Intermittent (*tai* 代) pulse: pulse normal with regular pauses; onset of pulse after the pause slightly retarded.[17] Indicates debility

---

[16] High blood pressure is a condition in modern medicine only; these two disorders are definitely mixed in character. Note that the basic finding is high blood pressure and that traditional manifestation types are used to distinguish two types. Modern diseases are frequent in this book's discussions of diagnosis.

[17] Regular intermittences in the pulse were used in the early classics to indicate directly how many of the visceral systems were being adequately supplied with *ch'i*. See TS, *14* (5): 265 = LS, *2*

of visceral system *ch'i*, fearfulness, and injury from falls. This pulse may also be observed after copious vomiting or diarrhea, and after childbirth.

These three pulses may also be seen in all sorts of heart disorders, such as rheumatic or coronary heart disease.

2. *Soft pulse*

Floating, small, and soft. Like cotton floss in water, it may be found by pressing lightly, but is lost under heavy pressure. The soft (*ju* 濡) pulse determines moist heteropathy and the depletion manifestation type, and may thus be observed in edema, *ch'i* and blood depletion and debility, and so on.

3. *Weak pulse*

Sunken, small, and soft. The weak (*jo* 弱) pulse indicates *ch'i* and blood insufficiency.

4. *Subtle pulse*

Extremely small and soft. It is difficult to be sure of its presence, and its rise and fall are indistinct. The subtle (*wei* 微) pulse determines extreme depletion. In prolonged disorders this pulse is a grave sign.

5. *Large pulse*

The wave form is larger than normal, but lacks the onrush configuration of the swollen pulse. Indicates preponderance of heteropathy. Large (*ta* 大) pulse lacking strength is the depletion manifestation type.

6. *Hollow pulse*

Floating, large, but hollow—with sides but no center, like pressing on the stem of a scallion. Indicates considerable loss of blood. The hollow (*k'ou* 扎 , literally, "scallion-stalk") pulse is often observed in victims of aplastic anemia.

---

(5): 15 and *Nan ching*, problem 11. From *Nan ching* (probably 2d century A.D.) on, the word *tai*, "intermittence," was generally replaced by *chih* 止 , "pause," in discussions of this technique.

6.4.1.3. Conclusion

The three components of the healthy pulse are equable beat, neither floating nor sunken; strength within calm onset of the beat; and sunken reading distinct.[18]

Combinations of pulse phenomena are clinically more common than simple phenomena. The disorders they determine are combinations of their individual correlations. In some disorders a pulse will appear singly and only in one section, as when in headache the floating pulse may be observed alone in the Inch Section, while the other sections remain normal.

Use of the pulse in diagnosis depends on identifying divergences from the healthy pulse. It is necessary to keep in mind that the latter varies considerably with age, sex, physical condition, and body weight. In old people the anatomical location of the radial artery may shift considerably.

There is a general correlation of pulses with manifestation types—floating pulse with outer type, sunken with inner, accelerated with hot, retarded with cold, vigorous pulses with repletion, and pulses lacking strength with depletion. In a small number of cases pulse and symptomatic manifestations do not correspond,

---

[18] This is a summary of the more diffuse conclusion in the original, which I have supplemented with table 6.2. The second member of each yin-yang pair is marked with a plus sign. This table additionally provides manifestation types listed in Li Shih-chen's annotations to his *Pin-hu mai hsueh*, pages 1–16. Comparison indicates the extent to which the discussion in the *Revised Outline* diverges from classical doctrine (full forms of the Chinese names for the pulses are given, where they differ from the simplified forms, for convenience in referring to the sixteenth-century work). I have also listed for comparison the translations of pulse designations given in Porkert 1983, pages 210–24. The Latin names (which are Porkert's standards) differ to some extent from the summary list in P30–31 (1974). I differ from Porkert mostly in the interest of more colloquial English and to some extent for the sake of more indicative and less literal translations. His Latin translations are generally excellent. Xie Zhufan and Huang Xiaokai ed. 1984: 72–76 give an exceptionally comprehensive list of pulse types, but the English translations are often imprecise.

Table 6.2
Pulse Types in the Revised Outline and Other Sources

Type Above	Manifestation Type Above	Manifestation Type in Pin hu mai hsueh	Translation in Porkert
Moderate (*huan*)	Normal or moist heteropathy	Yin, defensive *ch'i* preponderance†	Languid, *pulsus languidus*
Floating (*fu*)	Outer	Yang, outer	Superficial, *pulsus superficialis*
+Sunken (*ch'en* 沉)	Inner	Yin, inner	Submerged, *pulsus mersus*
Retarded (*ch'ih* 迟)	Cold	Yin, cold	Slowed-down, *pulsus tardus*
+Accelerated (*shuo* 数)	Hot	Yang, hot	Accelerated, *pulsus celer*
Empty (*hsu* 虚)	Depletion	Yin, depletion, inner	Exhausted, *pulsus inanis*
+Full (*shih* 实)	Repletion	Yang, repletion	Replete, *pulsus repletus*
Smooth (*hua* 滑)	Moist	Yin within yang, yin *ch'i* or *hsueh* preponderance	Slippery, *pulsus lubricus*
+Rough (*se* 涩)	Stasis	Yin, *hsueh* or *ching* depletion	Grating, *pulsus asper*
Swollen (*hung*)	Repletion	Yang, yang preponderance, yin depletion	Flooding, *pulsus exundans*
+Small (*hsi*)	Depletion	Yin, depletion	Minute, *pulsus minutus*
Strung (*hsuan*)	Yin depletion, yang excess	Yin within yang, varied	Stringy, *pulsus chordalis*
Tense (*chin*)	Cold	Yang, cold	Tense, *pulsus intentus*
Hurried (*ts'u*)	Repletion hot	Yang, yang preponderance	Agitated, *pulsus agitatus*
Hesitant (*chieh*)	Yin preponderance	Yin, yin preponderance	Adherent, *pulsus haesitans*
Intermittent (*tai*)	*Ch'i* debility	Yin, debility	Intermittent, *pulsus intermittens*
Soft (*ju*)	Moist, depletion	Yin, *hsueh* depletion	Frail, *pulsus lenis*‡
Weak (*jo*)	*Ch'i* and blood insufficiency	Yin, *ch'i* depletion	Infirm, *pulsus invalidus*
Subtle (*wei*)	Depletion	Yin, prolonged depletion	Evanescent, *pulsus evanescens*
Hollow (*k'ou*)	Blood loss	Yang, stasis or *hsueh* loss	Onion-stalk, *pulsus cepacaulicus*
Large (*ta*)	Heteropathy preponderant	Not separately listed	Large, *pulsus magnus*
Number of Pulses Listed	20	27	31

†In *Pin-hu mai hsueh* (pages 6, 9), unlike *Revised Outline* and many other sources, the normal pulse is not the moderate pulse but the long (*ch'ang* 长) pulse. See above, note 11, page 318.

‡Porkert translates the name of the *juan* 软 pulse, which he distinguishes but which *Pin-hu mai hsueh* and other sources consider synonymous, as "soft, *pulsus mollis*" (page 219).

and evaluation must proceed from an analysis of the overall situation. Accelerated pulse persisting after the disappearance of appendicitis symptoms, for example, indicates the need for continued therapy to prevent a recurrence. Sometimes a pulse alteration appears before other symptoms, and can be used for early diagnosis.

6.4.2. Tactile examination

This includes palpating the chest and abdomen to discern whether they are soft or hard and whether there are tender spots or lumps; palpating the joints for fractures and dislocations; palpating the skin to determine whether it is warm or cool; and pressing lightly along the circulation tracts to discern the presence of pathological reactive corpuscles.

6.4.2.1. Abdominal palpation

Abdominal pain which diminishes when pressed is depletion manifestation type; if it increases when pressed it is repletion manifestation type. Softening of the site of pain indicates depletion manifestation type; hardening means repletion type.

6.4.2.2. Skin palpation

The main concern is changes in temperature. When the backs of the hands are warm it indicates hot sensations of external origin. When the palms and soles of the feet are warm it indicates yin depletion internal hot manifestation type. Cold extremities is yang depletion. In children, hot sensations of great intensity with cold fingertips indicate likelihood of convulsions. When the bowels are loose, if the pulse is small and weak and the extremities are cold, the diarrhea will be comparatively difficult to stop; if the hands and feet are warm it will be easier to stop.

6.4.2.3. Circulation tract palpation

One palpates the acupuncture loci along the circulation tracts, searching for pathological reactive corpuscles as a basis for diagnosis or therapy. Wherever a node or ropy corpuscle is felt, therapeutic massage, acupuncture, or drug injections at the loci (4.3.3) may be applied.

6.5. Conclusion

[Omitted from translation.]

7. Manifestation Type Determination

Characterization of a disorder as the basis for therapy requires that the case history, symptoms, physical signs, and other data from the examination be meticulously analyzed and integrated. This process, requisite to correct diagnosis, is called "manifestation type determination" (*pien cheng* 辨 证). It demands that one be concerned not only with the common characteristics of a disease but with characteristics of the individual case; that one be concerned not only with local pathological changes but also with changes involving the patient's whole body; that one be concerned not only with the growth and diminution of heteropathy but also with the rise and fall of the organism's power of resistance.

It is a practice of Chinese physicians to use the [homophonous] words *cheng* 症 and *cheng* 证 to denote two distinct concepts. The former refers to individual symptoms, such as headache and hot sensations [and is thus translated "symptom"]. The latter refers to a complex of determinate symptoms and physical signs [and is translated as "manifestation type" or, when signs and symptoms are merely being enumerated, as "manifestations"]. The manifestation type is a synthesis of pathological and clinical phenomena expressed in such a way as to imply therapeutic principles. It is in effect the diagnosis of the traditional physician.[1]

Let us take the "large intestine system moist hot" manifestation type as an example. In addition to explaining that the location of pathological changes is the large intestine system, and that the external heteropathies that brought about the disorder are of the moist and hot types (5.1.3, 5.1.4), it also indicates that the therapeutic principle of "clearing the hot heteropathy and freeing the moist" (*ch'ing li shih je* 清 利 湿 热 , 12.5) should be selected. Another example is the "splenetic-stomach system deple-

---

[1] See the discussion of manifestation type determination in the introductory study, pages 109–11.

tion cold" manifestation type. This explains that the pathological changes are located in the splenetic and stomach systems, that the cause of the disorder was cold heteropathy, and that the orthopathic energy of the body was debilitated. At the same time it shows that treatment on the principle of "warming the splenetic system and strengthening the stomach system" (*wen p'i chien wei* 溫 脾 健 胃 , 12.4) should be undertaken. Thus the concept of manifestation type usually involves multiple aspects such as etiology, location of pathology, and reactions of the organism.

What must be done to clearly and correctly determine the manifestation type? Chinese physicians, on the basis of long clinical experience, have gradually formed an ensemble of methods, the most important of which are based on the Eight Rubrics (*pa kang* 八 綱), the visceral systems of function (chapter 8), and the defensive *ch'i*, active *ch'i*, constructive *ch'i*, and blood sectors (9.1). Among these the Eight Rubrics provides the overall framework, in accord with which one sums up the location of the pathological changes, their character, and the circumstances of the struggle between the organism and the heteropathy.[2] On that foundation, in order to further clarify the special nature of the disorder, one must use one of the other methods to determine the attributes of the heteropathy, the visceral system in which the disorder is found, and the extent to which it has damaged the organism. Thus, often one must use several methods to supplement each other if the diagnosis is to be completely satisfactory.[3]

---

[2] The Eight Rubrics, often considered the most important system of manifestation types, does not go back to the early canons, but was first used in the mid-twelfth century and was popularized in such works as *I hsueh hsin wu* 醫 學 心 悟 (1732), *1*: 18a-19a. This was an improvement on the Eight Essentials (*pa yao* 八 要) of *Pen-ts'ao yen i* 本 草 衍 義 (1119), *1*: 6. The latter conception, rather than making a summary distinction between yin and yang, divided manifestations into those due to heteropathic *ch'i* and those due to a defect in orthopathic *ch'i*. These are not, however, diagnostically independent entities.

[3] The three methods of classification discussed in the last paragraph are not the only ones that have been important in classical practice. They are emphasized here because they are combined in a comprehensive system for making therapeutic decisions. This combination is neither ancient nor universal.

Only by comparing can one make distinctions. In manifestation type determination one not only must have a sound grasp of each type's clinical manifestations, but must also be attentive to the distinctions between one type and another, in order to diagnose correctly.

The Eight Rubrics comprise outer and inner (*piao li* 表里), cold and hot (*han je* 寒 热), depletion and repletion (*hsu shih* 虚 实), and yin and yang. The manifestation type is determined by using these four pairs of contradictions to sum up the various special features of all disorders. Outer and inner are used to distinguish the location of the pathological changes; cold, hot, depletion, and repletion to distinguish their character, and then yin and yang to provide a general characterization. The clinical employment of the Eight Rubrics is usually in that order. Using these paired opposites as units for comparison and distinction helps one to recognize the various characteristics and special features of medical disorders. At the same time, because the pairs of rubrics are related and mutually reinforcing, when the manifestation type is being determined they should not be considered in isolation.

Coverage varies considerably in handbooks of the last couple of decades. Nan-ching Chung-i hsueh-yuan ed. 1958: 130–50 gives priority to the Six Warps method, which is described only briefly below (9.5) despite its great authority in early times. Among important recent textbooks, Hu-pei Chung-i hsueh-yuan 湖 北 中 医 学 院 ed. 1978: 68–97 discusses an additional ch'i-blood system; Shang-hai Chung-i hsueh-yuan 上 海 中 医 学 院 ed. 1979–80: I, 21–23 merely introduces the Six Warps and Warm Factor systems; Nan-ching Chung-i hsueh-yuan 1983: 60–93 discusses the same schemata as the *Revised Outline*. In evaluating this diversity it is well to keep in mind the increasing frequency with which traditional physicians are using Western diagnostic techniques and categories (see the introductory study, page 28, note 23). This trend may render the choice of manifestation type systems in textbooks beside the point.

7.1. Outer and Inner

Outer and inner refer to the depth at which the pathological changes are located and the seriousness of the disorder. In general, a disorder in the peripheral flesh (*chi piao* 肌 表) belongs to the outer manifestation type; the disorder is mild and its locus shallow. A disorder in the visceral systems belongs to the inner manifestation type; the disorder is more severe and its locus deeper.

7.1.1. Outer manifestation type

This is generally seen in the early stages of disorders of external origin. The main clinical manifestations are fever, abnormal sensitivity to cold (or to wind or fresh air), headache, sore or painful extremities, stuffy nose and light cough, tongue coating thin and white, pulse floating, and so on. Among these, fever, abnormal sensitivity to cold, and floating pulse are the special features of the outer manifestation type.

It is divided into outer cold, outer hot, outer depletion, and outer repletion subtypes. On the basis of the symptoms mentioned above, if the aversion to cold is strong, fever mild, and pulse floating and tense, it is called the outer cold manifestation type, and is treated by "flushing the outer aspect with pungent and warming drugs" (*hsin wen chieh piao* 辛 溫 解 表 , 12.1.1.1). If the aversion to cold is mild, the fever serious, and the pulse floating and accelerated, it is called the outer hot manifestation type, and is treated by "flushing the outer aspect with pungent and cooling drugs" (*hsin liang chieh piao* 辛 凉 解 表 , 12.1.1.2). Outer manifestations without sweating are called the outer repletion manifestation type, and may be treated with comparatively strong drugs for "venting the outer aspect" (*fa piao* 发 表 , 12.1.0). With profuse sweating they are called the outer depletion type, for which such drugs may not be too freely used. When the outer type is found in old people or people with weak constitutions, while flushing the outer aspect one should pay heed to "reinforcing orthopathic *ch'i*" (*fu cheng* 扶 正 [by use of replenishing drugs, 12.16.0]).

7.1.2. Inner manifestation type

This is mostly seen in the intermediate and advanced stages of all kinds of disorders of external origin. By this time the outer manifestations have already dissipated, and the heteropathy has passed to the inner aspect and involved the visceral systems. In addition, all sorts of disorders due to internal disturbance (*nei shang* 内 伤) are of the inner manifestation type. Its clinical manifestations are extremely varied; not only is it divided into cold, hot, depletion, and repletion subtypes, but it differs according to the visceral system affected. Its concrete manifestations will be discussed in detail in connection with visceral system (chapter 8) and Heat Factor Disorder (chapter 9) manifestation type determination. Generally, in the inner manifestation type, abnormal sensitivity to wind or fresh air and aversion to cold are lacking, the pulse is sunken, there are alterations in the tongue tissues, and the tongue coating is yellow or black.

For instance, when a case of pneumonia begins there are abnormal sensitivity to cold, fever, aches in the head and body, pulse floating and accelerated, and similar symptoms; this condition belongs to the outer manifestation type. With further development the patient exhibits high fever with flushed face, lack of abnormal sensitivity to cold, thirst, chest pain, intense coughing, expectoration of rust-colored mucus, agitation, pink tongue with yellow coating, swollen and accelerated pulse, and other symptoms of pulmonary system hot heteropathy; this condition belongs to the inner manifestation type.

Not only are there cold, hot, depletion, and repletion subtypes, but when there have been complicated pathological changes one must distinguish depletion cold type from repletion cold type, and depletion hot from repletion hot type, as explained separately under each rubric below (7.3.1, 7.3.2). In addition, a disorder neither inner nor outer but on the borderline between the two is called the half-outer half-inner manifestation type (*pan piao pan li cheng* 半 表 半 里 证). Its principal symptom is alternating fever and cold sensations, and it is treated by the "mediating and flushing" (*ho chieh* 和 解) technique (12.7.0).

7.1.3. Combined inner and outer manifestation type

Sometimes it is possible for the outer and inner aspects to be simultaneously disordered. For example, in the first stage of acute bacillary dysentery [Shigellosis, and symptomatically indistinguishable disorders] there are not only such symptoms of the inner manifestation type as abdominal pain, pus and blood in the stool, thirst, and yellow or whitish tongue coating, but also such outer manifestation type symptoms as abnormal sensitivity to cold, fever, sore or painful extremities, and pulse floating and accelerated. This is called a "combined inner and outer" disorder (*piao li t'ung ping* 表 里 同 病). Such disorders are ordinarily seen in two circumstances. One is when in a disorder of external origin the outer manifestations have not yet dispersed but the heteropathy has already passed to the inner aspect. In the other, the patient originally has a disorder due to internal disturbance and newly contracts one of external origin. The former should be treated by "flushing both the outer and inner aspects" (*piao li shuang chieh* 表 里 双 解 , 12.7.0), and the latter by giving priority to the new disorder.

Main points in distinguishing the outer from the inner manifestation type: Generally among disorders of hot character it is most important to distinguish clearly whether the fever is accompanied by abnormal sensitivity to cold, whether the tongue tissues are pale or normal pink, whether the tongue coating is whitish or yellow, and whether the pulse is floating or sunken. Fever with sensitivity to cold, pale tongue with whitish coating, and floating pulse belong to the outer manifestation type; fever without abnormal sensitivity to cold, tongue pink and coating yellow, pulse sunken (and in some cases accelerated) belong to the inner manifestation type.

7.2. Cold and Hot

Cold and hot refer to the character of the disorder—"hot if yang is predominant, cold if yin."[4] Cold and hot essentially are concrete

---

[4] This saying may seem to imply that in the Eight Rubrics the cold/hot pair is not independent of the yin/yang pair. Clinically that is not the case. Note that the cold/hot pair originated in a manifestation type system that did not include the yin/yang pair; see note 2 above.

manifestations of yin and yang imbalance. The distinction between disorders of the hot and cold manifestation type can thus serve as a basis for use of warming or heating drugs as against chilling or cooling drugs.

7.2.1. Cold manifestation type

There are both outer cold and inner cold types; we will be concerned mainly with the latter. Its main manifestations are sensitivity to cold, ice-cold hands and feet, insipid taste in the mouth unaccompanied by thirst, preference for hot drinks, protracted voiding of clear urine, thin stool, pale complexion, tongue whitish, coating moist and whitish or black, and pulse sunken and retarded. Certain patients with chronic wasting diseases often exhibit symptoms of this kind. Treatment uses the technique of "expelling the cold heteropathy" (*ch'ü han* 祛寒 , 12.4.0).

7.2.2. Hot manifestation type

There are both outer hot and inner hot types; we will be concerned mainly with the latter. Its main manifestations are fever, abnormal sensitivity to heat, agitation, preference for cold drinks, urination brief with urine tinged scarlet, constipation, face flushed, tongue pink, coating dry and yellow or black, and pulse accelerated. Disorders of hot character regularly exhibit symptoms of this kind. Treatment uses the technique of "clearing the hot heteropathy" (*ch'ing je* 清热 , 12.2.0).

7.2.3. Cold and hot intermeshed

"Cold and hot intermeshed" (*han je chiao-ts'o* 寒热交错) refers to the simultaneous appearance of hot and cold manifestations. For example, abnormal sensitivity to cold, fever without perspiration, head and body pains, labored and noisy breathing, agitation, thirst, tongue pink with yellow or whitish coating, and pulse floating and tense are called the outer cold-inner hot manifestation type. Fever, headache, coughing up of yellow mucus, dry throat and distended abdomen, and watery stool are the outer hot-inner cold type (seen in people suffering from depletion [inner] cold heteropathy in the intestinal and stomach systems [5.1.2.2] as well as wind-hot heteropathy of external origin [5.1.1.2]). Headache, inflamed eyes or toothache, and mouth sores with chills and pain in the lower abdomen are the upper hot-lower cold manifestation type (seen in sufferers from depletion [inner] cold heteropathy in the lower *chiao* system [2.1.6] with hot heteropathy in the cardiac and stomach systems). Pain in the stomach cavity, belching with putrid odor and sour liquid disgorged in the back of the mouth, insipid taste in the mouth, poor appetite, and frequent, harsh, and painful urination are the upper cold-lower hot manifestation type (seen in sufferers from stomach system cold heteropathy with moist-hot heteropathy in the lower *chiao* system, 5.1.4.1.3).

7.2.4. Hot and cold: true and false

In clinical practice one may often encounter situations in which the essential character of the disorder is that of the hot manifestation type but it exhibits phenomena of the cold type, called the "true hot-false cold" (*chen je chia han* 真 热 假 寒) type, and vice versa. Unless one grasps the essential character, one may be confused and the diagnosis or therapy may be incorrect. For instance, in the case of a child with measles which are about to erupt or are not erupting freely, outwardly the child seems completely fatigued, languid in speech and movement, with cold extremities, sallow complexion, and sunken, small, and accelerated pulse. On careless examination this seems to be the cold manifestation type. But from the child's hot exhalation; burning heat in the chest and abdomen; foul mouth odor; thirst with great liquid intake and preference for cold drinks; pink tongue with yellow, dry coating; and sunken, small, accelerated, and vigorous pulse, one may see that the essential character nevertheless is that of the hot manifestation type. Traditional physicians believe that the more deeply seated the internal stasis of circulation due to hot heteropathy, the chillier the peripheral extremities, as in the saying "the deeper the hot heteropathy, the deeper the contraversion" (*chüeh* 厥 [dysfunction of circulation leading to cold extremities; P38]). This true hot-false cold type may often be observed in disorders of hot character in which the peripheral circulation is unhealthy. For therapy one uses chilling or cooling drugs to "clear the hot heteropathy and flush out the toxicity" (*ch'ing je chieh tu* 清 热 解 毒, 12.2.1.2).

The symptoms of a patient suffering from a chronic wasting disease who feels hot sensations in his body, as well as intermittently flushed cheeks, agitation, black tongue coating, and floating and large pulse, on the surface would appear to be those of hot phenomena. But if the patient prefers hot food and drink, dresses warmly, sleeps with limbs drawn up, and presents a pale or whitish tongue with black, moist coating, although the pulse is full and large it will lack vigor; one can see that the essential character is that of the cold manifestation type, so this condition is called true cold-false hot. Therapy uses warming or heating drugs to "warm the yang and expel the cold heteropathy" (wen yang ch'ü han 溫 陽 祛 寒 , 12.4.0).

Main points in distinguishing the cold from the hot manifestation type: It is most important to distinguish whether or not there are thirst and preference for or aversion to hot or cold, and what are the circumstances of any alterations in elimination, complexion, tongue phenomena, pulse phenomena, and so on.

Insipid taste in the mouth without thirst, preference for hot drinks, protracted voiding of clear urine, thin stool, facial pallor, pale tongue with whitish, moist coating, and retarded pulse belong to the cold manifestation type; thirst and preference for cold drinks, urination brief with urine tinged scarlet, dry and hardened stool, flushed face, pink tongue with yellow, dry coating, and accelerated pulse belong to the hot manifestation type.

In addition, do not equate elevated body temperature with the hot manifestation type.[5] The latter refers to a set of symptoms and body signs which involve hot phenomena; high temperature is only one such item. At times elevated body temperature may not be the hot manifestation type, and body temperature may not be elevated in every instance of the hot manifestation type. For example, in the outer cold manifestation type, although the patient's temperature is elevated, because there are preponderant sensitivity to cold, no thirst, tongue coating whitish and moist, and other cold phenomena, it is still diagnosed as the cold manifestation type. Another example is inner hot manifestation type. Although the

---

[5] Note that in this chapter and elsewhere in the Revised Outline, references to hot sensations felt by the patient are less frequent than mentions of fever in the sense of elevated body temperature. This is another instance of a tacit shift from a traditional to a modern diagnostic entity. See the introductory study, page 106.

patient's temperature is not high, there are thirst, constipation, flushed face, pink tongue with yellow, dry coating, accelerated pulse, and other hot phenomena, so that it is still diagnosed as the hot manifestation type.

When cold and hot are both observed, or when it is difficult to distinguish which is true and which false, the reason is generally a complex condition. In diagnosis, in addition to paying heed to symptoms, pulse, and tongue, one must also refer to the patient's previous medical history, constitutional tendencies toward cold or hot, and experience of illness and therapy, in order to see past the immediate phenomena and grasp the essential character of the disorder, clarifying the primacy and true or false status of cold and hot manifestation types, and thus carrying out the correct therapy.

7.3. Depletion and Repletion

"Depletion" and "repletion" refer to levels of the orthopathic and heteropathic *ch'i* lower and higher than normal [depletion is envisioned as less *ch'i* or a lower level of function than normal, and repletion as the opposite]. Generally speaking, depletion refers to insufficiency of the body's orthopathic energy (3.1.1, 5.7) and weakening of its power of resistance; repletion refers to preponderance of heteropathic energy and to the violence of the struggle between orthopathy and heteropathy.

7.3.1. Depletion manifestation type

This generally occurs [during or] after serious or protracted disorders, when the body is debilitated and the orthopathic energy insufficient. Among its manifestations the most important are facial pallor, lethargy, languor, regular throbbing of the heart and shortness of breath, perspiration without external cause and nocturnal sweating, soft tongue without coating, and small, weak, debilitated pulse. Therapy uses the technique of "replenishing" (*pu* 補 , 12.16). The depletion manifestation type is divided into the yin depletion (depletion hot), yang depletion (depletion cold), *ch'i* depletion, blood depletion, and visceral system depletion subtypes.

7.3.2. Repletion manifestation type

The repletion manifestation type is generally associated with new and comparatively threatening medical conditions. This is a result of the violence of the struggle between the orthopathic and heteropathic *ch'i*, on the one hand because the heteropathic *ch'i* is preponderant—as in preponderant external heteropathy, mucus associated with stasis of moisture (3.5), *ch'i* stasis and blood coagulation, Overnight Food Accumulation Disorder (*shih chi* 食 积 [=*su shih*, 6.3.2]), worm infestations, and so on—and on the other because the organism's vital capacity for resistance is high.

The special clinical features of the repletion manifestation type are the comparatively brief course of the disorder, relatively strong reaction of the organism, mental overexcitement, loud voice and harsh breathing. Some cases also include high fever and flushed face or no fever and sallow complexion, congestion of the pulmonary system (*t'an hsien yung sheng* 痰 涎 壅 盛),[6] intense pain aggravated by pressure, comparatively thick tongue coating, swollen and vigorous pulse, and so on.

The repletion manifestation type is also divided into cold and hot types. For instance, cases that involve abscesses in the pulmonary system; fever with thirst; coughing and harried, difficult breathing accompanied by chest pains; congestion of the pulmonary system by pus and mucus (*nung t'an yung sheng* 脓 痰 壅 盛); pink tongue and yellow, thick coating; and smooth, accelerated, and vigorous pulse are of the inner hot repletion manifestation type. Treatment uses drugs for "clearing the hot heteropathy and draining the pulmonary system" (*ch'ing je hsieh fei* 清 热 泻 肺 , 12.2.0). Another example is intestinal contractions [enterospasms] in which the patient suffers intense paroxysmal abdominal pain, and tosses about and moans, with loud voice and harsh breathing; pale face and cold extremities; whitish, thick tongue coating; and sunken, tense, and vigorous pulse. This belongs to the inner cold repletion manifestation type, and is treated with drugs for "warming the medial aspect and dispersing the cold heteropathy" (*wen chung san han* 温 中 散 寒 , 12.4.0). [See table 7.1.]

---

[6] This term implies congestion due to constraint on circulation, with copious expectorate and feelings of lodged phlegm. I am grateful to Drs. Lu Gwei-djen and Fu Xiaoyan for consultation.

Table 7.1
Essential Points in Manifestation Type
Determination by the Eight Rubrics

Type	Main Phenomena	Tongue Phenomena	Pulse Phenomena	Therapy
Outer	fever, aversion to wind and cold	coating thin, whitish	floating	"flushing the outer aspect" (12.1)
Inner	absence of outer manifestations, but with symptoms of pathological changes in the visceral systems, varying according to whether hot, cold, depletion, or repletion	changes	not floating	varies according to whether hot, cold, depletion, or repletion
Cold	sensitivity to cold, hands and feet cold, insipid taste without thirst, preference for hot drinks, protracted voiding of clear urine, thin stool, complexion pale	pale, coating whitish or black, and moist	retarded (or tense)	"expelling the cold heteropathy" (12.4)
Hot	sensitivity to heat, fever, thirst with preference for cold drinks, agitation, urination brief, urine tinged scarlet, constipation, flushed complexion	pink, coating yellow or yellowish-black and dry	accelerated	"clearing the hot heteropathy" (12.2)
Depletion	manifestations of somatic debilitation: pale complexion, lethargy, languor, throbbing of the heart with shortness of breath, perspiration without external cause, nocturnal sweating	pale, tender with little or no coating	debilitated (empty)	"replenishing" (12.16; distinguish type of depletion)
Repletion	strong reactions of the organism, mental overexcitement, loud voice and harsh breathing, sometimes high fever and flushed face, or no fever and pale face, or intense abdominal pains aggravated by pressure	roughened and hard, coating thick	vigorous (full)	"attacking and driving out" (12.3–12.5), "dispersing" (12.10), or "draining and bringing down" (12.9)
Yin	complexion darkened but colorless, body drawn in, extremities cold, short breath and drawling speech, urine clear, stool thin	pale, tender, coating white and moist	sunken, retarded, small, weak	"replenishing with warming drugs" (12.16)
Yang	face flushed, body hot, mental agitation, harsh breathing, thirst with preference for cold drinks, urine tinged scarlet, constipation	pink, coating yellow and thick	swollen, large, smooth, accelerated	"clearing the hot heteropathies," "draining the repletion" (12.2)

7.3.3. Depletion and repletion intermixed (*hsu shih chia-tsa* 虚 实 夹 杂)

Clinically it often happens that both repletion and depletion manifestations are present. For instance, in cirrhosis patients with abdominal fluid [ascites, etc.] the whole body is emaciated, with anemia, languor, and decreased intake of food; these are basically depletion manifestations. But at the same time there are a large volume of abdominal fluid, abdominal swelling (here, of the spleen, *p'i k'uai* 痞 块), pain in the rib and abdominal regions, and other symptoms of the repletion manifestation type. Therapy should combine attack (*kung* 攻 [on the heteropathy]) and replenishment [of the orthopathy], giving precedence as the situation dictates (10.3.3).

7.3.4. Depletion and repletion: true and false

A disorder with the essential character of the depletion type, but with clinical manifestations which appear to be of the repletion type, is called "false repletion" (*chia shih* 假 实). The inverse case is called "false depletion" (*chia hsu* 假 虚). [Examples of their general features appear in table 7.2].

Main points in distinguishing the repletion from the depletion manifestation type: It is most important to consider such aspects as whether the disorder is of long or short duration, whether the voice and breathing are strong, whether the pain is worsened by pressure, whether the tongue is roughened and hard or fat and soft, and whether the pulse is vigorous. In general, if the course of the disorder has been short, if the voice is loud and breathing harsh, the pain aggravated by pressure, the tongue tissues roughened and hard, and the pulse vigorous, it is the repletion manifestation type, and vice versa.

7.4. Yin and Yang

Outer and inner, cold and hot, depletion and repletion: generally the rubrics yin and yang may be used to provide a summary of these, with outer, hot, and repletion belonging to the yang manifestation type and inner, depletion, and cold belonging to the yin type. Thus yin and yang are the most general classifications among the

Table 7.2
False Repletion and Depletion

Type	Apparent Symptom	Actual Characteristics
False repletion	Abdominal distension	Not the unabating distention of the repletion manifestation type, but rather comes and goes
	Abdominal pain	Not aggravated by pressure as in the repletion type, but the pain instead lessens under pressure
	Fever	Tongue is soft and pulse empty
False depletion	Patient remains silent	When he speaks it is generally in a loud voice with harsh breathing
	Patient does not want to eat	At times he can take food
	Bowels are loose	Great feeling of relief after elimination
	Distension and fullness in the chest and abdomen	Local pressure gives rise to pain which is sometimes fixed in location

Eight Rubrics, and any manifestation of medical disorder may be assigned to one of the two.

7.4.1. Yin manifestation type

General manifestations are lethargy, darkened complexion, cold sensations in the body and extremities, preference for sleeping with limbs drawn up, shortness of breath and drawling speech, low and indistinct voice, preference for quiet, lack of thirst or preference for hot drinks, abdominal pain temporarily diminished by pressure, thin stool, protracted voiding of clear urine, tongue tissues pale and soft, tongue coating moist and slippery, and pulse usually sunken, retarded, small, or weak.

7.4.2. Yang manifestation type

General manifestations are mental overexcitement, flushed face, hot sensations in the body and extremities, preference for sleeping with limbs extended, harsh breathing, talkativeness, resonant voice, preference for activity, thirst sometimes accompanied by preference for cold drink, abdominal pain aggravated by pressure, dry and hardened stool, urination short and urine tinged scarlet, tongue red or crimson and hard with yellow, dry coating, and pulse usually swollen, accelerated, or vigorous.

7.4.3. Yin depletion

This refers to insufficiency of the yin aspect. "Yin depletion gives rise to internal hot heteropathy" (*yin hsu sheng nei je* 阴 虚 生 内 热); this is the depletion hot manifestation type often referred to (7.3.1). Main manifestations are a hot sensation in the palms of the hands or soles of the feet, intermittent hot sensations after noon, emaciation, nocturnal sweating, mouth and throat dry, urination short with urine tinged scarlet, stool dry and scanty, tongue pink with little or no coating, pulse small, accelerated, and debilitated, and other symptoms of the depletion hot manifestation type. These may be seen in pulmonary tuberculosis and other chronic wasting diseases.

7.4.4. Yang depletion

This refers to insufficiency of yang *ch'i*. "Yang depletion gives rise to [internal] cold heteropathy" (*yang hsu tse sheng han* 阳 虚 则 生 寒); this is the depletion cold manifestation type often mentioned (7.3.1). Main manifestations are languor, shortness of breath and drawling speech, aversion to cold with chills in the extremities, sweating without external cause, facial pallor, protracted voiding of clear urine, thin stool, tongue pale and soft with whitish coating, pulse retarded and weak or large but debilitated, and other symptoms of the depletion cold type. It is often seen in various disorders in which there is a decline in the functioning of the organism and a fall in basal metabolism. It is also observed in aged patients with weak constitutions.

7.4.5. Yin *ch'i* failure and yang *ch'i* failure manifestation type

"Failure of yin *ch'i*" (*wang yin* 亡 阴) and "failure of yang *ch'i*" (*wang yang*) refer to grave manifestations which appear with sudden and considerable loss of yin fluids and yang *ch'i*, as in profuse sweating, high fever, violent vomiting or diarrhea, and excessive loss of blood. In such cases one must make a timely and accurate diagnosis and actively work for immediate relief. In addition to all sorts of serious manifestations of the precipitating disease, failure of yin and yang *ch'i* have these special features:

Yin ch'i failure manifestation type. The most important manifestations are perspiration hot, salty, but not sticky; extremities warm; respiration comparatively harsh; dry mouth and throat with desire to drink; intermittently flushed face; tongue pink and dry; and pulse empty, large, accelerated, and debilitated.

Yang ch'i failure manifestation type. The most important manifestations are cold perspiration, neutral in taste, sticky, profuse and unceasing; coldness in the peripheral extremities due to contraversion (*chüeh leng* 厥 冷 , 7.2.4); indistinct and weak respiration; lack of thirst; greyish white complexion; tongue pale or whitish and moist; and pulse subtle, as though about to cease.

According to clinical observation, profuse sweating, vomiting, or diarrhea may lead to either the yin or yang failure type. Damage to the yin aspect in hot disorders, as in profuse bleeding, may bring on the yin failure type. Damage to yang by cold heteropathy may bring on the yang failure type. Because of the common roots of yin and yang, yin failure type may lead to yang failure type and vice versa. But there are variations in priority and severity. Generally speaking, yin failure leading to yang failure is more frequently seen. In therapy, cases of yin failure type should be treated speedily by the technique of "relieving the yin and producing dispersed body fluids" (*chiu yin sheng chin* 救 陰 生 津 , 12.16.0 and 12.17.0), and yang failure cases by prompt use of the "restoring the yang and relieving the backflow" method (*hui yang chiu ni* 回 陽 救 逆 , 12.4.0).

7.5. A Medical Case History

[Only one of three is translated.]

Hsieh *X*, male, twenty years old. The patient was of strong constitution. A few days earlier he had squeezed some edematous sores on his head, bringing on aversion to cold, high fever, and pain over his whole body. At the time he entered the hospital for examination his white corpuscle count was 28,500, with 90 percent neutrophils and 10 percent lymphocytes. Staphylococcus aureus was cultured from his blood, with positive coagulase reaction. The diagnosis was septicemia. On the afternoon of the third day after entering the clinic, the patient began dripping sweat and his temperature abruptly fell to 35.6 degrees C (98.0 degrees F). His face was pale, extremities ice cold, blood pressure 88/54mm Hg, tongue pale and moist, and pulse subtle, small, and weak. A Western-style physician's diagnosis was shock.

Analysis. Because of the patient's head boils, the Fire toxicity [i.e., internal heteropathy] became predominant in intensity. When he squeezed the boils the heteropathic toxicity spread, invaded the constructive *ch'i* and blood and, moving inward, attacked the visceral systems. The traditional physician calls this situation "boils running yellow" (*ting-ch'uang tsou huang* 疔 疮 走 黄 [so-called because after the boil aborted the pus was thought to disperse through the body]). Then because the orthopathy was unable to overcome the heteropathy, the patient dripped sweat and his yang *ch'i* became very deficient, giving rise to the yang failure manifestation type. Treatment required a combination of Chinese and Western medicine. The traditional physician promptly applied the technique of "restoring the yang and relieving the backflow," after which an infusion for "supporting the inner aspect and penetrating the pus" (t'o li t'ou nung t'ang 托 里 透 膿 湯 , 14.3.2) was administered to get rid of the pus, and the patient was given drugs for "cooling the blood" (liang hsueh 涼 血 , 12.13.1.1) and "flushing out the toxicity" (chieh tu 解 毒 , 12.2.1.2).[7]

7.6. Conclusion

The Eight Rubrics provides a method for diagnosis through distinguishing eight different aspects of medical disorders. Although it must be used in conjunction with visceral system manifestation type determination and other approaches in order to be entirely satisfactory, it provides a foundation for all of them through its concern for essentials.

Any of the eight types under certain conditions may evolve into another. Generally the change from outer to inner type indicates an increase in the severity of the condition; from inner to outer, a turn in the direction of recovery. A change from hot to cold type or from repletion to depletion type means that the orthopathic ch'i is deficient, and the inverse change indicates that it is gradually reviving.

Few of the manifestation types encountered frequently in clinical practice are simple. Most are combinations of outer and inner, cold and hot, and depletion and repletion, and at times complex and false types appear. This situation demands that in the process of manifestation type determination we conscientiously investigate each case, form a coherent pattern on which to reason, and concentrate our efforts on finding the principal contradiction [i.e., the most essential aspect of any dialectical process, 10.4]. Only in this

---

[7] "Supporting the inner aspect" refers specifically to therapeutic methods that replenish the orthopathic ch'i in order to expel pus. Note that this medical case history, meant to illustrate a chapter on manifestation type determination, is not based on traditional diagnosis, and omits an account of signs and symptoms that would be of interest to traditional physicians. There is in fact no sign that they were involved in the diagnosis. This account suggests that their involvement began with interpreting modern diagnostic data in a way that would allow them to take part in an eclectic program of therapy. The modern component of that program is not recorded here, rendering the history valueless.

way is it possible to reach a correct conclusion; otherwise a sound analysis is impossible.

As to the pathological and physiological foundations of the Eight Rubrics, further research is needed. It is generally believed that the outer manifestation type is mainly seen in the early stages of infectious diseases, and is a kind of defensive response of the organism to the factors that cause the disorder. The inner manifestation type is mostly seen in the middle and advanced phases of infectious diseases, and when there is constitutional or functional damage from non-infectious diseases. It is a result of attack on the visceral tissues or organs by the factors that cause the disorder. Often its most important characteristic is serious hindrance to the energy metabolism and the functioning of the central nervous system and organs associated with it. The appearance of symptoms that indicate damage to the visceral systems [i.e., the inner aspect] at a point in the process when the manifestations of the outer types have not yet disappeared is called "combined inner and outer disorder."

As for the hot manifestation type, most people believe that it is related to a high level of physiological function in the body, with a rise in energy metabolism and increased reactivity against the causative factors. The resulting symptoms include overproduction of heat, rise in body temperature, increase in rate of respiration, increased cardiac heat volume, cutaneous vasodilation, speeding up of blood flow, increase in excitability of the cerebral cortex, as well as sweating due to the high temperature. These lead to such manifestations as loss of body fluids. Most people believe the cold manifestation type to be related to a decrease in the level of physiological function, and lowered energy metabolism and reactivity against the causative factors, with opposite results.

The depletion manifestation type generally refers to pathological conditions involving a fall in the power of resistance of the organism or a decrease in or failure of physiological functioning. Among these conditions are functional hindrances of the stomach and intestinal systems, drooping of the internal organs [splanchnoptosis] and hypothyroidism. The repletion manifestation type generally refers to pathological conditions involving strong reactivity of the organism and hyperfunction of tissues or organs, as in various infections, tumors, accumulations of fluid in the thoracic and abdominal cavities, hematomas, and purulent swellings, as well as other perceptible pathological changes. All of these problems deserve our further study.

8. Visceral System Manifestation Type Determination and Therapy

Manifestation type determination and therapeutic reasoning in which the visceral systems provide the system of rubrics is the foundation of diagnosis and therapy in the various clinical specialties. Because the functions of each visceral system are diverse, and the relations between yin and yang visceral systems and their relations to tissues and organs are complicated, the phenomena corresponding to disorders in the visceral systems are extremely varied. In clinical manifestation type determination it is imperative to see past the immediate phenomena, grasp the essential character, seek out the principal contradiction, and from among the complicated symptoms grasp the key manifestations (in italics below) for analysis. As an aid to study, in connection with each manifestation type we adduce several Western diseases. The reader can infer others by analogy. (The same Western disease may appear in traditional medicine under several headings; these are differences of type, not duplications.)

8.1. Cardiac and Small Intestine Systems (2.1.1)

The main physiological functions of the cardiac system are control of the blood circulation (*hsueh mai* 血 脉) and control of the consciousness. Thus pathological reactions of this system are in the main reflected in abnormalities in the circulation and in the state of mind. According to clinical observation, manifestations that belong to control of the circulation include cardiac system yang depletion, cardiac system yin depletion, and "cardiac system blood coagulation obstruction" (*hsin hsueh yü tsu* 心 血 瘀 阻). Those that belong to control of the state of mind include "internal disturbance from mucus and Fire" (*t'an huo nei jao* 痰 火 内 扰), "phlegm clogging the orifices of the heart" (*t'an mi hsin ch'iao* 痰 迷 心 窍),

349

and so on. As for the small intestine system, a common manifestation of disorder is transfer of hot heteropathy by the cardiac system to the small intestine system. Entry of hot heteropathy into the Cardiac Envelope Junction system falls within the scope of heat factor disorders, and will be discussed in 9.1.3.4.

8.1.1. Cardiac system yang insufficiency (cardiac yang lacking vigor)

Main manifestations.[1] Cardiac yang insufficiency *(hsin yang pu-tsu* 心 阳 不 足) includes cardiac system *ch'i* depletion, cardiac system yang depletion, and cardiac system yang depletion prostration. Their main common manifestations are *regular throbbing of the heart, shortness of breath* (worsened by physical activity), *perspiration without external cause,* and tongue pale with whitish coating.

Cardiac system ch'i depletion. One additionally observes languor, facial pallor, *a tendency to exhale long breaths, tongue fat and soft,* and empty pulse.

Cardiac system yang depletion. One additionally observes cold in the body and extremities, *distress and pain in the cardiac region,* and pulse small and weak and in some cases hesitant and intermittent.

Cardiac system yang depletion prostration (hsin yang hsu shuai 心 阳 虚 衰 *or hsin yang hsu t'o)* 心 阳 虚 脱). One additionally observes *profuse and incessant perspiration, coldness in the extremities due to contraversion* (7.2.4), lips virid or purplish, respiration weak and indistinct, or even sudden unconsciousness or coma, and *pulse subtle as though about to cease.*

---

[1] *Note in the original.* There is often some variation in the terminology used by Chinese physicians for manifestation types given here and in chapter 9. Here and below we append equivalent and similar names for reference.

Translator's note. The therapeutic discussions at the end of each subsection are of little relevance to the topic of this book, and are not very useful without reference to the extensive formulary in chapter 12. I omit most of them, retaining a few representative examples. Note that in some instances the authors equate manifestation types with modern diseases.

Pathology. In cardiac *ch'i* depletion, because motive power for propulsion in the blood vessels by the cardiac *ch'i* is insufficient, such symptoms appear as regular throbbing of the heart, shortness of breath, and empty pulse. In cardiac yang depletion, because of yang exhaustion, cold phenomena are observed. In cardiac yang depletion prostration, the cardiac *ch'i* is inadequate; at the same time there is yang depletion in the cardiac system, and the condition is more serious. Thus one observes throbbing of the heart and subtle and small pulse. Because the yang aspect is greatly depleted, there are copious sweating and coldness in the extremities. If the disorder develops a step further the state of mind may be affected, leading to coma and other dangerous symptoms.

Therapy. For cardiac system *ch'i* depletion one replenishes the cardiac *ch'i* and calms the mind. For the former, Four Gentlemen Infusion (*ssu chün-tzu t'ang* 四 君 子 汤 [12.16.0; on compounding see 11.2.2]) is used, adding seeds of sour jujube (*suan-tsao jen* 酸 枣 仁 [Zizyphus jujuba var. spinosa, 12.15.0]), Chinese senega root (*yuan-chih* 远 志 [Polygala sibirica or P. tenuifolia, 12.15.0]), fruit of schisandra (*wu-wei tzu* 五 味 子 [Schisandra chinensis, 12.17.1]), or other drugs to nourish the cardiac system and calm the mind. For cardiac yang depletion, the motion of the cardiac yang *ch'i* should be freed; Trichosanthes, Chives, and Cassia Infusion (*kua-lou hsieh-pai kuei-chih t'ang* 似 蒌 薤 白 桂 枝 汤 , 12.12.2.1) may be used. If there is also obstruction due to coagulation, Breaking into Laughter Powder (*shih hsiao san* 失 笑 散 , 12.13.2.6) should be added to vivify the blood and get the coagulum moving. In cardiac yang prostration, the technique is "restoring the yang and relieving the backflow" (7.4.5, 12.4.0) by prompt moxibustion at the *pai-hui* (TM19) and *tsu-san-li* (V36) loci and perhaps also at the *yung-ch'üan* 涌 泉 (R1) locus. Fourfold Backflow Infusion (*ssu ni t'ang* 四 逆 汤 , 12.7.0), with the addition of tangshen root (*tang-shen* 党 参 [Codonopsis pilosula or C. tangshen, 12.16.1], or ginseng root from Jilin, *Chi-lin shen* 吉 林 参 [Panax ginseng, 12.16.1]) is to be prepared without delay and administered to the patient.

For neuroses which belong to cardiac system *ch'i* depletion, therapeutic methods that replenish the cardiac *ch'i* (12.16) may be used. For heart failure that belongs to cardiac yang depletion prostration, the therapeutic technique of "restoring the yang and relieving the backflow" may be used. For angina pectoris that belongs to cardiac yang depletion, the method of "replenishing the cardiac system yang" (12.16.1.4) should not be used alone, but on the principle that "if [the circulation is] free (*t'ung* 通) there can be no pain (*t'ung* 痛)," drugs which "free the motion of the mucus" (*t'ung t'an* 通 痰) and "vivify the blood" (*huo hsueh* 活 血) are added to the prescription. For the former one uses whole tricosanthes (*kua-lou* 瓜 蔞 [T. kirilowii, 12.11.1.2]) and white of Chinese chive (*hsieh-pai* 薤 白 [Allium chinense]), which also free the motion of the yang *ch'i*, 12.12.1.2. For vivifying the blood, pollen and root of cat-tail (*p'u-huang* 蒲 黃 [Typha orientalis or angustifolia, 12.13.1.2]), guano (*wu-ling-chih* 五 灵 脂 [dung of bats, 12.13.1.5]), root of red-rooted sage (*tan-shen* 丹 参 [Salvia miltiorrhiza, 12.13.1.5]), cordyalis tuber (*yen-hu-so* 延 胡 索 [C. yanhusuo et al., 12.13.1.5]), and so on may be used. For irregular heart rhythm in which the pulse is hesitant or intermittent, Infusion of Roasted Licorice Root and Stem, with proportions adjusted to the case (*chih kan-ts'ao t'ang chia chien* 炙 甘 草 汤 加 减 [Glycyrrhiza uralensis, 11.3.2, 12.16.2.3]) is used. Presystolic contraction, pale tongue with whitish, moist or unctuous coating, and hesitant pulse indicate that the cardiac yang is blocked by phlegm. Gall Bladder System Warming Infusion (*wen tan t'ang* 温 胆 汤 , 12.11.0) with tangshen root added is used to eliminate the mucus and free the motion of the yang *ch'i*.

8.1.2. Cardiac system yin insufficiency

Main manifestations. Cardiac yin insufficiency may be divided into cardiac system yin *ch'i* depletion and cardiac system blood depletion. Main manifestations of both are *regular throbbing of the heart, worry and mental upset*, tendency to be frightened easily, insomnia, and absent-mindedness.

Cardiac yin depletion. One additionally observes moderate fever, nocturnal sweating, dry mouth, *tip of tongue red* with thin and whitish coating or no coating, *pulse small and accelerated*, and so on.

Cardiac blood depletion. One additionally observes dizziness, facial pallor, insipid taste in the mouth, tongue pale and soft, pulse small and weak, and so on.

Pathology. Because the cardiac *ch'i* is insufficient the cardiac yang *ch'i* becomes excessive; because of the yin-yang imbalance there are throbbing of the heart, worry, and mental upset. The cardiac yin depletion type is mostly caused by emotional exhaustion which consumes the cardiac yin *ch'i*; thus the manifestations of the

yin depletion internal hot manifestation type (7.4.3). The cardiac blood depletion type is mostly due to inadequate sustenance of the blood; thus the manifestations of blood depletion (3.2).
[Therapy omitted.]

8.1.3. Cardiac system blood coagulation obstruction

Main manifestations. Regular throbbing of the heart; heart pains (in the anterior part of the heart, or pricking or oppressive pains behind the breastbone), intermittent but disturbing when serious; bluish or purplish nails; perspiration; cold extremities; *tongue dull red or spots of coagulated blood on the sides of the tongue,* with scanty but moist coating; and rough pulse.

Pathology. When the cardiac system is clogged by blood coagulum, the *ch'i* and blood are unable to move freely, so that there are cardiac throbbing and pain. Because of the coagulation of blood in the cardiac system, there is a loss of free flow in the blood vessels all over the body. Thus the color of the blood is dull instead of vivid, there are spots of coagulum on the tongue, and the nails are bluish or purplish. Because the cardiac yang *ch'i* is insufficient, it is unable to warm the extremities, so they are cold. Because the yang *ch'i* is unable to defend the periphery of the body and prevent penetration of the outer aspect, there is perspiration. This manifestation type is often seen in coronary heart disease and cardiac infarction.
[Therapy omitted.]

8.1.4. Internal disturbance from mucus and fire

Main manifestations. Derangement, manic agitation and behavior, raving, intermittent laughing and crying, or even cursing and assaulting people, *red tongue with yellow, unctuous coating,* and *smooth, accelerated pulse.*

Pathology. Because the state of mind is disturbed by mucus and Fire there are derangement and mania. The unctuous tongue coating and the smooth pulse are due to the etiological role of mucus. The red tongue, yellow coating, and accelerated pulse are due to that of Fire.

Therapy. One should "clear the Fire and dissolve the mucus" (*ch'ing huo hua t'an* 清 火 化 痰), for which Mica-schist Mucus-

boiling Pellets (*meng-shih kun t'an wan* 礞 石 滚 痰 丸 ,
12.11.0) or Black Ferric Oxide Potion (*sheng-t'ieh-lo yin* 生 铁 落
饮 , 12.15.2.1) is used. Schizophrenia, manic-depressive psychosis,
hysteria, and similar disorders in which mucus and Fire manifestations are observed may be so treated.

8.1.5. Phlegm clogging the orifices of the heart

Main manifestations. Dementia, clouded perception, vomiting of
mucus, and in some cases coma, sound of phlegm in the throat,
tongue stiff and incapable of speech, *coating whitish and unctuous*,
and *pulse smooth*. If there is also mucous hot heteropathy, the
tongue is red with yellow coating and the pulse smooth and accelerated.

Pathology. Because the cardiac system is beclouded by mucus,
the consciousness in unclear, leading to dementia, clouded perception, and similar symptoms, and coma in serious cases. If there is
also hot heteropathy, although it would then be similar to the
preceding manifestation type (8.1.4), the difference of degree calls
for different therapy.

Therapy. "Eliminating the mucus and freeing the orifices" (*ch'u
t'an t'ung ch'iao* 除 痰 通 窍) with Mucus Guiding Infusion (*tao
t'an t'ang* 导 痰 汤 , 12.11.0). In case of coma, the "warming
and opening" technique (*wen k'ai fa* 温 开 法 , 12.14.0) uses
Storax Pellets (*su-ho-hsiang wan* 苏 合 香 丸 , 12.11.0). If the
coma is due to mucous hot heteropathy, the technique of "cooling
and opening" (*liang k'ai fa* 凉 开 法 , 12.14.0) is recommended,
using Perfect Treasure Elixir (*chih pao tan* 至 宝 丹 , 12.14.2.1)
or Cow Bezoar Pellets (*niu-huang wan* 牛 黄 丸 , 12.14.0).[2]
For hysteria and schizophrenia in which the tongue coating is
whitish and unctuous and the pulse smooth, Mucus Guiding Infusion
may be used for "eliminating the mucus and freeing the orifices,"
supplemented by Storax Pellets for rousing the mind. For
cerebrovascular accident in which the phlegm is clogging the cardiac

---

[2] "Opening" refers to prescriptions that relieve mucous blockages
responsible principally for mental confusion. "Warming and
opening" and "cooling and opening" are subtypes of the general
method called "opening the passages" (*hsuan ch'iao* 宣 窍 ,
12.14).

orifices and there is coma, the "warming and opening" method may be used. For such clogging in which the tongue is red, its coating yellow, and the pulse smooth and accelerated, use the "cooling and opening" technique. That is, for hot tendencies use "cooling and opening," and for cold use "warming and opening." If cerebrovascular accident develops "collapse" manifestations (*t'o cheng* 脱 证 : loss of natural palmar flexion at rest, open mouth, closed eyes, enuresis, perspiration, pulse subtle and weak, coma), in no circumstances may these methods of "opening the orifices" be used (so as to avoid accelerating the collapse on account of yang *ch'i* loss); instead perform moxibustion at the *shen-ch'üeh* 神 阙 (JM8) and *tsu-san-li* (V36) loci, determine the manifestation type, and treat as for Wind Attack Disorders (3.5). As for hepatic coma, diabetic coma, uremic coma, and so on, they are assigned to the mucous hot manifestation type. They may be treated with "cooling and opening" medicines of the Cow Bezoar Pellet type. At the same time acupuncture should be performed at the *jen-chung* (TM25) and *yung-ch'üan* (R1) loci. After recovery of consciousness, manifestation type determination and therapy should proceed according to the circumstances of each disorder.

8.1.6. Flaming up of the cardiac Fire; transfer of hot heteropathy by the cardiac system to the small intestine system (small intestine system repletion hot manifestation type)

Main manifestations. Sores in the mouth and on the tongue (usually recurrent), *mental upset and worry*, thirst, urination brief with yellow urine, or sometimes difficult with pricking pains or with blood in the urine, *tip of the tongue red* and coating yellow or white, and *pulse accelerated*.

Pathology. The cardiac system is vented in the tongue (2.1.1.1.3), so that when the cardiac Fire flames up (5.1.6.1) one observes mouth sores, mental upset and worry, thirst, tip of the tongue red, and similar manifestations. Because of the transfer of hot heteropathy to the small intestine system one observes urinary symptoms.

[Therapy omitted.]

8.1.7. Small intestine system *ch'i* pain

Main manifestations. Acute pains in the lower abdomen extending to the back and the testicles, whitish tongue coating, pulse sunken and strung or strung and tense.

Pathology. Mainly brought on by lack of moderation in eating and drinking, disproportion of cold or moisture, or static congelation of vital *ch'i* in the belly.

Therapy. "Setting the *ch'i* in motion and dispersing the congelation" (*hsing ch'i san chieh* 行 气 散 结) using Orangeseed Pellets (*chü-ho wan* 橘 核 丸 , 14.3.3) or Allspice Powder (*wu yao san* 烏 药 散 , 12.12.1.1).

8.1.8. Important points in cardiac and small intestine system manifestation type determination and therapy

[Recapitulation omitted.]

Because of the common roots of yin and yang (7.4.5), when cardiac system yin or yang depletion develops to a certain degree, it can bring on simultaneous depletion of yin and yang, *ch'i* and blood. At such times both yin and yang aspects should be treated, or drugs given for the more serious condition. For instance, when there are both yin and yang depletion but the balance is tipped in the direction of blood depletion, drug therapy should concentrate on replenishing the latter.

When the cardiac Fire flames up, giving rise to sores in the mouth and on the tongue, the method should be "clearing the hot heteropathy and draining the Fire" (*ch'ing je hsieh huo* 清 热 泻 火 , 12.2.1.1). When the cardiac system transfers hot heteropathy to the small intestine system, with frequent and painful urination, the method should be "clearing the hot heteropathies and freeing the moist heteropathies" (*ch'ing je li shih* 清 热 利 湿 , 12.5.0). For small intestine system *ch'i* pain or colic, the method should be "setting the *ch'i* in motion and dispersing the congelation."

8.2. Hepatic and Gall Bladder Systems (2.1.2)

The main physiological functions of the hepatic system are upward and outward dispersion (2.1.2.1.1) and storage of blood (2.1.2.1.2). The pathological changes are mainly due to abnormalities in the dispersion function, which bring on hepatic system *ch'i* stasis (*kan yü* 肝 郁), hepatic system Fire preponderance (*kan huo sheng* 肝 火 盛), hepatic system yang rising in excess (*kan yang shang k'ang* 肝 阳 上 亢), hepatic system yin insufficiency (*kan yin pu tsu* 肝 阴 不 足), and similar pathological changes. Defects in dispersion, or preponderance of hepatic Fire (5.1.6.1), may affect the hepatic system's blood storage function, bringing about hemorrhage manifestations. The most commonly observed manifestations of gall bladder system disorder are of the gall bladder system hot type.

8.2.1. Hepatic system *ch'i* stasis (hepatic *ch'i* not flowing freely)

Main manifestations. Agitation and irritability, depression in some cases, dizziness, *distension and pain* or furtive pains *in the rib region,* belching, poor appetite, bitter taste in the mouth or vomiting, abdominal pains, loose bowels, irregular menstruation, tongue coating whitish and moist, and *strung pulse.* Prolonged stasis induces blood coagulation, so that one also observes local swellings (of the liver or spleen), spots of coagulated blood on the sides of the tongue, and strung or rough pulse.

Pathology. Because of the hepatic system *ch'i* stasis (*kan ch'i yü chieh* 肝 气 郁 结 , *kan ch'i pu shu* 肝 气 不 舒) upward and outward dispersion is not possible; agitation and irritable disposition ensue. Because of the stasis of *ch'i* and blood in the circulation tracts associated with the hepatic system, there are distension and pain in the rib region. Because the *ch'i* of the hepatic system is unable to overcome this stasis, the *ch'i* backs up and invades the splenetic and stomach systems, and may give rise to pain in the rib region and abdomen, loose bowels, belching, poor appetite, vomiting, and other symptoms. In women, lack of free flow of the *ch'i* and blood in the hepatic circulation tract (H) affects the highway and conception (JM) tracts and induces irregular menstruation. The strung pulse is a common pulse phenomenon in hepatic system disorders.

[Therapy omitted.]

8.2.2. Hepatic yang rising in excess (yin depletion inducing intense heteropathy in the hepatic system)

Main manifestations. Headache, dizziness, irritability, in some cases indistinct vision, pain in the rib region, bitter taste in the mouth, edges of the tongue reddened, whitish tongue coating, and *strung pulse.* If the manifestations observed are *intense headache,* dizziness, ringing in the ears, deafness, *reddened and painful eyes, irritability,* restless sleep, vomiting of blood, nosebleed, pain in the rib region, pain in the arms, *tip and edges of the tongue red,* coating yellow or sometimes yellow, thick, and dry, *pulse strung, accelerated, and vigorous,* the manifestation type is preponderance of fire heteropathy in the hepatic system. If this condition advances to the point that "hepatic Wind stirs within" (*kan feng nei tung* 肝 凤 内 动 [i.e., internal wind manifestation type develops, 5.1.1.2]), it can induce a Wind Attack Disorder (cerebrovascular accident) leading to hemiplegia, inability to speak, deviation of the mouth or eyes, and in some cases muscle spasms, coma, and other symptoms. For symptoms of hepatic Wind stirring within due to extreme intensity of Fire heteropathy, see chapter 9 [especially 9.1.3] on Heat Factor Disorder manifestation type determination and therapy.

Pathology. Hepatic yang rising in excess is due to excessive upward dispersion of hepatic yang *ch'i,* so that there is a preponderance of yang *ch'i* in the head and eyes; thus headache, dizziness, spots before the eyes, rise in blood pressure, and similar symptoms are observed. Bitter taste, rib pain, reddened edges of the tongue, and strung pulse are commonly seen manifestations of disorders that involve the circulation tracts (H, VF) associated with the hepatic and gall bladder systems. In hepatic Fire preponderance (repletion due to Fire heteropathy in the circulation tracts associated with the hepatic system, *kan huo chih sheng* 肝 火 炽 盛 , *kan ching shih huo* 肝 经 实 火), in addition to the usual manifestations of hepatic yang excess there are others that correspond to imbalance in favor of Fire or hot heteropathy. For instance, in "Fire preponderant above" (*huo sheng yü shang* 火 盛 于 上 [i.e., Fire heteropathy risen to the head]) there are intense headache and such other symptoms as reddened eyes and ringing in the ears. When preponderance of hepatic Fire affects the blood storage function, the hot heteropathy "forces the blood into uncontrolled motion" (*pi hsueh wang hsing* 迫 血 妄 行), which may give rise to vomiting of blood, nosebleed, and other symptoms. When the hepatic Fire impairs the sinews it can induce arm pains.

Reddening of the top and sides of the tongue, yellow tongue coating, and strung, accelerated pulse are all manifestations of Fire or hot heteropathy.
[Therapy omitted.]

8.2.3. Hepatic system yin insufficiency

Main manifestations. *Dizziness, persistent headache,* ringing in the ears or deafness, indistinct vision and night blindness, *insomnia and a tendency to dream,* in some cases numbness or tremor of the hands and feet, *tongue red and saliva scanty,* coating scanty or absent, pulse strung and small or small and accelerated.

Pathology. The hepatic system relies on the water of the renal system (2.1.5.1.4) for sustenance. Hepatic yin insufficiency is often brought about by renal yin insufficiency, in which the *ching* (3.3) is not transformed into blood, and blood cannot nourish the hepatic system. Hepatic yin insufficiency can also bring on "hepatic yang rising in excess." (This is, however, the depletion manifestation type, and is not the same as the repletion type discussed above [8.2.2]. It is not at all the same as the hepatic Fire preponderance which belongs to the repletion hot manifestation type. Although headache, dizziness, ringing in the ears, and deafness are also observed in the present type, the headache is persistent rather than intense, the dizziness is such that the patient does not want to open his eyes, and the aural symptoms are gradual in onset, unlike the sudden ringing in the ears associated with hepatic Fire heteropathy; in addition, the voice is low and indistinct. These symptoms can be diminished by pressure of the hands [on the ears].[3] An even clearer distinction is that in the present type the tongue and pulse

---

[3] The Chinese is unclear about where pressure is applied, but Dr. Ma Boying kindly clarified this point. Most of the modern handbooks do not discuss this manifestation type under this name or the alternative name *kan hsueh pu-tsu* 肝血不足 . Those that discuss it vary considerably in their enumeration of symptoms. All of those I have consulted, for instance, omit mention of low and indistinct voice and of hand pressure; e.g., Hu-pei Chung-i hsueh-yuan ed. 1978: 78, Pei-ching Chung-i hsueh-yuan ed. 1978: 120, and Chiang-su sheng wei-sheng-t'ing 江苏省 工生斤 ed. 1980: 145.

phenomena are those of yin depletion.) The tremors and numbness of the hands and feet come about because the yin dispersed body fluids are inadquate to sustain the hepatic system.

[Therapy omitted; modern diseases said sometimes to exhibit this manifestation type include hypertension, central retinitis—exact type unspecified—and chronic or protracted hepatitis.]

8.2.4. Gall bladder system hot heteropathy (hepatic and gall bladder system moist-hot heteropathy)

Main manifestations. Intense rhythmic pains in the rib region on the right side, yellow jaundice, urination brief with urine tinged yellow or scarlet, bitter taste in the mouth, dry throat, hot-cold alternation (6.1.1.2), and in some cases nausea and vomiting, distended abdomen but little food intake, *red tongue with yellow coating,* and *strung, accelerated pulse.*

Pathology. Because a hot heteropathy in the gall bladder system has brought about a failure of upward and outward dispersion in the hepatic and gall bladder systems, there is great pain in the right rib region. Hot heteropathy in the gall bladder tract brings about the bitter taste, dry throat, and hot-cold alternation. Since there is moist heteropathy in addition to hot, the heteropathy becomes static and "steams" (*yü cheng* 郁 蒸). Thus the jaundice and brief urination with tinged urine. The hepatic *ch'i* invades the stomach system ("hepatic and stomach system disharmony," 6.4.1.2.6); thus one observes nausea and vomiting, abdominal distension with little food intake, and other splenetic and stomach system symptoms. The tongue and pulse manifestations are of the hot type.

[Therapy omitted; modern diseases said sometimes to exhibit this manifestation type include acute cholelithiasis (gallstones) and acute and chronic cholecystitis.]

8.2.5. Important points in hepatic and gall bladder system manifestation type determination and therapy

1. Hepatic system disorders mostly belong to the yang excess manifestation type. If they are prolonged, they tend to debilitate the hepatic yin, giving rise to yin depletion-yang excess manifestations. The therapeutic technique is "replenishing the hepatic yin"

(*yang kan yin* 养 肝 阴 , 12.16.0) and "calming the hepatic yang" (*p'ing kan yang* 平 肝 阳 , 12.15.0).

2. Most hepatic system depletion manifestations belong to the yin depletion type. "The hepatic and renal systems have a common source"; thus therapy should nourish the *ch'i* of both.

8.3. Splenetic and Stomach Systems (2.1.3)

The main physiological functions of the splenetic system are control of transmission and assimilation of food and governance of the blood. As for pathological changes, disorders of the splenetic system are mostly of the moist and depletion types (mostly yang depletion manifestation type), and those of the stomach system mostly of the hot and repletion types (its depletion manifestations are mostly of the stomach system yin depletion manifestation type). The splenetic and stomach systems are the "root of the postnatal vitalities."[4] Once depletion occurs it can affect all five of the yin visceral systems. Its relation with the cardiac, renal, and pulmonary systems is particularly close (pulmonary and splenetic system simultaneous depletion manifestations will be discussed in connection with the pulmonary system, 8.4.6).

8.3.1. Splenetic system yang depletion (splenetic and stomach system depletion cold manifestation type)

Main manifestations. Face yellow and deficient in luster; distension and pain in the stomach cavity or belly, with the *pain temporarily diminished by heat or pressure;* drooling a clear liquid [ptyalism]; poor appetite; *thin stool* or in some cases protracted diarrhea; *languor; lack of warmth in the extremities; protracted voiding of clear urine;* or in some cases *scanty urination and edema; emaciation; pale tongue with whitish, moist coating;* and *moderate or weak pulse.*

---

[4] *Hou t'ien chih pen* 后 天 之 本 ; see 2.3.4. The point is that the splenetic and stomach systems perform a central function in the assimilation of energy from food and inspired air, contrasted with the renal system's role with respect to the inborn primordial *ch'i* (8.5.0).

Pathology. The splenetic yang depletion (depletion cold manifestation type) causes a weakening of the transmission and assimilation functions of the splenetic and stomach systems, thus the yellow and lusterless face, poor appetite, thin stool, and stomach cavity and belly distension and pain diminished by heat or pressure (diminution of pain by heat indicates the cold manifestation type, and by pressure, the depletion manifestation type). The splenetic system governs the extremities and the flesh; when the splenetic yang *ch'i* is inadequate, the extremities lack warmth and are languid, and the flesh is emaciated. In splenetic yang depletion the transmission and assimilation of liquids is inadequate, so that one observes protracted voiding of clear urine or scanty urine accompanied by edema. The tongue and pulse phenomena are those of yang depletion.
[Therapy omitted.]

8.3.2. Splenetic and stomach system *ch'i* depletion (insufficiency of the medial *ch'i*, 3.1.2)

Main manifestations. Face yellow; *fatigue; poor appetite; pain in the stomach cavity temporarily diminished by pressure, or distress in the stomach cavity and abdominal distension;* belching; vomiting a sour liquid; *thin stool; tongue pale and soft and sometimes bearing toothmarks;* tongue coating whitish; pulse empty; and so on. If soft voice, shortness of breath, sensation of a drop in energy (*ch'i*) during activity, or abdominal or renal droop, prolapse of the anus or uterus and similar symptoms are noted, this is an even greater depletion in the active *ch'i* sector (9.1.2) called "sinking of the medial *ch'i*" (or "sinking of the splenetic *ch'i*"; 2.1.3.3). Simultaneous depletion of *ch'i* and blood in the splenetic and stomach systems can bring about all sorts of hemorrhage symptoms, and fever (moderate or in serious cases intense) may be noted. *Ch'i* depletion in the splenetic and stomach systems, with "invasion of the stomach system by hepatic *ch'i*" (*kan ch'i fan wei* 肝 气 犯 胃 [due to backflow, disrupts digestion]) may bring about pains in the stomach cavity, distension and fullness in the rib and abdominal regions, vomiting of a sour liquid or gurgling in the intestine with loose bowels, tongue coating whitish and unctuous, strung pulse, and other symptoms of hepatic and stomach system disharmony (6.4.1.6).

Pathology. Languor, diminished food intake, stomach cavity pain diminished by pressure, thin stool, and empty pulse are consequences of the *ch'i* depletion in the splenetic and stomach systems. If the depletion is more severe, the splenetic system's elevating function (2.1.3.3) becomes insufficiently vigorous, which may induce ptosis; such symptoms as shortness of breath and softness of voice are also observed.

The diminution in food intake due to this disorder further induces simultaneous depletion of *ch'i* and blood. Since the splenetic system is not governing the blood, all sorts of hemorrhage manifestations may develop; or there may be fever without hemorrhage. Since such fever is not brought on by external stimuli (*wai kan* 外 感), it is called "fever due to internal disturbance" (*nei shang* 內 傷). The relation of hepatic to splenetic system is that of what restrains to what is restrained in the mutual conquest order (1.2.1). When the *ch'i* of the hepatic system is backed up, it may exercise restraint upon the splenetic and stomach systems and bring about digestive system dysfunction. When there are depletion and debility of the splenetic and stomach systems, invasion of the stomach system by the hepatic *ch'i* may result, bringing about symptoms of hepatic and stomach system disharmony.

[Therapy omitted; no modern diseases are mentioned in this subsection.]

8.3.3. Splenetic system blocked by moist heteropathy (splenetic system depletion with blockage by moist heteropathy, moist heteropathy blocking the splenetic yang *ch'i*)

Main manifestations. Diminished diet; fullness and distress in the stomach cavity or even nausea; *insipid taste in the mouth or viscous saliva,* with preference in some cases for hot drinks; *head heavy as though bound up; lassitude in the extremities;* sluggishness in speech and movement; in some cases edema, loose bowels, and White Band Disorder (5.1.4.1); and in most cases *tongue coating thick and unctuous,* and *pulse moderate.*

Pathology. "Splenetic system blocked by moist heteropathy" (*p'i wei shih k'un* 脾 為 濕 困) means that the transmission and assimilation functions of the splenetic system are obstructed by moist, turbid heteropathy (*shih cho* 濕 濁 , 2.1.1.2, 5.1.4.2); thus such symptoms as decrease in diet, fullness and distress in the stomach cavity, and nausea and vomiting. Because the splenetic system governs the extremities, one observes lassitude. With the moist heteropathy creating a blockage within and the pure yang *ch'i* [refined from food] unable to disperse upward, the head is heavy. Because the moist heteropathy becomes concentrated below, in most cases there are loose bowels and White Band Disorder. The oral, tongue coating, and pulse phenomena are manifestations of serious moist heteropathy. Fat, soft tongue and empty pulse indicate splenetic system depletion in addition to the blockage by moist heteropathy. In most cases splenetic depletion first makes it impossible for the moisture to be assimilated, and blockage by moist heteropathy is the next step.

[Therapy omitted; modern diseases said sometimes to exhibit this manifestation type include chronic gastritis, chronic enteritis, chronic dysentery, chronic hepatitis, and dropsy.]

8.3.4. Moist-hot heteropathy collecting in the splenetic system

Main manifestations. Scleral or general jaundice, sometimes accompanied by general itching; local swelling and general distension in the stomach cavity and rib region; *lack of interest in eating; bodily fatigue; scarlet or yellow urine;* in some cases thirst or bitter taste in the mouth; fever; thin stool; yellow, unctuous tongue coating; and soft, accelerated pulse.

Pathology. Moist-hot heteropathy collecting in the splenetic and stomach systems (*shih je nei yun* 湿 热 内 蕰) may affect the upward and outward dispersion functions of the hepatic and gall bladder systems (2.1.2.1.1). The gall bile overflows into the skin, producing yellow jaundice and itching skin. Abnormality in the transmission and assimilation functions brings about lack of interest in eating, thin stool, and tinged urine. If the balance favors the hot heteropathy, thirst, bitter taste, fever, and similar symptoms are observed. The tongue and pulse manifestations are characteristic.

Therapy. "Clearing the hot heteropathy and freeing the moist heteropathy" (*ch'ing je li shih* 清 热 利 湿), using Capillary Artemisia Infusion (*yin-ch'en-hao t'ang* 茵 陈 蒿 汤 , 12.5.1.4) or Capillary Artemisia Fourfold Ling Infusion (*yin-ch'en ssu ling t'ung*

茵 陈 四 苓 汤).[5] Infectious hepatitis, leptospirosis, and acute cholecystitis associated with this manifestation type may be so treated.

8.3.5. Cardiac and splenetic system depletion; splenetic and renal system yang depletion

Main manifestations. In the cardiac and splenetic depletion manifestation type, *faded yellow complexion, regular throbbing of the heart and absent-mindedness, insomnia, languor, diminished appetite,* distended abdomen, thin stool, tongue coating whitish and moist, and pulse small and weak. In the splenetic and renal yang depletion type, *mental lethargy,* weak breathing and drawling speech; in some cases sounds of phlegm or asthmatic symptoms; *cold or lack of strength in the extremities; thin stool;* sometimes predawn loose bowel movement, *cold loins with aversion to low temperature;* edema over the whole body or on the abdomen; *whitish, moist tongue coating;* and *small, weak pulse.*

Pathology. Both of these manifestation types occur due to the influence of pathological changes in one visceral system upon a related system, or heteropathy functioning in two visceral systems at once. For instance, in the cardiac and splenetic system depletion manifestation type, one notes not only such cardiac system *ch'i* depletion manifestations as throbbing of the heart, insomnia, and absent-mindedness, but also such splenetic depletion manifestations as diminished appetite, abdominal distension, thin stool, and languor. Whitish, moist tongue coating and small, weak pulse are manifestations of cardiac and splenetic system yang depletion. Splenetic and renal system yang depletion similarly combines manifestations.

[Therapy omitted.]

---

[5] This prescription is named after one of its ingredients, the sclerotium of China-root (*fu-ling* 茯 苓 [Poria cocos]). It is an adaptation of a four-ingredient formula, hence the name. The composition given in the *Revised Outline* (12.5.0) is for a powdered medicine (*san* 散), not an infusion, but this prescription is prepared in both forms.

8.3.6. Stomach system Fire preponderance (heteropathic Fire disturbing the stomach system, stomach Fire blazing); stomach system yin depletion

Main manifestations. In stomach system Fire preponderance type, there are *fever, constipation,* toothache, *bleeding gums,* vomiting of blood, nosebleed, agitation, dry mouth, *bitter taste in the mouth, red tongue with yellow coating,* and *accelerated pulse.* In the stomach system yin depletion type there are *diminished diet* or even complete loss of appetite; and in some cases hectic, intermittent, or moderate fever; constipation; *red tongue* with little or no coating; and *small or small and accelerated pulse.*

Pathology. In stomach system Fire preponderance, since yang *ch'i* is preponderant the heteropathy is hot, thus the fever. Because Fire or hot heteropathy damages the dispersed body fluids there are agitation and constipation. Since it is characteristic of Fire to flame upward and force the blood into uncontrolled motion there are vomiting of blood and nosebleed. The upward rush of stomach system Fire along the stomach's yang brightness circulation tract (V, table 4.1) can bring about swelling and pain in or hemorrhage of the gums. The preponderance of stomach system Fire heteropathy is responsible for the appearance of the bitter taste and dry mouth, yellow tongue coating, accelerated pulse, and other manifestations of Fire or hot heteropathy.

Stomach system yin depletion may also bring about hot manifestations—the so-called "yin depletion giving rise to internal hot heteropathy" (7.4.3)—but this is not the same as the repletion hot manifestation type (7.3.2). Although there is fever or hectic fever, the degree is not great; although there is constipation the tongue coating is not yellow and thick, but rather scant or absent; although there is diminution of diet, it is not due to stomach system *ch'i* depletion (inadequate digestive function) but is instead induced by yin dispersed body fluid insufficiency (diminished digestive juices). Stomach system Fire preponderance may impair the yin aspect, and stomach system yin depletion may give rise to hot heteropathy, but the former is repletion Fire manifestation type and the latter is depletion type. Their essential character is thus different.

[Therapy omitted; modern medical conditions said sometimes to exhibit this manifestation type include high fevers, ulcers (mainly gastrointestinal), periodontitis, blood disease (not further defined), tuberculosis, chronic gastritis, diabetes mellitus, and dysentery.]

8.3.7. Important points in splenetic and stomach system manifestation type determination and therapy

1. Disorders of the splenetic system mostly involve moist heteropathy. Regardless of whether the manifestation type is cold or hot, depletion or repletion, moist heteropathy usually plays an integral part in the disorder. It may be that preponderance of moist heteropathy blocks the splenetic system, or that splenetic depletion precedes the blockage. In therapy, in accord with the characteristic tendency of splenetic depletion and repletion to evolve into each other or often to be intermixed, one should demark the type in which there is more of repletion than depletion from its opposite, and flexibly employ the method of "vaporizing the moist heteropathy" (*hua shih* 化 湿 , 12.5.0) in the one case and that of "strengthening the splenetic system" (*chien p'i* 健 脾 , 12.16.0) in the other.

2. In the splenetic system depletion manifestation type, depletion of the cardiac or renal system is often also noted; both affected systems should be treated. Protracted pulmonary depletion may also give rise to the splenetic depletion manifestation type. One uses the "replenishing the splenetic *ch'i*" method (12.16.0) to bring the pulmonary *ch'i* to an adequate level; this is called the technique of "cultivating Earth to produce Metal," 1.2.2).

3. The splenetic and stomach systems form an "inner-outer" relation (2.1.3.3). Clinically the cold and depletion manifestation types belong to the splenetic system, and the hot repletion types to the stomach system. Yang depletion belongs to the splenetic system and yin depletion to the stomach system.

8.4. Pulmonary and Large Intestine Systems (2.1.4)

The main physiological functions of the pulmonary system are control of the *ch'i* (2.1.4.1.1) and of clearing away and carrying downward (2.1.4.1.2). The majority of pathological changes are disorders of the respiratory system. The repletion and cold manifestation types include "phlegm obstructing the pulmonary system" (*t'an cho tsu fei* 痰 浊 阻 肺) and coughing and labored breathing due to pulmonary system cold heteropathy. The repletion and hot manifestation types include coughing and labored breathing due to pulmonary system hot heteropathy. Among those which belong to the depletion manifestation type are pulmonary system *ch'i* depletion, pulmonary system yin depletion, pulmonary and splenetic system depletion, and pulmonary and renal system depletion. The most commonly noted manifestation type of large intestine system disorder is the large intestine system moist-hot heteropathy type.

8.4.1. Phlegm obstructing the pulmonary system (mucus invading the pulmonary system)

Main manifestations. Coughing and labored, noisy breathing; sound of phlegm in the throat; *sticky, thick, and profuse mucus;* fullness, distress, and pain in the chest and rib regions; inability to lie horizontally; *turbid, unctuous tongue coating;* and *smooth pulse.* If hot or cold heteropathy is involved, corresponding manifestations and pulse phenomena appear.

Pathology. The phlegm obstructing the pulmonary system (*t'an cho tsu fei, t'an yin fan fei* 痰 浊 阻 肺   痰 饮 犯 肺) keeps the pulmonary *ch'i* from flowing freely; thus the series of respiratory symptoms. The tongue coating and pulse phenomena are manifestations of the mucous type (3.5). If there is also pulmonary cold heteropathy, the mucus is thin and usually foamy, tongue pale, coating unctuous, and pulse sluggish and smooth; if hot heteropathy, the mucus is mostly thick and yellow, there is fever in some cases, the tongue is red and its coating yellow, and the pulse is smooth and accelerated.

[Therapy omitted.]

8.4.2. Coughing and labored breathing due to pulmonary cold heteropathy (wind-cold heteropathy constricting the pulmonary system)

Main manifestations. Frequent and intense coughing; forced respiration; mucus viscous, white, and profuse, and in some cases thin but not easily coughed up; in serious cases, asthmatic cough and chest distress; inability to lie horizontally; in some cases fever and abnormal sensitivity to cold; *tongue coating whitish and smooth;* and *pulse floating and tense* or tense.

Pathology. The pulmonary system contains cold heteropathy or cold mucus, so the pulmonary *ch'i* is unable to clear away and carry downward; thus the coughing with profuse mucus, and in serious cases thoracic distress, forced respiration, and inability to lie flat.

In disorders brought on by cold heteropathy, fever and sensitivity to cold are also noted. The whitish, smooth tongue coating and tense pulse are cold manifestations.

[Therapy omitted; modern medical conditions said sometimes to exhibit this manifestation type include acute and chronic bronchitis, asthmatic bronchitis, and bronchial asthma.]

8.4.3. Coughing and labored breathing due to pulmonary hot heteropathy

Main manifestations. Coughing; gasping, forced breath; yellow, viscous, and thick mucus; in some cases coughing or vomiting purulent blood; rank or foul breath; throat or chest pain; in some cases abnormal sensitivity to cold accompanied by fever; *red tongue with yellow or yellow and unctuous coating;* and *accelerated or smooth and accelerated pulse.*

Pathology. There are repletion hot manifestations in the pulmonary system and adhesion by mucous hot heteropathy (*t'an je chiao chieh* 痰 热 胶 结), so that the pulmonary *ch'i* is unable to move freely; thus coughing and labored breathing are both observed. When there is obstruction by mucous hot heteropathy preventing free circulation in the tracts associated with the pulmonary system, fullness of the chest may be observed. When hot heteropathy is predominant and there is blood coagulation, the blood and flesh decay; there may be vomiting of purulent blood, and cold sensitivity and fever may also be noted. The tongue and pulse phenomena are those of the hot and repletion manifestation types.

[Therapy omitted; modern medical conditions said sometimes to exhibit this manifestation type include acute and chronic bronchitis, bronchial asthma, the initial and middle stages of pneumonia, bronchodilatation, and pulmonary abscess.]

8.4.4. Pulmonary system *ch'i* depletion

Main manifestations. Coughing and shortness of breath; in serious cases, gasping, forced breath or respiratory difficulties; mucus profuse, clear, and thin; fatigue; drawling speech; *soft, indistinct voice;* aversion to cold; perspiration without external cause; facial pallor; *tongue pale and soft;* and *pulse empty or weak.* If chest pain and spots of coagulated blood on the sides of the tongue are also noted it is *ch'i* depletion combined with blood coagulation.

Pathology. In pulmonary *ch'i* depletion, because of the *ch'i* insufficiency there are coughing and shortness of breath, and soft, indistinct voice. Because it is *ch'i* depletion, mucus is produced, thus the profuse, clear, and thin mucus. In pulmonary *ch'i* insufficiency, the surface of the body is no longer normally impermeable; for this reason there are aversion to cold and perspiration without external cause. The tongue and pulse phenomena are those of the depletion manifestation type. The pale face indicates pulmonary *ch'i* insufficiency.

[Therapy omitted; modern medical conditions said sometimes to exhibit this manifestation type include chronic bronchitis, pulmonary tuberculosis, pulmonary emphysema, and bronchial asthma.]

8.4.5. Pulmonary yin depletion (pulmonary system dryness due to yin depletion)

Main manifestations. Coughing without mucus or with scanty, viscous mucus, sometimes bloody; *hectic or intermittent fever;* nocturnal sweating; *hot sensation in the palms of the hands and the soles of the feet; flushed cheeks in the afternoon;* insomnia; dry mouth and throat; in some cases hoarse voice; *tongue red and soft with little coating;* and *pulse small and accelerated.*

Pathology. Since the dispersed body fluids are insufficient, there is coughing with little or no mucus; because of the inability of these fluids to nourish with their moisture the circulation tracts associated with the pulmonary system, it is easy for the circulation tracts to be damaged by coughing, so that the mucus bears blood. Yin depletion produces internal hot heteropathy; thus the fever and dryness of mouth and throat. Since in yin depletion Water cannot constrain the Fire, internal Fire heteropathy creates a disturbance which forces the dispersed body fluids to drain out, giving rise to nocturnal sweating, and which disturbs the mind and brings about insomnia. The tongue and pulse phenomena are characteristic of yin depletion, and flushed cheeks in the afternoon are frequently seen in the pulmonary system yin depletion manifestation type.

[Therapy omitted; modern medical conditions said sometimes to exhibit this manifestation type include pulmonary tuberculosis, chronic bronchitis, and bronchodilatation.]

8.4.6. Pulmonary and splenetic system depletion; pulmonary and renal system depletion

Main manifestations. Pulmonary and splenetic system depletion mostly belongs to the *ch'i* depletion manifestation type. Its main manifestations are *protracted coughing; profuse, clear, thin mucus;* complexion deficient in luster; emaciation; *languor; diminished diet; distended abdomen and thin stool; tongue tissues soft and pale in color* with whitish coating; and *pulse small, or empty and large.*

Pulmonary and renal system depletion mostly belongs to the yin depletion manifestation type. Its main manifestations are *coughing with scanty mucus, shortness of breath during activity, pale complexion with flushed cheeks,* hectic or intermittent fever or mental upset accompanied by hot sensations in the Five Hearts (heart, palms of hands, soles of feet), *emaciation,* insomnia, *nocturnal sweating,* dry mouth in the evening, *aching loins and flabby legs,* involuntary loss of sperm [spermatorrhea], *tongue red with scanty coating,* and *pulse small and accelerated.*

Pathology. The splenetic and pulmonary systems and the pulmonary and renal systems contribute to each other's vitality; depletion in one system is likely to bring about depletion and manifestations of medical disorder in both. For instance, in pulmonary and splenetic system *ch'i* depletion there are such symptoms of the pulmonary *ch'i* depletion manifestation type as protracted coughing with profuse, clear, thin mucus, as well as such manifestations of the splenetic depletion manifestation type as fatigue, emaciation, diminished diet, and abdominal distension and thin stool. Pulmonary and renal system depletion, in addition to manifestations of pulmonary yin depletion, exhibits such manifestations of renal yin depletion as dry mouth in the evening, aching loins and flabby legs, and involuntary loss of sperm.

[Therapy omitted; certain refractory cases of tuberculosis are associated with this manifestation type.]

8.4.7. Large intestine system moist-hot heteropathy

Main manifestations. Abdominal pain; loose bowels; in some cases *tenesmus* (6.1.2.4) and *a viscous fluid or pus and blood* in the stool; or in some cases bloody bowel movement; bleeding piles; red tongue with white, thick or yellow, unctuous coating; and pulse sunken and accelerated.

Pathology. When moist-hot heteropathy collects in the large intestine system, heteropathy and orthopathy contend; thus the abdominal pain and loose bowels. If the heteropathy is relatively preponderant, the damage extends to the *ch'i* and blood, and the turbid *ch'i* weighs downward; thus the tenesmus. If the heteropathy invades the circulation tracts, the stool will carry pus and blood; if a moist-hot stasis develops in the blood vessels there is bloody stool or bleeding piles.

[Therapy omitted; no modern diseases are mentioned in this subsection.]

8.4.8. Important points in pulmonary and large intestine system manifestation type determination and therapy

1. The pulmonary system controls clearing away and carrying downward; the most important therapeutic method for pulmonary disorders is "clearing downward the pulmonary *ch'i*" (*ch'ing su fei ch'i* 清肃肺气 [for reversing an upward pulmonary *ch'i* backflow, 12.11.0]). If, however, the pulmonary *ch'i* is so inadequate that phlegm is not easily coughed up, or if the pulmonary *ch'i* is greatly depleted, one should "replenish the *ch'i* by elevation" (*sheng t'i pu ch'i* 升提补气 [i.e., via the splenetic system, 8.3.2, 12.16]).

2. Pulmonary system repletion hot and yin depletion manifestation types can both bring on coughing and spitting of blood, but the two types differ in character. It is necessary to heed tongue and pulse phenomena and other observed manifestations in order to distinguish the two.

3. The pulmonary and large intestine systems form an "inner-outer" relation and can affect each other, so in therapy attention should be paid to both. For instance, in treating the pulmonary system repletion hot manifestation type one should also use drugs which drain the large intestine [i.e., laxatives], since this is beneficial to the "clearing away and carrying down" function of the pulmonary *ch'i*. As another instance, in constipation due to *ch'i* and dispersed body fluid insufficiency (habitual constipation), rather than the technique of draining one should use drugs that replenish the pulmonary *ch'i* and moisten the large intestine system.

8.5. Renal and Urinary Bladder System (2.1.5)

"The renal system is the root of the prenatal endowment" (*hsien t'ien chih pen* 先 天 之 本 , cf. 8.3.0). Its physiological functions are control of the storage of *ching* (3.3) and control of water. In the renal system are stored the primordial yin and yang energies (3.1.1), which should be kept intact, avoiding their outward leakage. Pathological changes in this system are mostly of the depletion manifestation type, and are generally divided into the broad renal yin depletion and yang depletion classes, which include a variety of diseases of the reproductive, urinary, nervous, and endocrine systems. The most commonly observed manifestation type of urinary bladder system disorder is the urinary bladder moist-hot heteropathy type.

8.5.1. Renal system yin depletion

Main manifestations. Dizziness accompanied by disturbances of vision; ringing in the ears or deafness; *loose or aching teeth; insomnia; dry mouth at dusk;* mental upset accompanied by hot sensations in the Five Hearts [i.e., heart, palms of hands, soles of feet]; nocturnal sweating; *aches and pains in the hips and knees;* in some cases, pain in the shinbones; pain in the heels; *involuntary loss of semen; red, dry tongue,* sometimes with peeling coating; and *small, accelerated pulse.* If accompanied by reddening of the cheeks and lips, excessive sexual desire, brief urination with urine tinged scarlet, mouth extremely dry in the middle of the night, and acclerated pulse or strung, small, and accelerated pulse, it is yin depletion with intense Fire heteropathy (*yin hsu huo wang* 阴 虚 火 旺 , 2.1.5.1.4).

Pathology. In renal yin depletion the dispersed body fluids are insufficient, and the Ministerial Fire (*hsiang huo* 相 火)[6] waxes intense (also called "renal Fire waxing intense," (*wang sheng* 旺 盛); thus the Five Hearts symptom and the dry mouth at dusk (dusk belongs to yin, which is why the mouth dryness is more pronounced then). When there is a yin depletion the yang is in ex-

---

[6] *Note in the original.* This term denotes the internal Fire heteropathy stirred in the hepatic system by anger or, as in this case, in the renal system by lust.

cess; thus the visual, aural, and sleep symptoms. The control of the bones by the renal system is responsible for the bone aches and pains. "The teeth are the outcrop of the bone"; bone and marrow are inadequately nurtured by the circulation, thus the loose or aching teeth. In renal yin depletion the *ching* and dispersed body fluids are no longer immune to loss outward; thus the sweating and involuntary loss of semen. In more serious yin depletion the depletion Fire heteropathy (5.1.6.2) is intense, producing such manifestations of body fluid loss due to internal hot heteropathy (3.4) as flushed cheeks and lips, excessive sexual desire, and brief urination with urine tinged scarlet. The tongue and pulse phenomena are characteristic of yin depletion.

[Therapy omitted.]

8.5.2. Renal yang depletion

Main manifestations. Dull complexion, falling hair, *aversion to cold, lack of warmth in the hands and feet,* shortness of breath and noisy breathing, *mental fog,* ringing in the ears or deafness, loose teeth, aches and pains (or joint limpness) in the hips and knees, scanty urine and edema or profuse urine at night, *thin stool,* perspiration without external cause, *fat, soft tongue with whitish, moist coating,* and *pulse empty and floating, or sunken, retarded, and debilitated.* If the Fire of the Gate of Life (2.1.5.1.4) is weakened, impotence or "slipping semen" (*hua ching* 滑 精 , nocturnal emission without dreams), chronic diarrhea, cold extremities, sometimes shortness of breath and noisy breathing with perspiration, and weak or subtle, small, sunken, retarded pulse in the foot section (6.4.1.1), and so on, may appear. If the quantity of urine is great or if there are incontinence, profuse urination at night, persistent dripping after urination, "slipping semen" or premature ejaculation, soft tongue with whitish coating, and empty pulse with weak foot section, the renal *ch'i* is no longer immune to loss outward.

Pathology. The renal system is vented in the ears (2.1.5.1.6) and is manifested outwardly in the hair (2.1.5.1.7). The renal *ch'i* is inadequate, so there are ringing in the ears or deafness and falling hair. The renal system controls bone (2.1.5.1.3); since the renal yang *ch'i* is insufficient, aches and pains in the hips and knees and loose teeth may also occur. Because there is depletion in the renal system and it is unable to "admit *ch'i*" (*na ch'i kuei shen* 纳 气 归 肾 , 2.1.5.1.5), there are shortness of breath and difficult breathing. In renal yang depletion, general yang depletion ensues, and thus lack of warmth in the extremities, perspiration without external cause (in yang depletion the outer aspect is no longer impermeable), mental fog, and thin stool. Because of the flooding upward due to yang depletion (in renal depletion there is flooding upward, 2.1.5.1.2) there are scanty urine and edema. With the Fire of the Gate of Life weakened, the depletion cold manifestations become even more intense, so there are cold extremities, impotence, slipping semen, and predawn loose bowels. This weakening of the Fire of the Gate of Life is often accompanied by inability to admit *ch'i*, so that symptoms such as shortness of breath, difficult breathing, and perspiration are also noted. If the renal *ch'i* is no longer immune to loss outward it is no longer active in retaining the dispersed body fluids, so slipping semen, premature ejaculation, profuse urine, or urinary incontinence are noted. Generally in renal system yang depletion the pulse is empty and floating and the coating whitish and moist, but in yang depletion with flooding of Water the tongue is bound to be fat and soft and the pulse sunken and debilitated. If the pulse is sunken and retarded the balance has shifted far to the side of cold heteropathy.

[Therapy omitted; modern medical conditions said sometimes to exhibit this manifestation type include hypoadrenocorticism, hypothyroidism, sexual neurasthenia, chronic nephritis, and bronchial asthma.]

8.5.3. Renal yin and yang depletion

Main manifestations. Dull complexion; falling hair; teeth loose or painful; mouth dry; worry and mental upset; nocturnal sweating; cold extremities and aversion to cold; involuntary loss of semen; urine profuse at night; tongue pale, sometimes with fissures; coating thin; and pulse sunken and small or weak.

Pathology. Because of the mutual roots of yin and yang, protracted yin depletion may bring on yang depletion and vice versa. When this happens in the renal system, manifestations of both types are combined. In manifestation type determination one should, on the basis of the concrete situation, distinguish which depletion is the more serious and direct drug therapy accordingly.

[Therapy omitted; modern medical conditions that correspond to this manifestation type are those cited in 8.5.1 and 8.5.2.]

8.5.4. Cardiac and renal systems not in correspondence (*hsin shen pu chiao* 心 腎 不 交)

Main manifestations. Regular throbbing of the heart, worry and mental upset, dizziness, insomnia, absent-mindedness, ringing in the ears or deafness, aches and pains in the hips and knees, tongue soft and red, and pulse small or small and accelerated.

Pathology. The cardiac and renal systems interact, contribute to each other's vitality, and complement each other's functions. If their adjustment to each other is lost these symptoms appear.

[Therapy omitted; the only modern medical condition mentioned in this subsection is neurosis.]

8.5.5. Urinary bladder moist-hot heteropathy

Main manifestations. Hot sensations or abnormal sensitivity to cold; *frequent urination; excessive urge to urinate; painful urination;* in some cases urination difficult or unexpectedly terminated, urine turbid or bearing pus, blood, or sandy granules; *tongue coating yellow or yellow and unctuous;* and *pulse accelerated.*

Pathology. Because internal hot heteropathy is preponderant there are hot sensations; if these are accompanied by outer manifestations, sensitivity to cold is observed. The moist-hot heteropathy pours downward and causes interference with urination, thus the urinary symptoms. If the moist-hot heteropathy collects within for a long period, there will be sandy granules in the urine. If the heteropathy is in great preponderance there will be pus or blood in the urine. The tongue and pulse phenomena are characteristic of moist-hot heteropathy.

[Therapy omitted.]

8.5.6. Important points in renal and urinary bladder system manifestation type determination and therapy

1. In renal system disorders the repletion manifestation type is rare and the outer type is never found. The renal cold manifestation type is brought on by yang depletion, and the "renal Fire intense" condition by yin depletion. The root of the disorder is treated by replenishing the renal yang aspect or nourishing the renal yin aspect. Because the renal system controls the storage of *ching,* the

method of replenishing the yang aspect is usually to add yang-replenishing drugs to a yin-replenishing foundation. For instance, in Golden Casket Renal *Ch'i* Pellets (*chin kuei shen ch'i wan* 金 匱 腎 气 丸 , 12.16.0), a famous prescription for this purpose, Sichuan aconite root (*fu-tzu* 附 子 [Aconitum carmichaelii]) and Saigon cinnamon bark (*jou-kuei* 肉 桂 [Cinnamomum loureiroi]), which warm the renal yang, are added to the basic prescription for Six-ingredient Chinese Foxglove Pellets (*liu wei ti-huang wan* 六 味 地 黄 丸 , 12.16.0), which nourishes the renal yin. If the yang depletion is extremely pronounced one may depend entirely on reinforcing the yang aspect to match the yin (*fu yang i p'ei yin* 扶 阳 以 配 阴), but this method may be used only temporarily. If it is used for a long time the condition may turn into yin depletion.

2. The urinary bladder and renal systems form an "inner-outer" relation. For this reason the depletion cold manifestation type in the urinary bladder system is best treated at the root by replenishing the renal yang aspect. In treating urinary bladder system moist-hot heteropathy, one may proceed directly with "clearing and freeing" (12.5) the urinary bladder system.

8.6. Examples of Visceral System Manifestation Type Determination

[Omitted from the translation.]

8.7. Conclusion

Visceral system manifestation type determination is one of the traditional physician's most frequently used methods for determining the manifestation type. Conclusions reached by using it amount to a comprehensive and concrete diagnosis as a basis for therapy. In clinical applications the following points should be grasped:

1. On the basis of Eight Rubrics principles, concretely analyze the data from the four methods of examination, and correctly sum up the character of the disorder as yin or yang, cold or hot, depletion or repletion, and outer or inner.

2. On the basis of the special physiological and pathological characteristics of the visceral systems, considered jointly with the clinical observations, clarify the location and causes of the disease. (That is, clarify which circulation tract and system is affected,

whether the disorder is in the active *ch'i* or blood sector (9.1), and what heteropathy has brought it on.)

3. On the basis of the therapeutic principles of Chinese medicine, properly select and employ therapeutic techniques and drugs.

Thus when studying visceral system manifestation type determination and therapeutic reasoning, one should take a comprehensive view of the visceral systems and circulation tracts, the four methods of examination, the Eight Rubrics, etiology, therapeutic methods, materia medica, prescriptions, and so on. It is imperative to apply them all flexibly and learn by analogy.[7]

---

[7] Literally, "give three instances in reply to one."

9. Manifestation Type Determination and Therapy in Heat Factor Disorders

"Heat Factor Disorders" refers to acute disorders of which fever is the main characteristic, brought on by the exogenous Six Excesses (5.1) or pestilential *ch'i* [epidemic heteropathies, 5.2]. They include all sorts of infectious and non-infectious acute febrile disorders. Historically there have been three kinds of manifestation type determination for Heat Factor Disorders, one based on the six cardinal tract system (chapter 4); one based on the triple *chiao* system of functions (2.1.6); and one based on the defensive *ch'i*, active *ch'i*, constructive *ch'i*, and blood sectors (*wei, ch'i, ying, hsueh* 卫 气 营 血 , 3.1, 3.2, 3.1.3). Each has its advantages and disadvantages. This chapter will concentrate on the third system, but will introduce materials from the others as appropriate.[1]

---

[1] In this chapter only, in order to avoid confusion with the defensive and constructive *ch'i*, I translate the word *ch'i* as "active *ch'i*" when it denotes the second sector. The word "sector," which I have introduced to label the underlying concept of *fen* 分 , does not imply a simple geometrical or spatial division (9.1), but rather stages of the transmission of heteropathy between the outer and inner aspects of the body. No author localizes the four sectors; their relation to each other is not primarily spatial but sequential. The sense of "sector" is analogous to such common usages as "the industrial sector of the economy."

9.1. Manifestation Type Determination and Therapeutic Reasoning Using the Defensive *Ch'i*, Active *Ch'i*, Constructive *Ch'i*, and Blood Sectors

These four are part of the normal structure and functioning of the body, but when a heat factor disorder is contracted they successively undergo pathological changes in response. These changes follow definite rules. People have borrowed this set of four concepts to epitomize the manifestation types corresponding to four different stages of heat factor disorder, and adapted them to explain through the course of a disorder the depth at which the pathology is located, the seriousness of the illness, and its advance and retreat, thus providing a basis for therapy of heat factor disorders. Thus the pathological implications of the terms "defensive *ch'i*" "active *ch'i*" "constructive *ch'i*," and "blood" as used here differ from their implications in physiology.

There are four important points in this system of manifestation type determination and therapeutic reasoning.

1. Distinguishing the location of pathological changes. A defensive *ch'i* sector disorder in heat factor disorders is equivalent to the outer manifestation type in the Eight Rubrics system; disorders of the other three sectors are equivalent to the inner manifestation type. Defensive *ch'i* disorders mostly invade the pulmonary system's defensive *ch'i* (2.1.4.1.3), the extremities, and the head, nose, and throat; in the active *ch'i* sector they mostly invade the pulmonary, splenetic, stomach, large intestine, and gall bladder systems; in the constructive *ch'i* sector they mostly invade the cardiac and hepatic systems; and in the blood sector they mostly invade the cardiac, hepatic, and renal systems.

2. Demarking stages in the progress of the disorder. Heat factor disorders are divided into four stages according to the four sectors. The special features of defensive *ch'i* sector disorders are fever and abnormal sensitivity to cold, headache, tongue coating thin and whitish, and pulse floating or floating and accelerated. Those of the active *ch'i* sector are strong (that is, high) fever without abnormal sensitivity to cold, perspiration, dry mouth with desire to drink, red tongue with yellow coating, pulse swollen and accelerated or sunken and full. Those of the constructive *ch'i* sector are fever rising during the night, agitation, mind half-beclouded, raving, little thirst, in some cases a barely perceptible rash, tongue crimson with little or no coating, and pulse small and accelerated. Those of the blood sector are—on a foundation of those of the con-

structive sector—confused state of mind; sometimes agitation or manic behavior; clearly perceptible rash; and in serious cases vomiting of blood; blood in the stool or urine and other hemorrhagic symptoms; tongue tissues crimson or purple and dry; coating absent; and pulse sunken, small, and accelerated.

3. Recognizing the rules for transmission of pathological changes. Heat factor disorders usually begin in the defensive sector and follow the following sequence:

defensive sector

active *ch'i* sector

constructive *ch'i* sector

blood sector

From outer to inner and from mild to serious; this is the usual order of transmission. But sometimes changes do not appear in this order. The disorder may first appear in the active *ch'i* sector or even in the constructive *ch'i* or blood sector ("hidden heteropathy" [*fu hsieh* 伏 邪] of internal origin). It may be transmitted directly from the defensive *ch'i* sector to the constructive *ch'i* or blood sector. Two sectors may be affected simultaneously. The disorder may remain in the defensive *ch'i* and active *ch'i* sectors even after it has entered the other two, so that all four are affected at the same time. These various possibilities depend on the power of resistance of the body, its responsiveness, and the character of the heteropathy, and are sometimes related to the appropriateness of therapy and care.

4. Determining the therapeutic method. For disorders in the defensive *ch'i* sector, "flushing the outer aspect" (*chieh piao* 解 表 , 12.1.0) is recommended; for those in the active *ch'i* sector, "clearing the active *ch'i* sector" (*ch'ing ch'i* 清 气 , 12.2.2.1); for those in the constructive *ch'i* sector, "clearing the constructive *ch'i* and draining the hot heteropathy" (*ch'ing ying hsieh je* 清 营 泄 热 , 12.2.0); and for those in the blood sector, "cooling the blood and flushing the toxicity" (*liang hsueh chieh tu* 凉 血 解 毒 , 12.2.2.2).

Below we discuss manifestation type determination and therapy for each stage of heat factor disorders.

9.1.1. Defensive *ch'i* sector disorders

Defensive *ch'i* disorders are the initial stage of heat factor disorders. Their distinguishing features are *fever with abnormal sensitivity to cold*, headache and body aches, *thin, whitish tongue coating*, and *floating pulse*. In view of differences in the season of onset, character of the heteropathy, and responsiveness of the body, these disorders may be divided into five types.

9.1.1.1. Wind warm outer manifestation type

Main manifestations. Additionally, fever serious but sensitivity to cold mild, stuffed and running nose, coughing, *slight thirst, sides and tip of tongue slightly reddened*, and *pulse floating and accelerated*.

Pathology. This manifestation type occurs mainly in winter and spring, when wind-warm external heteropathy invades the pulmonary system's defensive *ch'i*. The warm heteropathy belongs to the hot type; thus the more serious fever, redness of the sides and tip of the tongue, and accelerated pulse. The hot heteropathy impairs the dispersed body fluids, thus the thirst. This is equivalent to the "outer hot manifestation type" in the Eight Rubrics system (7.2.2).

Therapy. [Beginning omitted.] The early stages of influenza, colds, acute conjunctivitis, acute tonsillitis, acute bronchitis, epidemic parotitis [i.e., mumps], and epidemic meningitis may be so treated when of this manifestation type.

9.1.1.2. Summer warm outer manifestation type

Main manifestations. Additionally, *heavy sensation in the body and distress in the stomach cavity*, with little or no sweat, *tongue coating whitish and unctuous, tongue slightly reddened*, and *soft and accelerated pulse*.

Pathology. This manifestation type mostly occurs in summer, due to prevalent heat heteropathy (5.1.3) or to availing oneself of cool air or cold drinks so that cold or moist heteropathy blocks the seasonal heat [, breaking the adjustment of the body to the regular climatic rhythms]. Cold heteropathy becomes static in the outer part of the flesh; thus the sensitivity to cold and lack of perspiration. The heat factor corresponds to Fire heteropathy, so there are fever and accelerated pulse. Heat heteropathy impairs the dispersed body fluids, thus the slight reddening of the tongue. Heat heteropathy is mostly accompanied by moist; thus the heavy feeling in the body, stomach cavity distress, and soft pulse.

Therapy. "Flushing the outer aspect and clearing the heat heteropathy," for which Newly Augmented Aromatic Madder Potion (*hsin chia hsiang-ju yin* 新加香薷饮 , 12.1.2.2) is often used. The early stages of influenza, colds, Japanese type B encephalitis, and other diseases may be so treated when of this manifestation type.

9.1.1.3. Moist warm outer manifestation type

Main manifestations. Additionally, *distended and heavy sensation in the head, heavy sensation in the extremities,* aches and pains in the joints, *whitish and unctuous tongue coating,* and *soft and moderate pulse.* This manifestation type usually occurs in seasons of copious rain, when moist and hot heteropathies invade the defensive periphery of the body. The nature of moisture is heavy, viscous, and sluggish, hence such symptoms as the heavy sensations and the whitish, unctuous tongue coating.

Therapy. "Flushing the outer aspect and vaporizing the moist heteropathy" (*chieh piao hua shih* 解表化湿), for which Three Kernel Infusion (*san jen t'ang* 三仁汤 , 12.5.0) with added stems and leaves of patchouli or agastache (*huo-hsiang* 藿香 [Pogostemon cablin or A. regosa]) and stems and leaves of eupatorium (*p'ei-lan* 佩兰 [E. japonicum or E. fortunei]) are often used. The early stages of typhoid fever, infectious hepatitis, leptospirosis, urinary infections, influenza, and colds may be so treated when of this manifestation type.

9.1.1.4. Autumn dry outer manifestation type

Main manifestations. Additionally, *dry cough;* dry mouth, throat, and nose; *tongue coating thin, whitish, and dry;* and *floating and small pulse.*

Pathology. This manifestation type mostly occurs in autumn, when dry heteropathy invades the pulmonary system's defensive *ch'i.* The pulmonary system and dispersed body fluids are readily impaired by dry heteropathy, thus the symptoms. Within the autumn dry manifestation type, when sensitivity to cold is more serious and the pulse is floating and tense, it is called the cool dry type; when the fever is more serious, there is thirst, and the pulse is floating and accelerated, it is called the warm dry type.

Therapy. [Beginning omitted.] Influenza, cold, infantile paralysis, and diphtheria may be so treated when of this manifestation type.

9.1.1.5. Wind cold outer manifestation type

This manifestation type corresponds to the *outer cold manifestation type of the Eight Rubrics system* (7.2.1); it is the "mature yang disorder" (*t'ai-yang ping* 太 阳 病) of the Six Warps system (9.5.1). It mostly occurs in the cold part of winter, when wind-cold heteropathic *ch'i* infiltrate the defensive periphery of the body. For therapy "flushing the outer aspect with pungent and warming drugs" (*hsin wen chieh piao* 辛 温 解 表 , 12.1.1.1) is recommended. For the outer cold repletion manifestation type, Ephedra Infusion (*ma-huang t'ang* 麻 黄 汤 , 12.1.0) or Chingchieh and Anisomeles Infusion for Flushing the Outer Aspect (*ching fang chieh piao t'ang* 荆 防 解 表 汤 , 14.1.1) is used; for the outer cold depletion manifestation type Cassia Twig Infusion (*kuei-chih t'ang* 桂 枝 汤 , 12.1.0) is used to regulate the defensive periphery of the body. Influenza, colds, and other disorders which exhibit symptoms of the wind cold outer manifestation type may be so treated.

Of the five types described above, the wind warm outer manifestation type is observed most often. The tongue coating turning from whitish to yellow is an important sign of transmission from the defensive *ch'i* to the active *ch'i* sector. The summer warm outer manifestation type (without admixture of cold heteropathy) is transmitted most quickly, so its course in the defensive *ch'i* sector is often very short. Next in order are the wind warm, moist warm, and autumn dry types; the wind cold outer type is transmitted most slowly.

9.1.2. Active *ch'i* sector disorders

This is the second stage of heat factor disorders. Its special features are *higher fever* without abnormal sensitivity to cold, thirst, reddened tongue with *yellow coating*, and *accelerated pulse*. When the heteropathy has entered the active *ch'i* sector, the heteropathic and orthopathic *ch'i* [due to their struggle, 7.3.2] are both at an abnormally high level. Excess of active *ch'i* is Fire, so the outcome is the active *ch'i* sector hot manifestation type. Except for the moist warm type, *all forms of defensive* ch'i *sector disorder, after they have passed into the active* ch'i *sector, are transformed into the hot manifestation type, so there is no need for further distinctions involving wind, cold, cool, and dry*. Six types are often clinically observed.

9.1.2.1. Active *ch'i* sector hot heteropathy preponderance (hot heteropathy in the active *ch'i* sector)

Main manifestations. Additionally, *great fever, great thirst, profuse perspiration, pulse swollen and large*, tongue coating yellow and dry, face flushed, and in some patients delusional speech and muscle spasms.

Pathology. The hot preponderance is responsible for the fever and flushed face. Internal hot heteropathies impel the dispersed body fluids, hence the profuse sweat. The fever and perspiration damage the body fluids, thus the thirst and tongue coating. Hot heteropathy disturbs the mind, thus the raving. Extreme intensity of hot heteropathy gives rise to [internal] wind heteropathy, thus the convulsions.

Therapy. [Beginning omitted.] Influenza and Japanese type B encephalitis often produce this manifestation type, and may be so treated.

9.1.2.2. Mucous hot heteropathy obstructing the pulmonary system

Main manifestations. Additionally, *coughing, chest pain, profuse yellow phlegm, labored and noisy breathing*, and *pulse smooth and accelerated*.

Pathology. In this manifestation type hot heteropathy impairs the pulmonary system and cooks down the dispersed body fluids to yellow phlegm. The pulmonary system loses its ability to carry out its circulation functions (*hsuan chiang* 宣 降 , 2.1.4.1.1, 2.1.4.1.2); thus the panting, coughing, and chest pain.

Therapy. [Beginning omitted.] Acute bronchitis, lobar pneumonia, and other disorders that exhibit these manifestations may be so treated.

9.1.2.3. Stomach and intestine system repletion hot manifestation type

Main manifestations. Intense fever or intense hectic fever; constipation, or bowels running a yellow, malodorous, thin liquid; distension and fullness of the abdomen; abdominal pain aggravated by pressure; agitation and raving; profuse perspiration of the hands and feet; *reddened tongue with yellow, dry coating, or grey or black coating with spikes; and pulse sunken, accelerated, and vigorous.*

Pathology. This manifestation type is formed when hot heteropathy enters the inner aspect and becomes involved in a stasis due to an Accumulation Disorder (6.1.3). With internal hot heteropathy preponderant the dispersed body fluids are impaired; thus the fever, sweat, and tongue phenomena. The hot heteropathy disturbs the mind; thus the raving. Excrement dries up and solidifies in the intestines; thus the abdominal distension, fullness, and pain, which may be accompanied by either constipation or loose bowels.

Therapy. "Draining and bringing down" (12.9) to drain the hot heteropathy; Great *Ch'i* Acceptance Infusion (*ta ch'eng ch'i t'ang* 大承气汤, 12.9.0) is usually used. When the abdominal distension and pain are comparatively serious, increase the amount of poncirus fruit (*chih-shih* 枳 实 [P. trifoliata]) and magnolia bark (*hou-p'o* 厚 朴 [M. officinalis]). If the drying and solidification of excrement is more serious, increase the rhubarb root (*ta-huang* 大 黄 [Rheum spp.]) and epsom salts (*mang-hsiao* 芒 硝 [MgSO$_4$· 7H$_2$0]); if the dry mouth and tongue are more serious, increase the raw Chinese foxglove root (*sheng ti-huang* 生 地 黄 [Rehmannia glutinosa]) and lily-turf root (*mai-tung* 麦 冬 [Ophiopogon japonicus or Liriope spicata]). In general, after one or two doses, when the draining has been accomplished, modify the therapy according to the manifestation type. The intermediate and advanced stages of influenza and Japanese type B encephalitis, if these symptoms appear, may be so treated.

***9.1.2.4. Active ch'i sector moist warm manifestation type
(internal hot heteropathy with moist heteropathy intermixed,
moist-hot heteropathy internal stasis)***

Main manifestations. Additionally, *heavy sensation in the body
and chest distress;* abdominal region distended and full; *dry mouth
and throat without desire to drink; apathy; loss of hearing; urination
brief and harsh* (not flowing freely); uncomfortable bowel movement;
red tongue; yellowish white, thick, unctuous coating; and *strung,
moderate pulse.* Some cases are likely to be accompanied by loose
bowels or skin jaundice, white heat rash, a red rash, or mental confusion and raving.

Pathology. This manifestation type is due to moist-hot
heteropathy blocking the active *ch'i* sector. The white heat rash is
sudamina, small millet-shaped white transparent vesicles that appear on the skin when, due to internal stasis of moist-hot
heteropathy, perspiration is not thoroughly excreted. It mostly occurs on the skin of the neck, abdomen, and chest. Prognosis is
favorable if the heat rash is full and lustrous, and unfavorable if it
is dried out, greyish, and dull. The mental symptoms and tongue
phenomena are due to obstruction of the cardiac orifices by phlegm
carried by the moist-hot heteropathy. This mental confusion is distinct from that caused by hot heteropathy entering the Cardiac Envelope Junction system (9.1.3.4).

Therapy. [Beginning omitted.] Typhoid, leptospirosis, infectious
hepatitis, and acute bacillary dysentery with indications of this
manifestation type may be so treated.

***9.1.2.5. Active and defensive ch'i simultaneous disorder (ch'i
wei t'ung ping*** 气 工 同 病 *)*

This has the specific features of active *ch'i* disorders and *at the
same time such manifestations of defensive ch'i disorders as abnormal
sensitivity to cold and body pains.* It comes about when an external
heteropathy passes into the active *ch'i* sector without having been
flushed from the defensive *ch'i* sector. Chinese doctors often say "so
much abnormal cold sensitivity means that much outer manifestation type," which shows the important significance of this symptom
in diagnosing the outer type. In therapy the technique of "flushing
the outer aspect" and "clearing the active *ch'i* sector" (9.1) are used.
For instance, for influenza patients whose symptoms indicate both

external and internal hot heteropathy, White Tiger Infusion (*pai hu t'ang* 白 虎 汤 , 12.2.0) and Honeysuckle-Forsythia Powder (*yin ch'iao san* 银 翘 散, 12.1.0) may be used. If the symptoms indicate external cold and internal hot heteropathy, use Hare's-ear and Kudzu Flesh-flushing Infusion (*ch'ai ko chieh chi t'ang* 柴 葛 解 肌 汤 , containing hare's-ear root [*ch'ai-hu* 柴 胡 , Bupleurum falcatum or B. scorzoneraefolium]; kudzu root [*ko-ken* 葛 根 , Pueraria lobata]; chianghuo root [*ch'iang-huo* 羌 活 , Noto-pterygium incisium]; Chinese angelica root [*pai-chih* 白 芷 , A. anomala or A. dahurica]; root of Baikal skullcap [*huang-ch'in* 黄 芩 , Scutellaria baicalensis]; peony root [*pai-shao* 白 芍 , Paeonia lactiflora]; root of balloon flower [*chieh-keng* 桔 梗 , Platycodon grandiflorum]; licorice root; gypsum [*shih-kao* 石 膏 , $CaSO_4 \cdot 2H_2O$]; fresh ginger root [*sheng-chiang* 生 姜 , Zingiber officinale]; and jujubes [*ta-tsao* 大 枣 , Zizyphus jujuba]). These are all techniques for "flushing both the outer and inner aspects" (*piao li shuang chieh*, 7.1.3).

9.1.2.6. Half-outer half-inner manifestation type

Main manifestations. Alternating fever and chills (6.1.1.2), full-ness and distress in the chest and rib regions, nausea, poor appetite, worry and mental upset, bitter taste in the mouth and dry throat, dull-ness of vision or spots before the eyes, whitish tongue coating, and strung pulse. This manifestation type is brought about when the heteropathy invades the circulation tract associated with the gall bladder system (VF), and heteropathy and orthopathy contend in the region between inner and outer. It corresponds to the "imma-ture yang disorder" (*shao-yang ping* 少 阳 病) of the six cardinal tract manifestation type determination system (9.5).

Therapy. [Beginning omitted.] Influenza, biliary duct infections, and malaria may be treated if their manifestations are of this type. For malaria, Chinese quinine root (*ch'ang-shan* 常 山 [Dichroa febrifuga or Orixa japonica]) and fruit of tsaoko cardamon (*ts'ao-kuo* 草 果 [Amomum tsao-ko]) may be added to the prescription [for Minor Hare's-ear Infusion, *hsiao ch'ai-hu t'ang* 小 柴 胡 汤 , 12.7.0] directed against this manifestation type.

9.1.3. Constructive *ch'i* sector disorders

Most of these disorders are transmitted from the active *ch'i* and defensive *ch'i* sectors, but in some cases as soon as the disorder occurs it is found in the constructive *ch'i* sector. If disorders of this type are treated in time, it is possible to vent (*t'ou* 透) the hot heteropathy into the active *ch'i* sector. Constructive *ch'i* sector disorders may go on to invade the cardiac and hepatic systems, giving rise to symptoms of "hot heteropathy entering the Cardiac Envelope Junction system" (*je ju hsin pao* 热 入 心 包 , 9.1.3.4) and "hot heteropathy activating hepatic wind" (*je tung kan feng* 热 动 肝 风, 5.1.1.2).

9.1.3.1. Constructive *ch'i* sector disorder (hot heteropathy in the constructive *ch'i* sector)

Main manifestations. Fever, stronger in the evening; not much thirst; *agitation* or raving; in some cases a barely perceptible rash; *crimson tongue without coating; small, accelerated pulse.*

Pathology. The hot heteropathy entering this sector impairs the constructive yin *ch'i;* thus the fever, aggravated in the evening, and the tongue and pulse phenomena [of yin character]. The heteropathy steams (*cheng* 蒸) the constructive yin *ch'i* upward, hence thirst is not great. As the hot heteropathy disturbs the mind there is agitation or raving, and as it has entered the circulation tract system the rash is barely visible.

Therapy. "Clearing the constructive *ch'i* sector and draining the hot heteropathy," for which Constructive *Ch'i* Clearing Infusion (*ch'ing ying t'ang* 清 营 汤 , 12.2) is often used. Japanese type B encephalitis, epidemic meningitis, and all sorts of other serious infections that exhibit constructive *ch'i* manifestations may be so treated.

9.1.3.2. Defensive *ch'i* and constructive *ch'i* sector simultaneous disorder (constructive *ch'i* sector hot heteropathy accompanied by outer manifestation type)

This is constructive ch'i *disorder with additional defensive* ch'i *symptoms such as headache, body pain, and abnormal sensitivity to cold.* Therapy uses "clearing the constructive *ch'i* sector and draining the hot heteropathy" (9.1.0) and "flushing the outer aspect with pungent and cooling drugs" (7.1.1), for instance with Constructive *Ch'i* Clearing Infusion combined with Honeysuckle-Forsythia Powder.

9.1.3.3. Active ch'i and constructive ch'i sector simultaneous disorder

This is *constructive* ch'i *disorder with active* ch'i *manifestations and crimson tongue with yellowish-white coating.* For therapy "clearing the active *ch'i* sector and cooling the constructive *ch'i* sector" (*ch'ing ch'i liang ying* 清 气 凉 营 , 12.2.2.1) is recommended; White Tiger Infusion combined with Constructive *Ch'i* Clearing Infusion, with proportions adjusted to the case, may be used.

9.1.3.4. Hot heteropathy entering the Cardiac Envelope Junction

Main manifestations. Accompanying the special characteristics of constructive *ch'i* disorders, *various degrees of disturbance to consciousness,* such as apathetic expression, an intricate, abstruse style of speech, slow or dulled responses, hallucinations of hearing or vision, clutching at the air or groping about the bed, mental confusion [including partial or complete loss of consciousness, *shen hun* 神 昏] and raving, or even deep coma, incontinence, and so on; *crimson tongue;* and *smooth, small, and accelerated pulse.* Some patients may have convulsions.

Pathology. This manifestation type is due to invasion of the Cardiac Envelope Junction system by hot heteropathy and blockage of the cardiac orifices. It may also be referred to as the "closure (*pi* 闭)" manifestation type.

Therapy. [Beginning omitted.] All sorts of encephalitis, meningitis, septicemia, and toxemic bacillary dysentery, as well as heat stroke, may be so treated if they exhibit manifestations of this type.

9.1.3.5. Hot heteropathy activating hepatic wind (extreme intensity of hot heteropathy giving rise to wind heteropathy [je chi sheng feng 热 极 生 风])

Main manifestations. High fever, agitation, convulsions, in some cases cramps in the extremities, *stiff neck,* convulsive backward arching of the spine, *deviation or quivering of the tongue, strung, accelerated pulse, tongue red* (belonging to the active *ch'i* sector) *or crimson* (belonging to the constructive *ch'i* sector); sometimes accompanied by coma.

This manifestation type may occur in the active *ch'i,* constructive *ch'i,* or blood sector, but is more common in the last two.

Therapy. [Beginning omitted.] Encephalitis, meningitis, and all sorts of infectious disorders complicated by toxemic cerebral symptoms that exhibit the above manifestations may be so treated.

9.1.4. Blood sector disorders

This is the grave stage of heat factor disorders, in which the heteropathy is still at an abnormally high level and the orthopathic *ch'i* deficient.

9.1.4.1. Blood sector disorder (hot heteropathy in the blood sector)

Main manifestations. High fever; hemorrhage (vomiting, spitting blood, nosebleed, blood in the urine or stool); *purple or black skin rash; manic agitation; delusional speech or mental confusion;* convulsions; *crimson or purple tongue without coating;* and *small, accelerated pulse.*

Pathology. Blazing hot heteropathy which has entered the blood sector is responsible for the fever and for the tongue and pulse phenomena. The heteropathy impels the blood into uncontrolled motion, hence the hemorrhage or clearly evident rash. It disturbs the mind, thus the mental symptoms. Extreme intensity of hot heteropathy gives rise to wind heteropathy, hence the convulsions.

Therapy. [Beginning omitted.] Rashes, whether the lesions are large or small, are prognostically favorable if red, lustrous, slackly filled with fluids, and loosely distributed, and unfavorable if purplish and dull, congested with fluid, and tightly distributed. Dull purplish or black rash which does not pale in color when pressed, accompanied by crimson tongue, is a sign that the hot heteropathy has entered the blood sector. Typhoid, miliary pulmonary tuberculosis, leptospirosis, septicemia, and other disorders accompanied by various types of hemorrhage and indicating this manifestation type may be so treated.

9.1.4.2. Hot toxicity in the outer and inner aspects (hot toxicity preponderant within)

Main manifestations. Shivering accompanied by high fever; intense headache; indistinct vision; intense pain over the whole body; respiratory difficulties; *agitation; delusional speech and manic agitation;* confused state of mind or convulsions in serious cases; sometimes accompanied by vomiting or spitting blood, nosebleed, or blood in the urine or stool; *purple or black rash; crimson tongue with scorched yellowish, spiky coating;* and *swollen, large, and accelerated, or sunken, small, and accelerated pulse.* This manifestation type mostly occurs when infectious (*wen i* 瘟 疫) hot toxicity abounds in both outer and inner aspects, so that all four sectors are disordered.

Therapy. Clearing and flushing the hot toxicity from the outer and inner aspects, the active *ch'i* and blood sectors, for which Infection-clearing Toxicity-overcoming Potion (*ch'ing wen pai tu yin* 清 瘟 败 毒 饮 , 12.2.2.2) is often used. The more sunken and small the patient's pulse, the more deeply entrenched is the hot toxicity shown to be, and the greater must be the dosage of medicine. "Broiling in the active *ch'i* and blood sectors" (*ch'i hsueh liang fan* 气 血 两 燔), with hot toxicity in both, manifested by high fever and thirst, rash or nosebleed, crimson tongue with yellow coating, and pulse accelerated or small and accelerated may be treated as for this manifestation type, or using Jade Maiden Decoction (*yü nü chien* 玉 女 煎 , 12.2.2.2) adjusted to the case (omitting achyranthes root [*niu-hsi* 牛 膝 , A. bidentata] and cooked Chinese foxglove root, and adding finely cut raw foxglove root and Ningpo figwort root [*hsuan-shen* 玄 参 , Scrophularia ningpoensis]). Septicemia, epidemic encephalitis, leptospirosis, and other serious infectious disorders that exhibit the above manifestations may be so treated.

9.2. Damage to the Yin and Yang Aspects in Heat Factor Disorders

Heat Factor Disorders readily damage the yin body fluids (3.4), the *chin* fluids in mild cases and the relatively yin fluids in serious cases, sometimes proceeding until failure of yin *ch'i* (*wang yin* 亡 阴) ensues. In therapy, attention always must be given to protecting and nurturing yin body fluids. That is what is meant by "so long as one bit of yin body fluid survives, that much life-sustaining function remains."

The general method for protecting the dispersed body fluids consists of this: in the defensive *ch'i* sector, it is not advisable to overuse the sweating method; in the active *ch'i* sector (repletion hot manifestation in the stomach and intestine systems) it is advisable to use the method of bringing down (10.3.2) without delay; when there are no signs of moist heteropathy, bitter and drying or warming and drying drugs should be used with caution.

Methods of treatment are as follows:

1. *Damage to chin fluids.* Observed in disorders of the defensive and active *ch'i* sectors and manifested by *dry mouth, thirst,* thick saliva adhering in strands, *tongue coating dry, pulse accelerated,* etc., seen in patients with high fever and great loss of fluids. In therapy, to prescriptions directed toward the manifestation should be added such drugs as reed rhizome (*lu ken* 芦 根 [Phragmites communis or P. Karka]), trichosanthes root (*t'ien hua fen* 天 花 粉 [T. kirilowii]), pear peel (*li p'i* 梨 皮 [Pyrus serrulata or P. betulaefolia]), and Chinese sugar cane juice (*kan che chih* 甘 蔗 汁 [Saccharum sinense]), which produce *chin* fluids. If the fever has abated but the mouth and tongue are still dry, appetite is poor, or there is a dry cough, Stomach *Ch'i*-augmenting Infusion (*i wei t'ang* 益 胃 汤 : adenophora root [*sha shen* 沙 参 (A. polymorpha or A. tetraphylla)], lily-turf root, raw Chinese foxglove root, and rhizome of Solomon's seal [*yü chu* 玉 竹 , *ping t'ang (cha)* 冰 糖 渣 (Polygonatum odoratum, P. sibiricum, etc.)])[2] or Adenophora and Lily-turf Root Infusion (12.6.2) may be used.

---

[2] *Ping t'ang cha*, not discussed in the section on drugs of the *Revised Outline*, is a higher-quality rhizome than *yü chu*; the Chinese text lists both. See Chiang-su hsin i-hsueh-yuan 江 蘇 新 醫 學 院 ed. 1977–78: II, 2043a, item 4157.

2. *Damage to yeh fluids.* Mostly seen in the terminal stage of blood sector disorders. Those who suffer from it exhibit *emaciation and fatigue; face flushed and body hot; palms of the hands and soles of the feet hotter still; mouth and tongue dry;* teeth dirty and lips cracked; pharynx painful and hearing diminished; loins painful; knees week; feet swollen; *tongue red or crimson, dry, and weak; pulse small, accelerated, and debilitated;* and other manifestations of Realized Yin [*chen yin* 真 陰 , or renal Water, 2.1.5.1.4] debility. Sometimes these symptoms are accompanied by regular or irregular throbbing of the heart, copious sweating and a tendency to be startled, hesitant or intermittent pulse, and other manifestations of cardiac circulation vessel depletion (observable in myocarditis), and sometimes by twitching or trembling of the hands and feet, cramps, tremor of the tongue, and other manifestations of yin depletion activating [internal] Wind heteropathy (5.1.1.2), as in the sequelae of Encephalitis B.[3]

When the yin fluids have been damaged it is advisable to nourish the yin. Modified Pulse-restoring Infusion (*chia-chien fu mai t'ang* 加 减 复 脉 汤 , 12.16.2.3) is often used in therapy. When damage to yin fluids is accompanied by cardiac circulation vessel depletion or yin depletion activating Wind heteropathy, Three-shell Pulse-restoring Infusion (*san chia fu mai t'ang* 三 甲 复 脉 汤) may be used. If the patient feels hot at night and cool in the morning, and can eat but remains emaciated, this is because the heteropathy is retained in the yin sectors. Wormwood Leaf and Turtle Shell Infusion (*ch'ing hao pieh chia t'ang* 青 蒿 鳖 甲 汤 , 12.2) may be used to "nourish the yin and clear the hot heteropathy" (*tzu yin ch'ing je* 滋 阴 清 热).

3. *Failure of yin ch'i.* Occurs when yin fluids are lost due to damage to the Realized Yin and heteropathic heat fails to abate, sometimes because the therapeutic methods of sweating and bringing down (10.3.2) have been used erroneously. Manifestations are *body hot; sweating profuse;* perspiration saline and lacking viscosity; *face flushed; dry mouth and thirst;* constantly bleeding gums; tongue red or crimson, dry, and weak; and pulse empty, accelerated, and debilitated. This is mostly seen in the late stages of grave infectious disease. It is advisable to administer quickly Modified Pulse-

---

[3] *Yin hsu feng tung* 阴 虚 风 动   is a misprint for *yin hsu tung feng;* cf. 5.1.1.2. "Realized Yin" is the yin *ch'i* of the renal system; on the term "Realized" see P171, s.v. "true *ch'i.*"

restoring Infusion augmented with ginseng from Jilin (*Chi-lin shen* 吉 林 参 , Panax ginseng), fossil bone (*lung-ku* 龙 骨), oyster shell (*mu-li* 牡 蛎 [Ostrea gigas et al.]), boy's urine (*t'ung pien* 童 便 , from interrupted urination by a child of five years or less; serves to nourish the yin and bring down the Fire [8.1.8] as well as to cool the blood and disperse coagulations) and similar drugs to "nourish the yin and augment the *ch'i*" (*tzu yin i ch'i* 滋 阴 益 气) and to "arrest sweating and prevent collapse of the retentive function" (*lien han ku t'o* 敛 汗 固 脱, 12.17.2.1).[4]

4. *Failure of yang ch'i.* May occur in the active *ch'i*, constructive *ch'i*, or blood sector, developing due to serious hot toxicity with heteropathic preponderance and depleted orthopathy. The feverish patient *abruptly drips oily, cold, tasteless sweat; the body and limbs turn cold;* respiration becomes faint; the tongue becomes pale or whitish and moist; and the pulse becomes subtle as though about to cease: these are manifestations of yang failure. They indicate that yang *ch'i* has suddenly been lost and the patient's life hangs in the balance. Yang failure is equivalent to secondary shock. It may be observed in fulminant epidemic encephalomyelitis and meningitis, septicemia, and toxic bacillary dysentery with supervening circulatory failure.

In therapy it is advisable to "restore the yang and relieve the backflow" (*hui yang chiu ni* 回 阳 救 逆) and to "replenish the *ch'i* and prevent collapse of the retentive function" (*pu ch'i ku t'o* 补 气 固 脱). Fourfold Backflow Infusion (*ssu ni t'ang* 四 逆 汤, 12.4.2.3) augmented with such drugs as Jilin ginseng, huangchi root (*huang-ch'i* 黄 芪 [Astragalus membranaceus and A. mongholicus]), fossil bone, oyster shell, and schisandra fruit (*wu wei tzu* 五 味 子 [S. chinensis]), is often combined with emergency application of acupuncture.

In addition, damage to yin or yang *ch'i* in Heat Factor Disorders may cause depletion and debilitation of the visceral systems and an imbalance of functions. Thus after recovery various conditions of depletion and debilitation often occur. The mucus (3.5) formed as a result of unbalanced visceral functions may obstruct the orifices and circulation tracts, bringing on coma, dementia, paralysis, deaf-

---

[4] *Ku* literally means "to seal against leakage," as when astringent drugs (12.17) are used to control excessive perspiration, urination, loss of semen, diarrhea, etc. *T'o* refers to general prostration in which the body is no longer able to retain vital fluids.

mutism, drooling, incontinence of urine or feces, and other sequelae. Therapy for the aftermath of damage to yin or yang *ch'i* or for such sequelae should also take into consideration the visceral system manifestation type, whether by replenishing the yin or yang *ch'i* or blood of the visceral systems, or by dissolving the mucus and unblocking the orifices and circulation tracts, in combination with acupuncture and moxibustion therapy.

9.3. Examples of Heat Factor Disorder Manifestation Type Determination

[Two short examples omitted from translation.]

Example 3. Infant Li *X*, two years old, a measles patient. On the sixth day after onset the patient presented fever; thirst; cold hands and feet; somnolence; coughing; yellowish, mushy, and putrid stool; urination brief, with urine tinged scarlet; body temperature 40.8 degress C (105.4 degress F); breathing rough and rapid (38 respirations per minute); mental lethargy; deep red skin lesions covering the head and trunk, with some coalescence of masses that lose their color when pressed; skin lesions thinly distributed on the extremities, with none below the elbows and knees; face gray and eyes red; profuse gummy secretion in the eyes; tongue crimson with brownish coating; lips dry and pharynx reddened; index finger purple up to the "*ch'i* pass" (6.2.3); and a smooth, accelerated pulse.

Analysis. The fever and crimson tongue mean that the disorder has entered the constructive *ch'i* sector. That the tongue is crimson but still has a brownish coating means that the heteropathy is not yet gone from the active *ch'i* sector. The deep red color of the spots, the high fever, and the purple finger veins means that the hot toxicity is grave. Absence of lesions below the elbows and knees means that the hot toxicity, not having been vented, has become static within. This hot stasis is relatively deep-seated, so that gray face, cold extremities, and other false cold manifestations (7.2.4) are seen.

To sum up, the diagnosis is "disorder in both the active and constructive *ch'i* sectors, with the measles toxicity static within." In therapy the method of "clearing the active *ch'i* sector, cooling the constructive *ch'i* sector, and venting the measles toxicity" (*ch'ing ch'i liang ying t'ou chen* 清 气 凉 营 透 疹) is indicated. Use Lac and Safflower Potion (*tzu ts'ao hung hua yin* 紫 草 黄 花 饮): gum lac (*tzu ts'ao [jung]* 紫 草 茸 [secretion of Laccifer

lacca]),[5] forsythia fruit (lien-ch'iao 连 翘 [F. suspensa]), safflower blossoms (hung hua 红 花 [Carthamus tinctorius]),
honeysuckle fruit (chin yin hua 金 银 花 [Lonicera japonica]),
woad leaf (ta ch'ing yeh 大 青 葉 [Isatis tinctoria]), Zhejiang
fritillary (che pei 浙 贝 [Fritillaria thunbergii]), violet root and leaf
(tzu hua ti ting 紫 花 地 丁 [Viola yedoensis et al.]),
lophatherum leaf (tan chu yeh 淡 竹 葉 [L. gracile]), tamarisk
twig (ch'ui ssu liu 垂 絲 柳 [Tamarix chinensis]), and licorice
root (kan ts'ao 甘 草 [Glycyrrhiza uralensis]); or Constructive Ch'i
Sector Clearing Infusion (ch'ing ying t'ang 清 营 汤 , 12.2.2.3)
combined with White Tiger Infusion (pai hu t'ang 白 虎 汤 ,
12.2.2.1), modified as necessary.

9.4. Conclusion

This chapter has introduced the principles of manifestation type
determination and therapy in heat factor disorders. In manifestation type determination tongue inspection is especially important.
By examining alterations in tongue coating one can distinguish
whether the disorder is in the defensive ch'i or active ch'i sectors,
and at the same time can assess the state of the body fluids. By examining changes in the tongue tissues one can distinguish whether
the disorder is in the constructive ch'i or blood sector, and can determine whether the yin fluids [blood, ching, and dispersed body fluids]
are at a level higher or lower than normal. As for symptoms which
appear in the different stages of heat factor disorders, such as
fever, thirst, perspiration, white heat rash, coma, and muscle
spasms, if in one's study one draws distinctions [within each type]
and recognizes their various special characteristics, manifestation
type determination will be greatly facilitated. Taking fever as an
example, there are fever with and without abnormal sensitivity to
cold, alternating fevers and chills, fever with abnormal sensitivity to

---

[5] Tzu ts'ao may also refer to the Asiatic groomwell root, Lithosper-
mum erythrorhizon, and at least six other species. The function
of venting toxicity in eruptive disorders of children is especially
noted for the insect secretion, but there has been some research
on the efficacy of the root in measles prevention. See Chiang-su
hsin i-hsueh-yuan ed. 1977–78: 11, 2342–46, 2365–66 (items
4863 and 4892).

heat, intermittent fever, fever highest at night, hot sensations in the palms of the hands and soles of the feet, fever at night and chills in the morning, and many other types, for which diagnosis and therapy differ.

In therapy, one should be attentive to the special tendency in heat factor disorders [for cold heteropathy] to "turn hot" (*je hua* 热 化). Except for the wind cold outer and yang *ch'i* failure manifestation types, pungent, warming, or heating drugs are contraindicated. Hot heteropathy in particular tends to impair the yin aspect, so in therapy one must at all times safeguard the yin fluids. Moist heteropathy tends to impair the yang aspect, so in treating moist warm disorders one may not make excessive use of bitter and chilling drugs or mistakenly use medicines which "nourish unctuousness" (*tzu ni* 滋 腻 , 12.16.1.2 [drugs for replenishing blood and the yin aspect generally]).

9.5. Appendix: Manifestation Type Determination Using the Six Warps and Triple Chiao Systems

9.5.1. Manifestation type determination using the Six Warps System

Manifestation type determination as applied to Heat Factor Disorders is generally divided into analyses based on the Four Sectors, Six Warps, and Triple *Chiao* systems. We have emphasized the Four Sectors method above because, according to our clinical knowledge and the publications of recent years, it is used most often. Here we briefly discuss the other two methods for the reference of our readers.

The Six Warps comprise mature yang, yang brightness, immature yang, mature yin, immature yin, and attenuated yin. These were originally the names of circulation tracts (4.0), but later they were borrowed to encompass six stages of change in the developmental process of Cold Damage Disorders.[6] The Six Warps became the basic organizing principle for manifestation type determination and therapeutic reasoning in Cold Damage Disorders.

---

[6] The original denotation of the Six Warps is far from certain. See the discussion in the introductory study, pages 80–87.

Mature yang disorders. Mainly divided into "tract manifestation" (*ching cheng* 经 证) and "visceral system manifestation" (*fu cheng* 腑 证) types.

In the mature yang tract manifestation type, the heteropathy has invaded the peripheral flesh. It is further divided into "Wind Attack" and "Cold Damage" types; the former is outer depletion type and the latter, outer repletion type.[7] In mature yang "Wind Attack," manifestations observed are fever, abnormal sensitivity to wind, perspiration, headache and stiff neck, and floating, moderate pulse. Therapy uses the method of "flushing the flesh and venting the outer aspect" (*chieh chi fa piao* 解 肌 发 表), for which Cassia Twig Infusion is effective.[8] In mature yang "Cold Damage," manifestations observed are abnormal sensitivity to cold accompanied by fever, no sweating, joint pains, and pulse floating and tense. Therapy uses the method of "inducing perspiration and flushing the outer aspect" (*fa han chieh piao* 发 汗 解 表), for which Ephedra Infusion is effective.

Mature yang visceral system manifestations are brought about when, heteropathy in the outer aspect not having been flushed away, it is transmitted inward to the urinary bladder system (2.1.5.2). If the manifestations observed are fever, abnormal sensitivity to wind, difficult urination, thirst with frequent urination (*hsiao k'o* 消 渴),[9] or liquid vomited as soon as drunk, they con-

---

[7] These subdivisions correspond to individual disorders in the Cold Damage group described in *Shang han lun* 傷 寒 論 .

[8] This paraphases the passage from the *Shang han lun* translated above, page 86.

[9] This term is often mistakenly identified with modern "diabetes," correctly translated as *t'ang niao ping* 糖 尿 病 . See, for instance, the valuable historical discussion in Needham 1970: 303–9. *Hsiao k'o* may refer, as here, to symptomatic polyuria accompanied by persistent thirst, but in traditional medicine it usually denotes a large group of disorders the common symptoms of which are thirst, polyuria, and cachexia, with sweet-tasting urine frequently cited for some members of the group. For disorders in the *hsiao k'o* group see *Chu ping yuan hou lun* 諸 病 源 候 論 (610), 5: 30–31, and *San yin chi i ping yuan lun ts'ui* 三 因 極 一 病 源 論 粹 (ca. 1174), 10: 136–42. I translate *hsiao k'o* in the wider sense as "Wasting Thirst Disorders" (6.1.3.1).

stitute the urinary bladder system "water accumulation" (*hsu shui* 蓄 水 type. If the manifestations are a hard, full feeling in the belly, easy urination, and manic behavior, they constitute the urinary bladder system "blood accumulation" (*hsu hsueh* 蓄 血) type.

Yang brightness disorders. The heteropathy is transmitted from the mature yang tract, and is manifested as repletion heat in the stomach and large intestine systems. These disorders are divided into two types. That signalled by high fever, great thirst, sweating, and swollen, large pulse is the yang brightness tract manifestation type. The method of "clearing hot heteropathy in the inner aspect" (*ch'ing li je* 清 里 热) is used, for which White Tiger Infusion is the effective prescription. That signalled by intermittent fever; sweating; a full, hard feeling in the belly; constipation; raving and mental confusion; compulsive stroking of clothing or bed; and sunken, full pulse is the yang visceral system manifestation type. The method of "freeing the yang visceral system and draining the hot heteropathy" (*t'ung fu hsieh je* 通 腑 泻 热) is used, for which Great *Ch'i* Acceptance Infusion is effective.

Immature yang disorders. The main symptoms are alternating hot and cold sensations, feelings of fullness and distress in the chest, worry and mental upset with a tendency to vomit, bitter taste in the mouth and dry throat, dizziness, whitish tongue coating, and strung pulse. Disorders between the mature yang and yang brightness stages are called "half-outer half-inner" gall bladder hot manifestations (7.1.2). For therapy the method of "mediating and flushing the outer and inner aspects" (*ho chieh piao li* 和 解 表 里) is used; Minor Hare's-ear Infusion is effective.

Minor yin disorders. The great majority are the result of pathological changes transmitted from the yang tracts, but in some cases external heteropathy directly attacks the mature yin tracts. When external heteropathy penetrates the inner aspect it changes into cold, moist heteropathy. Manifestations observed are fatigue in the extremities, irritability and aches in the flesh, distension and fullness in the stomach cavity, disinclination to eat or drink, diarrhea with thin stool, lack of thirst, pale tongue with whitish coating, and moderate pulse. Mature yin disorders are equivalent to depletion cold or moist manifestations in the splenetic system. For therapy the method of "warming the medial aspect and dispersing the cold heteropathy" (*wen chung san han* 温 中 散 寒) is used; Medial Aspect Reordering Infusion (*li chung t'ang* 理 中 汤 , 12.4) is effective.

Immature yang disorders. May be transmitted from other circulation tracts or may attack directly. They represent a grave stage of cardiac and renal depletion and weakness. The main symptoms are abnormal sensitivity to cold in the absence of fever; small, subtle pulse; overwhelming inclination to sleep (accompanied by inability to sleep); coldness in the hands and feet; and protracted voiding of clear urine. For therapy the method of "restoring the yang and relieving the backflow" is used; Fourfold Backflow Infusion is effective.

Attenuated yin disorder. The main symptoms are coldness in the hands and feet, interlocking (*chiao-ts'o* 交错) of hot and cold manifestations,[10] diarrhea with foreign matter accompanied by vomiting or retching, thirst with dry throat, and vomiting of roundworms. These manifestations indicate the late stage of Cold Damage Disorders, in which hepatic and Cardiac Envelope Junction dysfunction is preponderant, and the patient's situation is relatively complicated. For therapy the methods of warming and clearing (10.3.2) should be used in combination. In cases of Roundworm Contraversion Disorder (*hui chueh* 蛔 厥),[11] drugs such as Wumei Pellets [*wumei wan* 乌 梅 丸 , an anthelminthic prescription, 12.18.2] may be used.

In Cold Damage Disorders the general rules for transmission of pathological changes are: yang tract disorders mainly begin in the mature yang tracts and are then transmitted to the yang brightness or immature yin tracts. If orthopathic *ch'i* is inadequate, they may also pass into the yin tracts. Yin tract disorders usually begin in the mature yin tracts and then pass into the immature yin or attenuated yin tracts. But disorders may originate not only in the yang but also in the yin aspect. Not only are they transmitted in the regular sequence of the tracts, but they may skip tracts (as when a mature yang disorder is transmitted to mature yin). It is also possible to have a "combination disorder" in two tracts (for instance, mature yang and yang brightness combination disorder) or an

---

[10] That is, they are simultaneously present, for instance in the upper and lower parts or inner and outer aspects of the body.

[11] Intermittent abdominal pain and abdominal swelling accompanied by cold extremities, corresponding to modern ascariasis and other syndromes caused by parasites.

"overlapping disorder" (such as mature yang and immature yin disordered together).[12]

9.5.2. Manifestation type determination using the triple *chiao* system

Triple *chiao* typing borrows the name of the triple *chiao* system (2.1.6) to epitomize three types of manifestations during the process of development of Heat Factor Disorders.[13]

Superior chiao manifestations. Include the symptoms of pulmonary and Cardiac Envelope Junction disorders, such as fever with abnormal sensitivity to cold, cough, labored and noisy breathing, and floating pulse, which are symptoms of pulmonary system disorders. If the heteropathy is transmitted to the Cardiac Envelope Junction system, contrary to the normal course, such symptoms proper to the latter as mental confusion and raving, stiff tongue, and cold extremities may appear. This is the early stage of Heat Factor Disorders, corresponding to manifestations of the defensive *ch'i* sector or of abnormal transmission (*ni ch'uan* 逆 传) to the constructive *ch'i* or blood sector.[14]

---

[12] *Footnote in original:* Two or more tracts simultaneously disordered is called a "combination disorder" (*ho ping* 合 病); a condition in which a disorder in one tract has not ceased by the time it has emerged in another tract is called an "overlapping disorder" (*ping ping* 并 病). *Addendum by translator:* This translation is based on the current understanding, but the classical sense of the latter term might be better rendered as "annexing disorder." The point is that heteropathy in different stages of seriousness (as indicated by the development of symptoms) in different tracts will, with the passage of time, be "annexed" into one tract. See *Shang han hai ti yen* 傷 寒 海 底 眼 (ca. 1416), 2: 60.

[13] Note the word "borrows," which denies that the manifestations are actually situated in or controlled by the triple *chiao* system, the physical status of which is ambiguous, and especially ambiguous to those trained in modern anatomy.

[14] Although *ni* usually implies a direction of movement opposite to the normal course, or "backflow," the present usage refers to any transmission of heteropathy that does not follow the usual sequence, and especially one that skips one or more stages. The

Medial chiao manifestations. Include symptoms of stomach, intestine, and splenetic system disorders. Fever without abnormal sensitivity to cold, but sensitivity to heat instead; face flushed and eyes reddened; constipation and scanty urination; tongue coating brownish, and similar symptoms are those of hot heteropathy in the stomach and intestine systems. Moderate fever, distress and subjective feelings of blockage in the thoracic cavity, nausea, thin stool, fatigue and feelings of heaviness, greasy tongue coating, moderate pulse, and so on are symptoms of moist-hot disorders (5.1.4.1.3) in the splenetic system. This is the crisis stage in Heat Factor Disorders, equivalent to manifestations in the active *ch'i* sector.

Inferior chiao manifestations. Include symptoms of hepatic and renal system disorders. When heteropathic heat has consumed the renal yin, such symptoms as hot sensations in the palms of the hands and the soles of the feet, dry throat, and insomnia due to mental distress may be observed. When diminution of renal yin has induced hepatic yin diminution, so that the "hepatic Wind stirs within" (8.2.2), such symptoms as twitching hands and feet, icy cold in the extremities, and heart palpitations may be observed. This is the terminal phase of Heat Factor Disorders, equivalent to manifestations in the blood sector.

Triple *chiao* system manifestation type determination assumes that Heat Factor Disorders first invade the superior *chiao* and from there are transmitted to the medial and inferior *chiao*.

---

term occurs in *Wen je lun* 溫 熱 論 (ca. 1740?), 6: 36b (II, 750).

10. Therapeutic Principles

Chairman Mao has instructed us: "We must take vigorous action to prevent and treat the illnesses of the people and to expand the people's medical and health services." This is a glorious political responsibility for health workers. In order to carry out this responsibility, not only must we, in preventing and treating disease, resolutely carry out the Party's health care policy of "being geared to the needs of the workers, peasants, and soldiers, giving priority to prevention, uniting Chinese and Western physicians, and integrating medical work with mass movements"; we must also earnestly study the brilliant philosophical thought of Chairman Mao, using dialectical materialism to guide clinical experience, and in clinical therapy paying attention to and mastering the following points.[1]

10.1. Mobilizing the Initiative of Both, Correctly Work Out the Relation between Medical Workers and Patients

"Two initiatives are much better than one." In treatment of disease neither initiative on the part of medical workers alone nor on the part of patients alone will do. Only when the initiatives of both are fully mobilized can the disease be treated as well, quickly, and economically as possible. Medical workers must, through conscien-

---

[1] This statement, in its adulation of Chairman Mao and its emphasis on "red" aspects of public health—that is, on the integration of medical and political priorities rather than on "expert," professional aspects of medicine—is characteristic of the Cultural Revolution, and unlikely to be seen in handbooks and textbooks published since the late 1970s. The next subsection is similarly obsolete but historically significant—and interesting in the view of relationships between therapists and patients that it reflects.

tiously studying the books of Marx and Lenin and the works of Chairman Mao, serve the people wholeheartedly. They must break with idealistic apriorism and take as their model the materialist theory of reflection [i.e., that correct knowledge reflects material reality]. They must break with superstition and emancipate their thought, constantly improving their skills, daring to attack medical difficulties, daring to scale the heights of medicine, unceasingly discovering, inventing, creating, advancing. Patients must, through conscientiously studying the books of Marx and Lenin and the works of Chairman Mao, acquire an attitude of treating the disorder for the sake of the revolution, and staunch confidence in vanquishing the disease. They must actively participate in therapy, cooperating of their own accord with providers of medical care, completely changing a situation in which they passively accept therapy into a struggle alongside the providers of medical care against disease.

Seen from the viewpoint of advanced experiments in China on combined Chinese and Western therapy, mobilizing the two initiatives is an important characteristic of our country's unified new medicine. In combining Chinese and Western therapy, for instance, the integration of motion and immobility in treatment of fracture,[2] the integration of comprehensive therapy and tenacious physical exercise in treatment of palsy, and the integration of acupuncture, drugs, and appropriate physical activity in treatment of heart disease, can play an active role in accelerating recovery.

10.2. Emphasizing a Holistic Approach, Correctly Work Out the Relation between the Parts and the Whole

"When Marxist-Leninists consider problems, they see not only the parts but the whole."

The parts and the whole are related by the unity of opposites. If there were no parts there could be no whole, and vice versa. In performing therapy we can neither consider the parts at the ex-

---

[2] This refers to the Chinese use of flexible willow splints to limit immobilization of fractures, as well as manipulation in setting the bone and flexion exercises during healing. For an accessible account of an influential experiment in combined therapy for fractures see Shang Tien-yu 1977.

pense of the whole, treating the head for head pains and the feet for feet pains, nor the whole at the expense of the parts, providing general therapy and overlooking local treatment at the site of infection. The correct method is to proceed from the holistic conception, giving serious attention to the parts and even more serious attention to the whole, forming a dialectical synthesis of the two aspects. Methodologically, one is thus able to influence the whole body through local treatment and vice versa. In clinical practice, some therapeutic measures are desirable from the local point of view but damaging to the body as a whole, so that they must be used judiciously. In situations of mortal danger certain therapeutic measures are feasible when considered from the viewpoint of the general situation but, seen from the local perspective, are to some extent harmful. They should be used resolutely to avoid great losses in the hope of small gains, missing the critical moment for therapy.

Traditional physicians, taking the holistic conception as their point of departure, and basing themselves on the mutual relations of the visceral systems of function and the circulation tract system, consistently make use of the following therapeutic principles.

10.2.1. Use of drugs in clinical medicine

The relations of mutual production and mutual conquest (1.2.1), and those of outer and inner aspects (2.1.1.2, 7.1), which hold between the visceral systems, are regularly employed as principles governing replenishing depletions and draining repletions in therapy.

10.2.1.1. Harmonizing yin and yang

An excess of renal yang or an insufficiency of renal yin can produce a series of signs of yang excess (8.5). In therapy the method of "greatly replenishing the renal yin" (ta pu shen yin 大 补 肾 阴 , for example, by using Six-ingredient Chinese Foxglove Pellets [8.5.6] to nourish the renal Water [1.2.1] in order to control the renal Yang) is often employed. When the renal Water becomes adequate, the symptoms of renal Fire excess abate. Therapeutic methods of this kind are called "strengthening Water to control Fire" (chuang shui chih huo 壮 水 制 火). An excess of renal yin and depletion of renal yang can produce a series of yin cold manifestations. In therapy the method of "greatly replenishing the renal yang" (for instance, using Golden Casket Renal *Ch'i* Pellets (8.5.6) to augment the renal yang and "diminish the yin shadow," *hsiao yin i* 消 陰 翳) is frequently used. This makes the renal yang adequate, so that the cold, congealing manifestations of yin excess naturally abate. Therapeutic methods of this kind are called "augmenting Fire to reduce yin" (*i huo hsiao yin* 益 火 消 陰).

Neither of these approaches treats the aspect that is in excess. Their effectiveness is instead a matter of focusing on the whole, of proceeding from the connections between one phenomenon and others, to treat the insufficient aspect.

10.2.1.2. Indirect replenishing and draining

When a visceral system is debilitated, in addition to directly replenishing its *ch'i*, one may proceed holistically and replenish that of another system to which its relation is close (the "mother system" [*mu tsang* 母 臟 , which precedes it in the production order of the Five Phases, 1.2.1]). Therapeutic methods of this kind are usually referred to as "in depletion, replenishing the mother." For instance, for patients with Pulmonary Consumption Disorder (*fei lao ping* 肺 癆 病)[3] who have been under treatment for some time

---

[3] In contemporary traditional medicine this term applies to pulmonary tuberculosis and symptomatically indistinguishable chronic wasting diseases (e.g., lung abscess, bronchogenic carcinoma, and pulmonary embolism), but in classical medicine the relation is by no means so simple. In early nosology there was a large group of Depletion and Wasting Disorders (*hsu lao* 虛 勞), many of them anemic and neurasthenic. See, for instance, the 75 varieties in *Chu ping yuan hou lun*, 3: 17a; 4: 27b. The character *lao* 癆 and the term *lao chai* 癆 瘵 are used for contagious chronic wasting disorders generally—including Pulmonary Consumption Disorder—in *San yin chi i ping yuan lun ts'ui*, 10: 128–30. Not only are these large classes of disorders, but they are not the only classes in which the characteristic symptoms of pulmonary tuberculosis are prominent. Others include Possession Disorders (*chu* 注 , 疰 ; see above, pages 103–5) and the related Cadaver Vector Disorders (*ch'uan shih* 傳 尸) as well as Bone-

without recovering, therapy employing the method of "replenishing the splenetic system to augment the pulmonary system," i.e., that of "cultivating Earth to produce Metal," often brings good results (1.2.2).

When there is a disorder in a visceral system of function, one may treat it by draining its "child" [the next system in the mutual production order of the Five Phases, 1.2.1]. Therapeutic measures of this kind are usually called "in repletion, draining the child." For instance, when the hepatic yang rises in excess (8.2.2) or a hepatic *ch'i* stasis (2.1.2.1.1) is transformed into Fire heteropathy, with flushed face, headache, agitation and irritability, mental distress and sleeplessness, therapy that, in addition to "calming the hepatic system and latensifying the yang *ch'i*" (*p'ing kan ch'ien yang* 平 肝 潜 阳 , 12.15), uses the method of "draining the cardiac Fire" (8.1), often brings relatively good results.

10.2.1.3. Mutual therapy of outer and inner aspects

Between the yin and yang visceral systems of function there is a definite relation of outer and inner (2.1.1.3). If the outer and inner aspects share a disorder (7.6), one may choose the method of "mutual therapy of outer and inner aspects" (*piao li hu chih* 表 里 互 治). For example, in symptoms of the inner hot manifestation type (7.2.2), when dried and solidified stool leads to lung congestion due to constraint on circulation of the pulmonary *ch'i* (*yung sheng*, 7.3.2), because the pulmonary and large intestine systems are related as outer and inner aspects (2.1.4.3), "Diaphragm-cooling Powder" (*liang ko san* 凉 隔 散 , 12.2.2.1) is used to drain the Fire of the large intestine system and clear the pulmonary *ch'i*. In another instance, when hot heteropathy transfers from the cardiac to the small intestine system (8.1.6), with sores developing on the mouth and tongue; urination brief, harsh, and painful; and urine tinged scarlet, because the cardiac and small intestine systems are related as outer and inner aspect, "Scarlet-guiding Powder" (*tao ch'ih san* 导 赤 散 , 12.2.2.1) is frequently used to clear the car-

---

steaming Disorders (*ku cheng* 骨 蒸). For some practitioners these groups are distinct from *lao chai* as well as from each other; for some (e.g., *San yin chi i ping yuan lun ts'ui*) they overlap.

diac Fire and drain the hot heteropathy in the small intestine system.

10.2.1.4. Treating the five sense organs via the five yin visceral systems

The five yin visceral systems and the five sense organs are closely related (table 1.2); a disorder in the latter may be treated via the former. For example, an eye disorder of the repletion manifestation type may be treated with drugs that clear the hepatic system; one of the depletion manifestation type may be treated with drugs that replenish the hepatic system; sores on the mouth and tongue may be treated with drugs that clear the cardiac Fire, and so on.

10.2.2. Selection of loci in acupuncture and moxibustion

Traditional physicians, taking the holistic conception as their point of departure, often use the following principles when determining a course of acupuncture treatment. When the disorder is in the upper part of the body, loci in the lower part may be chosen, for instance *yung-ch'üan* (R1) or *t'ai-ch'ung* (H3) for hypertension of the "hepatic *ch'i* rising in excess" type (8.2.2). When the disorder is in the lower part of the body. loci in the upper part may be selected, as when in prolapse of the anus moxibustion is often applied to *pai-hui* (TM19). The right side may be treated by way of the left, or vice versa, as when in hemiplegia loci are often selected on the unaffected side. In addition there is equivalent selection of dorsal and ventral transmission loci (4.3.3.3.1), of primordial *ch'i* and nexic loci (4.3.3.3.2), or combined use of loci in the outer and inner, front and back, upper and lower, or left and right aspects.

10.3. Emphasizing Internal Causes, Correctly Work Out the Relation between Orthopathy and Heteropathy

"Dialectical materialism considers external causes to be the conditions of change and internal causes to be the basis of change; external causes operate through internal causes."

The process of medical disorder in the human body is actually a process of struggle between the powers of resistance of the body, orthopathic *ch'i* (internal causes), and their contradiction, the elements responsible for the disorder, heteropathic *ch'i* (external causes).[4] Therapy is a battle in which drugs and other therapeutic techniques (external causes) aid the organism (internal causes) to defeat the disorder, resolve the contradiction, and restore health. Therefore in clinical work it is essential to remain fully attentive to internal causes, to acknowledge the ability of the mental to react on the physical, to give full play to the body's own initiative, and to correctly handle the dialectical relation between "orthopathy" and "heteropathy."

The basic goal of the traditional physician in treating medical disorders lies in altering the comparative strength of orthopathic and heteropathic *ch'i*, and causing the disorder to turn in the direction of order and recovery. All of the many therapeutic measures that may be used were instituted according to two principles: reinforcing orthopathic *ch'i* (7.1.1) and expelling heteropathic *ch'i* (*ch'ü hsieh* 祛邪). In general, the following principles of therapy sum up the way these measures are carried out.

10.3.1. Reinforcing orthopathy in order to expel heteropathy

This is the use of drugs, nutrition, functional training [physical exercises and physical therapy to restore bodily functions], and other therapeutic methods, to reinforce orthopathic *ch'i*, strengthen the constitution, and increase the resistance of the organism and its ability to recover. Thereby the goals of expelling heteropathic *ch'i*, conquering the factors responsible for the disorder, and restoring

---

[4] Although this section uses the same terminology as section 5.0, the meanings differ. In traditional medicine *nei yin* 內因 and *wai yin* 外因 are best translated "inner causes" and "outer causes" to avoid confusion with the endogenous/exogenous distinction in modern medicine. Here their sense is not specifically medical, but comes from dialectical philosophy. The point is not etiology but the interaction of opposites or complements. The translation differs from that in chapter 5 in order to make this difference clear.

health are attained. This method is applicable in cases where, although there is external heteropathy (5.1), the principal contradiction is a depletion of orthopathic *ch'i*. In clinical practice techniques for replenishing orthopathic *ch'i* — "reinforcing the yang" (*chu yang* 助 阳), "nourishing the yin" (*tzu yin* 滋 阴), "augmenting the *ch'i*" (*i ch'i* 益 气), and "replenishing the blood" (*pu hsueh*, 12.16) — are employed according to the concrete circumstances of the case.

10.3.2. Expelling heteropathy in order to reinforce orthopathy

This is the use of drugs, manipulation,[5] acupuncture, moxibustion, cupping, and other therapeutic methods, to expel heteropathy and allow orthopathic *ch'i* to recover. This method is applicable to cases in which there is a preponderance of heteropathic *ch'i* but no apparent depletion of orthopathic *ch'i*, or in which, although there is orthopathic depletion, the heteropathic preponderance is the principal contradition [i.e., the aspect that demands priority in treatment]. In clinical practice, according to the concrete circumstances of the case, one may choose among the techniques of sweating (*han* 汗 , for heteropathy in the outer aspect), disgorging (*t'u* 吐 , for heteropathy in the inner aspect or in the upper part of the body), bringing down (*hsia* 下 , for heteropathy in the inner aspect or in the lower part of the body), mediating (*ho* 和 [to stop the transfer of] heteropathy partly in the outer and partly in the inner aspect), warming (*wen* 温 , for cold manifestation types), clearing (*ch'ing* 清 , for hot manifestation types), and dispersing (*hsiao* 消 , for repletion manifestation types with heteropathic accumulations). These seven techniques [of "attacking" heteropathy, *kung* 攻], along with the technique of replenishing [orthopathy, *pu* 补 , mentioned above (10.3.1)], make up what is called the "eight basic

---

[5] Although the authors use *shou-shu* 手 术 , the normal modern medical term for surgery, they seem to have physical manipulation — usually called *shou-fa* 手 法 — in mind.

methods of drug therapy" (*pa fa* 八法), which are fundamental to the therapeutic principles of traditional medicine.[6]

10.3.3. Joint application of attacking and replenishment

Because of the complexity of the patient's condition and the great mutability of the relations between orthopathic and heteropathic *ch'i*, it may be necessary to form a dialectical synthesis of the two phases of treatment "reinforcing orthopathy" and "expelling heteropathy" in order to adapt to changing circumstances while determining the correct course of therapy. If there is a preponderance of heteropathic *ch'i* and a depletion of orthopathic *ch'i*, and the heteropathic repletion is paramount, emphasis should be placed on expelling heteropathy, with orthopathy-reinforcing drugs added at discretion. But if the disorder has persisted for some time, with heteropathy not completely expelled and considerable depletion of orthopathic *ch'i*, emphasis should lie in reinforcing the latter, with heteropathy-expelling drugs added at discretion. In addition, depending on the circumstances of the case, one may choose to use the principle of first attacking and then replenishing, or vice versa, or that of jointly clearing and warming, or jointly dispersing and replenishing.

10.4. Grasping the Principal Contradiction, Correctly Work Out the Relation between the Phenomena and the Essential Character

"When we consider a matter, it is imperative that we consider what is essential about it, so that we see its phenomenal aspect as no more than a guide through the doorway. Once within the doorway we want to grasp the essence. This is the only reliable scientific method of analysis." Medical disorder is a complicated process in which orthopathy and heteropathy are joined in struggle. In this process the internal contradictions [i.e., opposed aspects] of the organism are often multiple, with both real and spurious clinical

---

[6] See the introductory study, page 185. For systematic descriptions of the eight methods see Porkert 1978: 42–51 and Nanching Chung-i hsueh-yuan ed. 1958: 192–201.

manifestations. The duty of medical workers is, following detailed examination and research work, to penetrate beyond the phenomena and grasp firmly the essential character of the disorder, clearly distinguishing its primary from its secondary contradictions, and to provide appropriate treatment. If we are unable to grasp the essential character and are distracted by false appearances, we may fail to grasp the principal contradiction and the most important aspects of contradiction, and become bogged down in secondary contradictions and aspects of secondary importance, and consequently commit diagnostic and therapeutic errors.

Traditional doctors, in putting forward the therapeutic principles of "root and ramification therapy in ordinary and urgent cases" and "normal and inverse therapy," were fundamentally expressing this viewpoint.

10.4.1. Root and ramification therapy in ordinary and urgent cases

"Root and ramification" (*piao-pen* 标 本) is a concept used to explain the relation of priority between the two sides of a contradiction in every manifestation of medical disorder. In terms of the relation between orthopathy and heteropathy, the orthopathic *ch'i* of the body is the root aspect, and the heteropathic *ch'i* responsible for the disorder is the ramification aspect. In terms of temporal order, an established illness is the root aspect, and recent complications are the ramification aspect. In terms of the occurrence of disorder, the causes of the disorder are the root aspect and the symptoms the ramification aspect. In terms of the location of the disorder, internal illness is the root aspect and external illness the ramification aspect. In terms of causes, inner causes are the root aspect and outer causes the ramification aspect (5.0).[7]

---

[7] *Piao* and *pen* literally mean "twigs at the end of a branch" or "branches at the top of a tree" and "root." They are applied to medicine in a sophisticated way, but without much elaboration, in SW, 18 (65): 323–24 (passage not in TS, but see *2* [1]: 3). Here they are used to designate the aspects of a disorder to which first and second priority are to be accorded in therapy. The underlying idea is that the doctor ordinarily gives chief attention to the ramifications only when their contributions to a disorder are

On the basis of differences in therapy of root and ramifications in the ordinary and urgent cases, we may outline three therapeutic principles.

10.4.1.1. In urgent cases, treatment of the ramification aspect

This technique is used when in the course of a disorder complications appear which, if not given emergency treatment, would develop so as to affect the patient's safety. Take, for example, a disorder of the hepatic system which manifests swelling due to abdominal fluid (cirrhosis in combination with ascites), and in which the patient breathes with difficulty, is unable to sleep supine, and has difficulty in both urinating and defecating. If at this state it is still possible to maintain the patient's orthopathic *ch'i*, instead of hastening to clean out the hepatic stasis or nurture the hepatic *ch'i* one should immediately give medication for "attacking and bringing down" the heteropathy, and thus eliminate the abdominal fluid.

---

pressing, and otherwise concentrates on the more fundamental aspects, the root. "Root and ramification" is thus a relational concept in which the ideas behind the two words are always complementary parts of a whole, and change as the whole—the way of looking at the disorder under consideration—changes. Note that the image on which the *piao-pen* concept depends is more spatial than temporal. It is not genetic; the point is not that the ramifications grow from the root. I interject the word "aspect" to remind readers that, although the ramification aspect is less fundamental and generally more dynamic than the root aspect, it has not necessarily developed from it. The implication of development might be avoided by translating *piao-pen* as "radical and peripheral," but this would introduce worse confusion. The dichotomy is sometimes used in a way reminiscent of such modern dualities as "internal and peripheral phenomena" and "radical and conservative therapy"; but neither of these corresponds to the range of meaning of the Chinese term. For instance, internal pains and their external cause, considered together "in terms of the occurrence of disorder," will be ramification and root, and not vice versa. Therapy aimed at the root aspect is often palliative rather than radical.

Having dealt with these manifestations of the ramification aspect, one can proceed to treat the root aspect.[8]

10.4.1.2. In normal cases, treatment of the root aspect

In the general run of situations, it is imperative to grasp the essential character of the disorder in order to treat it. For instance, in "Pulmonary Consumption Disorder," coughing is the ramification aspect and yin depletion the root aspect. In therapy the emphasis should not be on treating the ramification aspect by "stopping the coughing and expelling the mucus" (*chih k'o ch'ü t'an* 止 嗽 去 痰 , 12.11.0) but rather on treating the root by "nourishing the yin *ch'i* and moistening the pulmonary system" (*tzu yin jun fei* 滋 陰 润 肺 , 12.6.0). Only through increasing the resistance of the organism is Pulmonary Consumption Disorder (2.1.4.1.5) curable.

10.4.1.3. Joint treatment of the root and ramification aspects

This technique is chosen when the condition in both aspects is urgent. For example, in a patient who is coughing and has a sensation of fullness in the chest, pain in the loins, diminished excretion of urine, and generalized edema (acute nephritis), the root aspect of the disorder is renal *ch'i* depletion (8.5.2) with Water flooding upward (2.1.5.1.2), and its ramification aspect is wind-cold heteropathy constricting the pulmonary system (8.4.2). Since both are urgent, the therapeutic technique of "flushing both inner and outer aspects" (7.1.3) is used. On the one hand the outer aspect is

---

[8] In this example the conventional strategy responsive to the root aspect is replenishing orthopathic *ch'i* or improving its circulation by unblocking a stasis (8.2.1). The complications dictate that priority be given instead to expelling with the stool the abdominal fluid and the heteropathy that it embodies (using laxatives or other drugs that ease defecation). "Urgent" overlaps with, but is not identical to, "acute"; its opposite is not "chronic" but "normal, not exceptional."

flushed by inducing sweating, and on the other the edema is reduced by freeing the flow of liquid (12.1, 12.19).[9]

10.4.2. Normal and inverse therapy

Normal therapy (*cheng chih* 正 治), also called "opposition therapy" (*ni chih* 逆 治), uses heating drugs to treat cold heteropathy disorders, chilling drugs to treat hot heteropathy disorders, the technique of replenishing to treat depletion manifestation types, and that of draining to treat repletion manifestation types. This is the therapeutic principle commonly used in clinical medicine.

Inverse therapy (*fan chih* 反 治), also called "conformity therapy" (*ts'ung chih* 从 治), is a therapeutic principle which seems superficially to conform to [rather than oppose the character of] the symptoms, but which actually remains directed at the essential character of the disorder.[10]

For instance, in cases of subjective feeling of blockage and fullness below the heart [i.e., in the stomach cavity, *hsin hsia p'i man* 心 下 痞 满], one generally "disperses and guides away [the accumulation, usually of undigested food, 12.10] to let the *ch'i* circulate" (*hsiao tao hsing ch'i* 消 导 行 气); but if the essential character of the disorder is derived from *ch'i* depletion, it is advisable to replenish the *ch'i*. This is called "use of blockage when the cause is a blockage" (*sai yin sai yung* 塞 因 塞 闭). In

---

[9] The symptoms described might correspond to acute nephritis with coughing, either due to a lung infection with streptococci that affected the kidneys autoimmunologically, or connected with uremia.

[10] Normally traditional medicine uses therapy of dynamic character opposed to that of the heteropathy, and thus of the disorder, as in the examples given in the paragraph before last. This strategy needs no special designation except when it is contrasted to the unusual approach in which *simple* opposition is ruled out by special circumstances. Even in inverse therapy one is not precisely "treating like with like," but rather choosing drugs to oppose certain elements *other than the obvious ones* in a complicated diagnostic picture. Therapy of this kind does not, strictly speaking, violate the principle of opposition therapy that governs traditional clinical medicine.

treating loose bowels, in general the goal is to stop the diarrhea, for which drugs that "keep intact the retentive function" are used (*ku se shou lien* 固 涩 收 敛 , 12.17), but if the essential character of the disorder is derived from moist-hot heteropathy, it is advisable to use the technique of "clearing the hot heteropathy and dispersing the stasis" (*ch'ing je tao chih* 清 热 导 滞 , 12.5.1.4); this is called "use of freeing the flow when the cause is a free flow" (*t'ung yin t'ung yung* 通 因 通 用). When treating "true-cold false-hot" manifestations with hot heteropathy in the outer aspect and cold heteropathy in the inner aspect (7.2.4), warming and heating drugs should be used to treat the "true-cold" manifestations; this is called "use of heating when hot heteropathy is the cause" (*je yin je yung* 热 因 热 用) or "heating to treat hot" (*i je chih je* 以 热 治 热). In treating "true-hot false-cold" manifestations—inner hot manifestation type accompanied by contraversion (7.2.4) with extremities ice-cold—chilling and cooling drugs are used to treat the "true-hot" manifestations; this is called "use of chilling when cold is the cause" (*han yin han yung* 寒 因 寒 用) or "chilling to treat cold" (*i han chih han* 以 寒 治 寒).[11]

In addition, there is the "inverse collateral" (*fan tso* 反 佐) technique, which also lies within the scope of "use of heating when hot is the cause" and "use of chilling when cold is the cause." When normal therapeutic methods are used to treat manifestations of intense hot and cold heteropathy, sometimes ingesting the medicine brings on vomiting, so that it cannot be retained ("rejection due to circulation blockage," *ko-chü* 格 拒 . A little of a warming drug may be added to a strongly chilling prescription to serve an inverse collateral function (or chilling or cooling prescriptions may be administered hot), or a little of a cooling drug added to a strongly warming prescription (or warming or heating medicines ad-

---

[11] Here as in other examples Chinese physicians are concerned not only with free circulation of vital substances but with the retentive function that keeps *ch'i*, body fluids, and excreta from leaking out of a healthy body, and which results in incontinence and graver symptoms when it fails. If the *ch'i* circulation is not free the stasis must be unblocked; but uncontrolled escape of excreta must be stopped by "roughening" the passages with astringent drugs—just as one may "smooth" the intestinal passages in constipation—or, more fundamentally, by replenishing orthopathic *ch'i* responsible for the retentive function.

ministered cold). In these cases there is no rejection, and the efficacy of the drugs is better enabled to exert itself.[12]

10.5. Concretely Analyzing Concrete Problems, Correctly Work Out the Relation between Reliance on Principle and Flexibility

"Deviating from concrete analysis makes it impossible to recognize the special character of any contradiction." In treating illness we must carry out a concrete analysis of every patient and recognize the special character of each disorder, so that we may carry out therapy directed at that character. The principle in traditional medicine of therapy based on manifestation type determination is fundamentally a matter of analyzing the special character of the contradiction involved in the disorder. It requires that treatment be carried out according to the varying essential character of the disorder. It emphasizes the synthesis of reliance on principle and flexibility, and opposes stereotyped rules to cover every case.

10.5.1. Adjusting medication to the season, place, and individual

The changes of climate through the four seasons have a definite effect on the human body. In summer the pores and interstices between skin and flesh (*chi ts'ou* 肌 腠) in the body are open; in winter they contract. In treating colds due to wind-cold heteropathy (9.1.1.5), in the summer it is best not to use too much of pungent

---

[12] The doctrine of normal and inverse therapy is outlined in one of the late, spurious chapters of the *Inner Canon*, SW, 22 (74): 483–87. That of inverse collaterals is developed from early antecedents (including *Shang han lun* and the *Inner Canon*, where the term has more than one meaning) in *Ching-yueh ch'üan shu* (1624), *2*: 51a-52a ("Ch'uan chung lu," chapter 2). "*Ko*" occurs in TS, *6* (4): 87 = LS, *4* (17): 42 to mean a blockage of yin *ch'i* circulation due to yang preponderance. In the 1088 recension of *Shang han lun* 傷 寒 論 , *ko* (there the name of a pathological pulse type) is connected with vomiting and backflow (Chao K'ai-mei ed., *1*: 13a).

and warming drugs, to avoid outer depletion manifestations due to profuse sweating, which will damage the dispersed body fluids (3.4), producing internal dry heteropathy (*hua tsao* 化 燥 , 5.1.5.2) and, by further transformation, other symptoms. In the winter, for the same cold, in general one may use substantial amounts of pungent and warming drugs to flush the outer aspect, so that the disorder will be flushed out with the perspiration. This is called "adjusting medication to the season" (*yin shih chih i* 因 时 制 宜).

Our country is so broad that north, south, east, and west differ in their use of drugs. Because cold weather is common in the north, for disorders of external origin it is best to use heavy doses of pungent warming drugs which serve a diffusing function (*fa san* 发 散 [i.e., mild diaphoretics which cause perspiration to diffuse the heteropathy outward]). Because heat is common in the south, for the same disorders it is best to use light doses of pungent cooling drugs for this function. This is called "adjusting medication to the place" (*yin ti chih i* 因 地 制 宜).

The ages, sexes, and constitutions of patients vary. The circumstances of women are complicated by childbearing, menstruation, and vaginal discharges; the visceral systems of children are delicate; *ch'i* depletions and repletions are unstable. For all these reasons each case should be thoroughly pondered. Not only should the dosage of medicine be varied, but the therapeutic approach and type of prescription will sometimes differ. For instance, if the patient is normally sensitive to heat, his constitution has a hot tendency, and warming drugs should be used with caution. If the patient is normally sensitive to cold, his constitution has a cold tendency, and chilling drugs should be used with caution. This is called "adjusting medication to the individual" (*yin jen chih i* 因 人 制 宜).

10.5.2. Different therapy for the same disorder; the same therapy for different disorders

Although all instances of a given disorder follow a common pattern, in varying circumstances therapy must be dealt with differently. In asthma, for instance, asthma due to cold heteropathy (*han ch'uan* 寒 喘) should be treated with drugs of chilling or cooling character; that due to depletion should be treated with replenishing drugs.

Although different disorders all have their special characteristics, they also have common characteristics from which one can infer common principles for therapy: "whenever there is dispersion [of orthopathic *ch'i*], retain it; whenever there is a blockage [of heteropathic *ch'i*], disperse it; whenever there is dry heteropathy, moisten it; whenever there is tension, relax it; whenever there is hardness [i.e., masses unyielding to palpation, such as enlarged organs and growths], soften it; whenever there is fragility (*ts'ui* 脆), toughen it" and "whenever there is rising [*ch'i*—see examples below], restrain it; whenever there is sinking [*ch'i*], raise it; whenever there is an excess, diminish it; whenever there is an insufficiency, replenish it; whenever there is hardness, reduce it; whenever there is external heteropathy (*k'o* 客 , lit., "guest"), expel it; whenever there is a congelation, disperse it; whenever there is a stasis (*liu* 留), attack it."[13] For example, abdominal droop, prolapse of the uterus, movable kidney, and prolapse of the anus are all induced by sinking of the medial *ch'i* (2.1.3.3); all of these may be similarly treated with prescriptions for "elevating the *ch'i*" (*t'i ch'i* 提 气) or replenishing the *ch'i* (8.3.2). Hiccups, vomiting, coughing, and labored breathing are all brought on by *ch'i* backflow, and can all be treated with prescriptions for "bringing down the *ch'i*" (*chiang ch'i* 降 气 , 12.12).

10.6. Example of the Application of Therapeutic Principles

Patient *X*, a child of two and a half years, female, admitted after three days of fever, asthmatic coughing, and respiratory difficulty. The patient, normally in good health, three days earlier had suddenly fallen ill with high fever and headache, and had vomited

---

[13] The quotations are from the spurious chapter of SW cited in the last note, pages 467 and 482; see P56. In the *Inner Canon* the first set of rules is concerned with treating the results of unseasonable weather (P103–04), and the second with the principles of opposition therapy. Both refer to qualities of *ch'i*, not to symptoms directly. Here these passages are reinterpreted for a broader purpose, to illustrate the point that there are general types of abnormal activity that underlie the great diversity of symptoms and syndromes, and that these point to a limited number of consistent therapeutic approaches.

once. Upon admission, temperature was 39.8 degrees C (103.6 degrees F). The patient was coughing and breathing rapidly, about 40 respirations/minute, with spasmodic quivering of the wings of the nose, slight perspiration, thirst and agitation, and occasional small twitches on the face and extremities. The face was red with grey appearing about the lips, tongue coating whitish with some yellow, pulse 150 beats/minute, smooth and accelerated. There were dispersed rhonchi in both lungs, with faint moist rales in the upper right lobe. The heartbeat was accelerated, with no adventitious sounds. The abdomen was slightly distended, with some subjective feeling of blockage and fullness. The liver and spleen were slightly enlarged. Leucocyte count was 8,000, 75 percent neutrophilis. An X-ray photograph showed a pattern of general coarsening, with a relatively large laminar shadow in the right upper lobe.

A synthesis of the clinical findings and the epidemiology led the Western doctors to a diagnosis of viral pneumonia and the traditional doctors to a diagnosis of wind-warm heteropathy invading the pulmonary system (*feng wen fan fei* 风 温 犯 肺 , 9.1.1.1), and coughing and hurried, difficult breathing due to pulmonary hot heteropathy (*fei je ch'uan sou* 肺 热 喘 嗽 , 9.1.2.2).[14]

Analysis. The patient's illness was already in its fourth day. The toxicity had penetrated the organism, which was then mobilizing all its strength for the struggle. The current stage of the organism's situation was "repletion of heteropathy with preponderance of orthopathy," with the principal contradiction manifested as high fever (heteropathy having entered the *ch'i* sector, 9.1.2). Because the fever would not abate, the disorder could have developed into spasmodic Fright Disorders[15] (*ching chueh* 惊 厥 , extreme intensity of hot manifestation type giving rise to [internal] wind heteropathy, 9.1.2.1); coma; respiratory and circulatory failure, and so on. If it were possible without delay to control heteropathy and drive out the high fever, serious complications might be avoided. The therapeutic principle was to be "expel heteropathy and reinforce orthopathy," choosing medicines that would "clear hot heteropathy and flush out the toxicity (*ch'ing je*

---

[14] In this case, unlike that recorded in section 7.5, the signs and symptoms are more or less adequate to document the manifestation type determination.

[15] See 5.1.1.2, note 4 above.

chieh tu 清 热 解 毒 , 12.2.1.2), calm the fright and the wind" (*ting ching hsi feng* 定 惊 息 风 , 12.15.1.3).

Ephedra-apricot-gypsum-licorice Infusion (*ma hsing shih kan t'ang* 麻 杏 石 甘 汤 , 12.1) with added woad root (*pan-lan-ken* 板 蓝 根 [Isatis tinctoria]) and leaf (*ta-ch'ing-yeh* 大 青 叶) was used to "attack heteropathy and drain the hot factor" (*kung hsieh hsieh je* 攻 邪 泻 热). Ramulus and uncus of gambir vine (*kou-t'eng* 钩 藤 [Uncaris sinensis or U. rhynchophylla]), dried whitened silkworm (*chiang ts'an* 僵 蚕) and water buffalo horn (*shui-niu chiao* 水 牛 角) were used to "calm the hepatic system and the wind." With these were combined dendrobium (*shih hu* 石 斛 [D. spp.]) and adenophora root (*sha-shen* 沙 参 [A. polymorpha et al.]) to protect the dispersed body fluids. At the same time the patient was given fluid infusions, vitamin supplements, physical cooling, and so on.

After the patient had been treated as above for two days, body temperature fell to 38.2 degrees C (100.8 degrees), the flesh tremors abated, and there was a turn for the better in her general condition. But on the third day her spirits [i.e., vitality and alertness] deteriorated. She breathed with difficulty at about 50 respirations/minute, opening her mouth wide and straining her shoulders. The skin of her entire body was cyanotic, with a few points of hemorrhage. The heartbeat was accelerated and occasionally irregular. The pulse was 155 beats/minute, small, accelerated, and debilitated. There had also been a drop in blood pressure. The tongue was reddened and its coating dry. The liver was enlarged to about 4 cm (one and one half inches) under the costal arcus. The abdominal distension had become more serious, and defecation had ceased.

Analysis. Although the patient's temperature was now under control and there had been no Fright Disorder seizures, heteropathy had gradually penetrated deeply inward. Due to the invasion of toxicity, at the time the respiratory and circulatory systems were failing. In addition, the toxemia caused symptoms of intestinal paralysis to become evident. According to Chinese medical theory, when the pulmonary system of functions is closed off by heteropathy and the vital energy loses its motility, damage to the constructive *ch'i* and the blood results, with manifestations of yang *ch'i* deficiency in the pulmonary and cardiac systems. Therefore impediments to the respiratory and blood distribution functions develop. The current state of the patient's constitution was "heteropathic preponderance, orthopathic depletion." The principal contradiction had evolved into failure of the respiratory and circulatory functions. The therapeutic principle became "reinforcing orthopathy and expelling heteropathy."

Plain Ginseng Infusion (*tu shen t'ang* 独 参 汤 , 12.16) was used without delay to reinforce the orthopathic *ch'i*. The prescriptions given earlier, with ephedra and apricot pits omitted and Ningpo figwort root, tree peony bark (*tan-p'i* 丹 皮 [Paeonia suffruticosa]), and unpeeled peony root (*ch'ih shao* 赤 芍 [Paeoni lactiflora et al.]) added, were used to clear hot heteropathy in the blood sector (9.1.4). Acupuncture and moxibustion also were used to stimulate the respiratory and circulatory centers, assisted by necessary Western drugs, in order to clear and eliminate the mucus and maintain unimpeded circulation paths without delay. As for the abdominal distension and related symptoms, flesh of water snails (*t'ien-lo* 田 螺 [Viviparidae spp.]) was pounded in a mortar with the white part of scallions (*ts'ung pai* 葱 白 [Allium fistulosum]) and rubbed on the navel. Acupuncture was applied at *tsu-san-li* (V36) to replenish the orthopathic *ch'i*.

After four days' rescue work by a team of traditional and Western physicians, the patient gradually passed out of danger. Her temperature dropped to 37.3 degrees C (99.1 degrees F). Her cough was slight, heartbeat and respiration were gradually becoming normal, the abdominal distension was gone, and normal elimination was unimpeded. There was still mental fog. Appetite was not good. She tended to sleep a great deal. There was a slight rise in body temperature in the afternoons. The mouth and lips were strawberry-red, the tongue reddened with scanty coating, and the mouth dry and lips chapped. The pulse was small and slightly accelerated.

Analysis. The patient had passed through ten days' serious illness. Although for the time being she was in effect out of danger, heteropathy was not yet entirely gone, and orthopathic *ch'i* was still greatly depleted; this was the "orthopathy depleted and heteropathy causing confusion" (*cheng hsu hsieh luan* 正 虚 邪 恋) stage. According to traditional medical theory, warm heteropathy particularly tends to damage the yin *ch'i*, so the patient's principal contradiction for the immediate future was damage to the dispersed body fluids and loss of pulmonary yin *ch'i*. The therapeutic principle was "nourish the yin and clear the pulmonary system." Adenophora root, lily-turf root, rhizome of Solomon's Seal (*yü-chu* 玉 竹), and tricosanthes root (*hua-fen* 花 粉 [T. kirilowii]) were used to nourish the yin *ch'i* and produce body fluids. Hyacinth bean (*pien tou* 扁 豆 [Dolichos lablab]) and licorice root were used to replenish the *ch'i* of the splenetic and stomach systems. Mulberry root bark (*sang pai p'i* 桑 白 皮 [Morus alba]) and matrimony-vine root bark (*ti-ku p'i* 地 骨 皮 [Lycium chinense]) were used to clear yin heteropathy. Intensive nursing and attention to nutrition led to a gradual revival of the patient's orthopathic *ch'i*. After a little more than an additional week of recuperation, the disorder was cured and the patient discharged.

10.7. Conclusion

[*Translator's Note:* Since the conclusion mainly recapitulates technical terms, it is not included in this translation. Instead I will summarize what is especially significant about the chapter from the non-Chinese reader's point of view.

In this chapter the authors stress and identify with modern dialectic analysis the dialectical approach of traditional doctors as seen in their synthetic and holistic tendencies.[16] In the argument heavy weight is placed on the many indirect methods of treatment based on the assumption that the body is an interdependent system, itself the synthesis of a variety of subsystems, each of these with its part to play in the congeries of vital functions.

This argument is well supported with traditional examples, but it is not a traditional argument, and goes beyond the conceptual vocabulary of indigenous medicine. It is, in other words, an accurate description of the contemporary understanding and a sign of transition. It signals transition of two kinds. First is the technical reinterpretation of classical concepts that has broadened their scope, rendered them more consistently holistic than they originally were,[17] and made them useful in current practice. (I have remarked in the footnotes on examples of this changed understanding.) Second is the adaptation of classical thought to contemporary ideology, particularly to dialectical materialism. This process began more gradually over the last generation, but may be responsible ul-

---

[16] A considerable specialized literature of this kind has accumulated since the *Revised Outline* was published. Examples are four essays in Jen Ying-ch'iu and Liu Ch'ang-lin ed. 1982: 145–236.

[17] Martha Li Chiu 1986 has drawn attention to aspects of early classical doctrine that are not holistic.

timately for even greater departures from premodern medical doctrine. The dialectical term "principal contradiction" is especially prominent in chapter 10. The term is not accompanied by formal dialectical analysis, as one would expect of a fully developed Marxist theory of health and medical disorder. Instead, since Chinese readers can be expected to understand its basic sense, it is used in a stereotyped way to refer to the aspect of a disorder that demands priority in treatment. Stereotyped though it may be, it has come to play an important role in clinical reasoning, a role that is not discernible in books published a decade earlier. One can see from the extended example (10.6) that analysis of findings proceeds, or at least is recorded, according to a schema that begins with classifying the patient's pathological state under a traditional rubric (e.g., heteropathic preponderance, orthopathic depletion), and goes on to identify therapeutic priorities (the principal contradition), to formulate a therapeutic strategy (summarized in "therapeutic principles"), and finally to arrive at tactical decisions about particular prescriptions and other measures. Although one can see in this recent systematization some influence from the ideal schemas of modern medicine, the latter's great battle-cry, "Find the lesion," has remained unheard.

The case study is perhaps the most valuable in this book for the glimpse into the traditional doctor's mind that it provides. But it omits too much to allow readers to evaluate fully the reasoning of the doctor when faced with the complexity of a sick child. The information given is mainly that useful in traditional diagnosis and therapeutic evaluation. It is mostly derived from close observation of signs and symptoms. The laboratory results that most modern physicians would depend on to judge the case are not fully recorded. They were obviously available, since the authors note in passing that Western therapy was incorporated into the treatment. Indeed the data on fever, the white blood cell count, X-rays, and so on, are anything but conventional in traditional medicine, and point to a synthesis of the traditional and modern systems that the authors acknowledge but pass over superficially. The book gives practically no detailed information about what "Western" drugs and therapeutic methods were used. It is thus impossible to estimate the role that traditional and modern medicine each played in the recovery of this patient. Here, as in section 7.5, their participation does not appear to be balanced. On the other hand, the purpose of this book is not to make such estimates possible, but to provide an introduction to the traditional healing art.

It is also clear from this chapter, even more than others, that the book is not a systematic compilation by a single group. A number of prescriptions and therapeutic principles mentioned here are not given in the chapter on drug therapy (12), and even a few of the drugs are not included in the enumeration there.]

APPENDIX A

Representative Textbooks and Handbooks of Traditional Chinese Medicine

This list includes thirty-five works published in the People's Republic of China from 1958 on that were chosen for use in this study from the limited number available. Titles are listed chronologically in English translation, followed by the name of the author or editor. Most of these books give only the name of the compiling organization—in most cases a college of Chinese medicine or a hospital. For full references see bibliography B under author or compiler and year. The purpose of each book is indicated here. The number of copies printed is noted when known. The form "12/900,000" means "twelfth printing, 900,000 copies to date."

1958. *Outline of Chinese Medicine.* Nan-ching Chung-i hsueh-yuan. Textbook for colleges of Chinese medicine.
1960. *Lectures on Acupuncture and Moxibustion.* Shang-hai Chung-i hsueh-yuan. Textbook for colleges of Chinese medicine.
1964. *Outline of Chinese Pharmacology.* Li Hsiang-chung. For secondary schools of medicine and pharmacology. 1/15,000.
____. *Lectures on Chinese Pharmacy.* Nan-ching Chung-i hsueh-yuan. For colleges of Chinese medicine.
1970. *Barefoot Doctor's Handbook.* Shang-hai Chung-i hsueh-yuan. For basic training of and advanced study by barefoot doctors.
____. *Handbook of Acupuncture and Moxibustion Therapy.* Shang-hai shih chen-chiu yen-chiu-so. For part-time and low-level medical personnel. *See also* Chang Sheng-hsing 1983.
1971. *Village Physician's Handbook.* Hu-nan i-hsueh-yuan. For practitioners above the barefoot doctor level. 12/996,600.

429

____. *Basic Knowledge about the Fatherland's Medicine, New Therapies, and Chinese Materia Medica.* Shang-hai ti-i hsueh-yuan. For mass education in a patriotic campaign; one of a set of ten introductory volumes.

____. *Simplified Teaching Materials on Chinese Medicine.* T'ien-chin i-hsueh-yuan. Based on a combination of Chinese and modern medicine, meant for barefoot doctors and others as part of a national patriotic campaign.

____. *Barefoot Doctor's Handbook.* Hu-nan Chung-i-yao yen-chiu-so ko-wei-hui. For basic training of and advanced study by barefoot doctors.

1972. *Simplified Chinese Medicine.* Chung-kuo jen-min chieh-fang-chün. Textbook for modern physicians and advanced classes of barefoot doctors.

____. *Revised Outline of Chinese Medicine.* Kuang-chou pu-tui. For modern physicians. 1/261,000.

____. *Lectures on Chinese Medicine.* Liao-ning Chung-i hsueh-yuan. For teaching and general study. Reflects movement for synthesis of Chinese and modern medicine.

1974. *Simplified Chinese Medicine.* Ho-pei hsin i ta-hsueh. Major revision of 1972 edition, for same use. 3/515,050.

____. *Foundations of Chinese Medicine.* Pei-ching Chung-i hsueh-yuan. Textbook for colleges of Chinese medicine. 1/200,000.

____. *Chinese Internal Medicine.* T'ien-chin shih Chung-i i-yuan. For clinical reference by barefoot doctors and basic medical workers. 1/65,000.

1975. *Practical Chinese Medicine.* Pei-ching Chung-i i-yuan. For modern physicians in study sessions in their hospitals as part of a campaign.

1976. *Chinese Internal Medicine.* Shan-tung Chung-i hsueh-yuan. For study by low-level health workers, including barefoot doctors. Largely based on T'ien-chin shih Chung-i i-yuan 1974.

1977. *Training Manual for Barefoot Doctors.* Chi-lin i-k'o ta-hsueh. For training of barefoot doctors in North China. 2/201,000.

____. *Training Manual for Barefoot Doctors.* Shang-hai shih. For training of barefoot doctors in South China. 9/797,700.

1978. *Chinese Pharmacology.* Ch'eng-tu Chung-i hsueh-yuan. For students of Chinese medicine and pharmacy in medical colleges. 2/220,000.

____. *Outline of Chinese Medicine.* Hu-pei Chung-i hsueh-yuan. For pharmacy students in colleges of medicine and pharmacy.

_____. *Foundations of Chinese Medicine.* Pei-ching Chung-i hsueh-yuan. Textbook for students of clinical medicine in schools of Chinese medicine and pharmacy. The virtually identical Shanghai ed. was published for use by modern physicians studying Chinese medicine. Revision of 1974 version, also using other materials.

1979. *Simplified Internal Medicine for Combined Chinese and Western Therapy.* Chang Hsueh-yung. Readership unspecified, but compiled by a military medical school and an affiliated hospital. Introduction to traditional concepts, including manifestation type determination, and Western diagnosis.

_____. *Pharmacy.* Kuang-chou Chung-i hsueh-yuan. For students of Chinese medicine and pharmacy in medical colleges. 3/ 180,000.

1979–80. *Internal Medicine.* Shang-hai Chung-i hsueh-yuan. For students of Chinese medicine in medical colleges. Vol. 1, 5/ 212,000; Vol. 2, 5/198,000.

1980. *Foundations of Chinese Medicine.* Chiang-su sheng wei-sheng-t'ing. For private study by basic medical workers in hospitals and as reference material in middle schools of public health. 1/34,600.

1981. *Foundation studies in Chinese Medicine.* Ku Chen-sheng et al. Uses modern diagnostic entities "in order to deepen the understanding" of modern physicians. 3(1984)/71,500.

1982. *Chinese Materia Medica.* Kan-su sheng hsin i-yao-hsueh yen-chiu-so. For study of traditional medicine by practicing physicians.

1983. *Handbook of Acupuncture and Moxibustion Therapy.* Chang Sheng-hsing. Revision of Shang-hai-shih chen-chiu yen-chiu-so 1970. Note changes in theoretical viewpoint. 1/50,700.

_____. *Chinese Medicine.* Nan-ching Chung-i hsueh-yuan. For modern physicians and others studying Chinese medicine. 1/ 13,500.

_____. *Handbook of Chinese Internal Medicine.* Che-chiang Chung-i hsueh-yuan. Reference material for "clinical workers" in Chinese medicine and combined Chinese-Western therapy. 2(1984)/61,000.

1984. *Chinese Materia Medica.* Ling I-k'uei et al. Textbook for colleges of Chinese medicine and pharmacy, designed for students of medicine, pharmacy, and acupuncture. 1/55,500.

_____. *Basic Theories of Chinese Medicine.* Yin Hui-ho and Chang Po-no. Textbook for students of general Chinese medicine and of acupuncture in colleges of medicine and pharmacy. 1/60,600.

_____. *Pharmacology.* Chou Chin-huang ed. Textbook for colleges of traditional medicine, combining traditional and modern drugs; presupposes some knowledge of organic chemistry. 2/29,350.

APPENDIX B

Untranslated Chapters of the
Revised Outline of Chinese Medicine

The excerpt from the *Revised Outline* translated above, about a fifth of the book, is concerned with the reasoning behind diagnosis and therapy. The translation is integral except for a few excisions explained in the preface, pages xiii-xiv. The remaining six hundred pages is in effect a reference handbook of preventive and therapeutic resources and their use. It almost exclusively discusses materia medica, although many other resources are described above. Its contents are set out below to provide a general view of the book's organization.

APPENDIX C

Some Hypotheses about the Circulation
of Vital Substances

There are many contentious issues in the historical study of Chinese medical theory, most of them due to reading modern presuppositions into documents of a tradition created by people who did not think about the body in the way moderns do. This appendix will discuss two sets of claims made by authors who in other respects have been exceptionally alert to the differences between Chinese and Western assumptions.

Circulation Tracts and Blood Vessels

Maruyama Masao and Lu and Needham have claimed that blood vessels (*hsueh-mai* 血 脉) were distinguished from *ch'i* circulation tracts (*ching-lo*) in the *Inner Canon* and later writings; see Maruyama 1977: 132–34 and CL25–30. Maruyama claims that the distinction ceased to be made in the eighth century; Lu and Needham do not specify temporal limits. Neither hypothesis is consistent with the evidence.

Lu and Needham provide in tabular form data from the *Inner Canon* about the relative proportions of *ch'i* and *hsueh* in the circulation tracts, not in two separate systems (CL48). The information in this table, by the way, is said to be derived from SW (7 [24]: 134 in the edition cited here), but if so it is incorrectly transcribed. The versions in TS, *10* (4): 151 and LS, *10* (65): 99, which are not cited, both differ from SW with respect to proportions of *ch'i* and *hsueh* in the yin tracts.

The authors equate *hsueh* with constructive energy (*ying ch'i* 營 气 , 3.1.3). They then read a famous passage, "the constructive [*ch'i*] is in the vessels (*mo*); the defensive [*ch'i*] is outside the vessels," to mean that the blood flows in blood vessels and the yang *ch'i* flows in the tracts. There is no warrant in the texts or commentaries for this reading, which they do not support by evidence. The usual understanding from the earliest scholiasts to the present is that given in the *Revised Introduction*, 3.1.3. For the passage in question, see TS, *12* (1): 3, a fragment in TIZ only, LS, *4* (18): 43 and other sources cited in CL29.

It is not difficult to find passages that put the constructive *ch'i* in tracts rather than vessels, such as "the *ch'i* that floats up and does not follow the course of the tracts (*ching*) is the defensive *ch'i*; the essential *ch'i* that travels in the tracts is the constructive *ch'i*"; see TS, *10* (7): 156 = LS, *8* (52): 83. Chang Chieh-pin 張 介 賓 , a commentator on whom Lu and Needham frequently rely, cites this passage in his *Lei ching* 類 经 (1624), *8* (23): 25b, as equivalent to that in the last paragraph. The only logical conclusion is that for the task of differentiating the two types of *ch'i* "tract" and "vessel" are interchangeable. See also pp. 135–36 and 157 above.

The Heart and Lungs as Pumps

CL30–32 attempts to prove that the heart is "a pump of some kind, working in systole to propel the blood through its system of tubes," and that the lungs are "responsible for pumping of the *chhi*" in traditional writings. The proof offered for the latter proposition is two classical statements that the *ch'i* "returns to the lungs," one that the *ch'i* "pertains to the lungs," and one that, grading the visceral systems hierarchically without mentioning *ch'i*, says (in the translation of Lu and Needham) "the heart (in the body) is like the monarch (in the State), fount of all clarity and brightness; the lungs are like the prime minister, from whom all control proceeds." The original context indicates that this statement (SW, *3* [8]: 49) is about all pulmonary functions, not about the respiration in particular. It appears to be saying that the pulmonary system's ability to regulate derives from the "directing influence" (P127) of the cardiac system, on behalf of which the entire somatic bureaucracy administers. The evidence concerning the lungs suggests that the pulmonary system does not provide the motive power but rather regulates the circulation of *ch'i* and *hsueh*, precisely as the *Revised Outline* explains in rather modernized language (2.1.4.1.1). The sources cited do not mention pumping.

As for the proposition about the heart as a pump, again no
evidence is provided for more than a regulatory function. The statement, attributed to SW, that "the heart presides over the circulation
of the blood and juices" is not from that source, but from a very free
1958 translation of the *Su wen* into modern Chinese.

Lu and Needham then quote SW, *13* (48): 238: "Asthma (*chia*
痃) will occur if there is no drumming in the vessel of the heart,"
adding that Wang Ping comments "if there is no working of the bellows (lit., drumming, *ku* 鼓) then the blood will not flow round."
The passage from SW cannot be so punctuated. The original sentence is "*Shen mai hsiao chi, kan mai hsiao chi, hsin mai hsiao chi,
chieh wei chia* 肾 脉 ·小·急 ， 肝 脉 小·急 ， 心 脉 ·小·急 ，
皆 為 痃 ." I would translate "if the renal, hepatic, or cardiac
pulse is small and hurried without drumming [*ku* is a technical term
for a strong beat on the 'floating reading,' 6.4.1], an intermittent,
indefinite abdominal mass (*chia*) is indicated." Wang's annotation,
read in its entirety, supports this understanding: "a small, hurried
[pulse] means that the cold heteropathy is strong. Absence of
drumming means *hsueh* is not flowing, and this means that the cold
heteropathy has formed a stasis (*po* 溥 = 搏). Thus the *hsueh*
congeals within as an abdominal mass." Wang understands SW to
be saying that the pulse, despite its acceleration, indicates a powerful stasis, a predisposing condition for growths. This quotation is in
fact taken from a canonical chapter on pulse phenomena. Other
commentators agree with Wang's understanding. See, for instance,
Yang Shang-shan 楊 上 善 (666/683?) in TS, *15* (5): 306; Wu
K'un 吴 焜 in *Nei ching su wen Wu chu* 内 经 素 問 吴 注
(1594), *13* (48): 196; Chang Chih-ts'ung 張 志 聰 in *Huang ti
nei ching su wen chi chu* 黄 帝 内 经 素 問 集 注 (1670), *5*
(48): 182; *Su wen ching chu chieh chieh* 素 問 集 注 節 解
(1677), *3*: 158; *Huang ti su wen chih chieh* 黄 帝 素 問 直 解
(1695), *4* (48): 325–26; and the annotation of Ma Shih 馬 蒔
(1586) in Ch'eng Shih-te 1982: 680n5.

As for late sources, twice on page 31 of CL, Lu and Needham
quote Chang Chieh-pin's *Lei ching* (1624), a topical rearrangement
of the *Inner Canon* with a valuable commentary. Chang's annotation does not say, as they claim, that the heart or cardiac system is
in some sense a pump. In one of the two places it says that "the
cardiac system governs the *hsueh* vessels, which respond to the motion of Fire and circulate [the *hsueh* and *ch'i*] throughout the entire
body" (*15* [25]: 5a, my translation). This might be taken to mean
that the pulsating vessels move the *ch'i* and *hsueh*, in resonance

with the cardiac *ch'i* (Fire, 5.1.6.1). Lu and Needham translate Chang's second statement as "the heart and pulse (*mai*) is not itself either *chhi* or blood (*hsueh*), but rather it is the bellows of the *chhi* and the *hsueh*." No word corresponding to "heart," however, is found in the original, *Lei ching*, 8 (23): 25b. The subject is not the phenomenon of the pulse but the circulation vessels; in fact Chang is commenting on the famous passage that puts the constructive *ch'i* in the vessels (*mai*) and the defensive *ch'i* outside them (see pages 437–38). Keeping this in mind, and translating the rest less freely, makes Chang's simile consistent with the first quotation: "The vessels themselves are not *ch'i* or *hsueh*, but it is as if they were the bellows-cases and airpipes (*t'o-yueh* 橐 籥) for *ch'i* and *hsueh*." Chang's collection *Ching-yueh ch'üan shu,* cited for additional support in CL31, note c, says merely "*hsueh* and *ch'i* are the bellows of man," without mentioning the cardiac system (2 [18]: 45b). This seventeenth-century medical scholar is certainly using technological imagery, but even that late in the evolution of medicine it is used only in an isolated simile for circulation vessels and as an undeveloped metaphor for the vital substances themselves. In none of these instances is propulsion traced to the cardiac system. The point of Lu and Needham's attempt is to prove that "the earliest reference to the heart as a pump is by a hairsbreadth Chinese" (CL34), but historians of medicine do not agree with them that Harvey argued that the heart is a pump "in the context of a general circulation" (note b). See the close analysis in Webster 1965, and the less critical discussion in Basalla 1962.

   To sum up, Lu and Needham's evidence merely confirms that Porkert and other writers, when they call the cardiac system's dominant function the regulation of the circulation vessels and pulses, are faithful to traditional physiology as a whole. The attempt by Lu and Needham to see mechanical models reminiscent of seventeenth- and eighteenth-century Europe in earlier Chinese sources goes even beyond the modernizing trend of such recent textbooks as the *Revised Outline*. The latter in this connection says merely that "the ability of the blood to circulate in the blood vessels depends entirely on its propulsion by the *ch'i* of the cardiac system" (1.1.1.1.2).

APPENDIX D

Curriculum of a Traditional Medical School

The list of subjects that follows is taken from the transcript of a recent medical school graduate, Shen Yü 沈 谕 . This five-year course was completed between 1978 and 1983 at the Beijing College of Traditional Chinese Medicine (Bei-ching Chung-i hsueh-yuan 北 京 中 医 学 院), a leading institution. Major courses are listed separately; subsidiary courses are grouped. For information regarding the medical classics listed as the topics of courses, see bibliography A.

Year 1

Foundations of Chinese Medicine
Medical Classical Chinese
Anatomy
Chinese Materia Medica
Philosophy, History of Medicine

Year 2

Chinese Pharmacy
Biochemistry
Physiology
Political Economy
Pathology
English
Huang ti nei ching, Latin, Microbiology

441

Year 3

Pharmacology
Shang han lun
Foundations of Diagnosis
Surgery

Year 4

Internal Medicine
Acupuncture and Moxibustion
Chinese Pediatrics
Chinese Traumatology, Obstetrics and Gynecology, EENT,
    Stomatology, X-ray Diagnosis, Electrocardiography

Year 5

Chin kuei yao lueh
Chinese Medical Doctrines
Warm Factor Disorders
Hygiene

Clinical Practice

Cardiovascular, Respiratory, Blood, and Digestive Disease in
internal; Surgery; Obstetrics and Gynecology; Acupuncture and
Moxibustion

APPENDIX E

Abbreviations for Acupuncture Loci

The European abbreviations follow the system of Otto Karow as given in Lu and Needham 1980: 53–59. There is no accepted standard in the P.R.C. for numbering loci. The numbers given here are those most commonly used, taken from Beijing College of Traditional Chinese Medicine et al. 1980. They coincide with, but are less extensive than, those in Shang-hai Chung-i hsueh-yuan ed. 1961, a monograph on loci.

Locus	Section	European	Chinese
Chang-men	4.3.3.2.2	H13	Liv13
Chao-hai	4.4.2.5	R6	K6
Ch'i-hai	4.2.5.3	JM6	Ren 6
Ch'i-men	4.3.3.2.2	H14	Liv14
Chien-ming	4.3.3.4	None	None
Chih-kou	4.4.2.1	SC6	SJ6
Ch'ih-tse	4.3.3.2.2	P5	Lu5
Chü-ch'ueh	4.4.2.1	JM14	Ren14
Ch'ü-ch'ih	4.4.2.2	IG11	LI11
Ch'ü-ku	4.4.2.5	JM2	Ren2
Chung-chi	4.4.2.5	JM3	Ren3
Chung-chu	4.3.3.2.1	SC3	SJ3
Chung-feng	4.3.3.2.2	H4	Liv4
Chung-fu	4.3.1	P1	Lu1
Chung-kuan	4.3.3.3.3	JM12	Ren12

Locus	Section	European	Chinese
Fei-shu	4.3.1	VU13	UB13
Feng-ch'ih	4.3.3.1	VF20	GB20
Feng-fu	4.2.5.2	TM15	Du16
Feng-lung	4.3.3.4	V40	St40
Feng-men	4.3.3.4	VU12	UB12
Feng-shih	4.3.3.4	VF31	GB31
Fu-liu	4.3.3.4	R7	K7
Ho-ku	4.3.3.2.1	IG4	LI4
Hsi-men	4.4.2.2	HC4	P4
Hsin-shu	4.4.2.2	VU15	UB15
Hsing-chien	4.3.3.2.4	H2	Liv2
Hsuan-chung	4.3.3.3.3	VF39	GB39
Jen-chung	4.2.5.2	TM25	Du26
Jen-ying	4.4.2.2	V9	St9
Kan-shu	4.3.3.2.4	VU18	UB18
Kao-huang	4.3.3.4	VU38	UB43
Ko-shu	4.3.3.3.3	VU17	UB17
Kuan-yuan	4.2.5.3	JM4	Ren4
Kung-sun	4.3.3.2.3	LP4	Sp4
K'ung-tsui	4.3.3.2.2	P6	Lu6
Lan-wei hsueh	4.3.1	None	Extra18
Liang-men	4.3.3.2.2	V21	St21
Lieh-ch'ueh	4.3.3.2.2	P7	Lu7
Mai-pu	4.3.3.4	None	None
Ming-men	4.2.5.3	TM4	Du4
Nei-kuan	4.3.3.4	HC6	P6
Nei-t'ing	4.3.3.2.1	V44	St44
Pai-hui	4.2.5.2	TM19	Du20
P'i-shu	4.3.1	VU20	UB20
San-yin-chiao	4.3.3.2.1	LP6	Sp6
Shan-chung	4.2.5.3	JM17	Ren17
Shang-chü-hsu	4.3.3.2.2	V37	St37
Shang-hsing	4.3.3.1	TM22	Du23
Shao-hai	4.4.2.7	C3	H3
Shao-tse	4.4.2.6	IT1	Si1
Shen-ch'ueh	8.1.5	JM8	Ren8
Shen-men	4.3.3.4	C7	H7

Locus	Section	European	Chinese
Shen-shu	4.2.5.3	VU23	UB23
Shih-ch'i-chui	4.4.2.2	None	Extra10
Shih-hsuan	4.4.2.2	None	Extra15
Shui-ch'üan	4.3.3.2.4	R5	K5
Ssu-feng	4.4.2.1	None	Extra14
Su-liao	4.2.5.2	TM24	Du25
Ta-ch'ang-shu	4.4.2.1	VU25	UB25
Ta-chu	4.3.3.3.3	VU11	UB11
Ta-chui	4.2.5.3	TM13	Du14
T'ai-ch'i	4.3.3.2.4	R3	K3
T'ai-ch'ung	4.3.3.2.2	H3	Liv3
T'ai-pai	4.3.3.2.4	LP3	Sp3
T'ai-yang	6.1.2.1	VF1	GB1
T'ai-yuan	4.3.3.2.2	P9	Lu9
Tan-nang-tien	4.3.1	None	Extra19
Tan-shu	4.4.2.6	VU19	UB19
T'ien-shu	4.4.2.1	V25	St25
T'ien-t'u	4.4.2.1	JM22	Ren22
Ting-ch'uan	4.3.3.4	None	Extra6
T'ing-ling	4.3.3.4	None	None
Tseng-yin	4.3.3.4	None	None
Tsu-san-li	4.3.3.2.2	V36	St36
T'ung-tzu-liao	6.1.2.1	VF1	GB1
Wei-chung	4.3.3.2.1	VU54	UB40
Wei-shu	4.3.1	VU21	UB21
Yang-ling-ch'üan	4.3.3.1	VF34	GB34
Yin-ling-ch'üan	4.3.3.2.4	LP9	Sp9
Yin-men	4.3.3.2.1	VU51	UB37
Yin-t'ang	4.3.3.1	Odd1	Extra1
Yung-ch'üan	8.1.1	R1	K1
Yü-chi	4.3.3.2.2	P10	Lu10

APPENDIX F

Summary Conversion Table for Pinyin and Wade-Giles Romanizations

This table is approximate. It ignores elements that are identical in the two systems.

	Pinyin	*Wade-Giles*
Initials	b	p
	c	ts'
	d	t
	g	k
	j	ch
	k	k'
	p	p'
	q	ch'
	r	j
	t	t'
	x	hs
	z	ts
	zh	ch
Finals	e	eh
	ian	ien
	ong	ung
	ui	uei
	o *or* uo	o
Syllables	ju	chü
	yi	i
	you	yu
	yu	yü

447

BIBLIOGRAPHIES

The two annotated bibliographies that follow include only books, essays, and manuscripts cited in this book. They represent only a fraction of the sources consulted.

The Chinese sources written before 1900 in bibliography A are cited in this book by title. Authoritative works were often given various names over the centuries; I cite books consistently by their oldest known titles, with cross-references from more familiar titles where necessary. The editions used are identified using the varied but unambiguous forms customary in Sinological writings. When possible I avoid citing editions printed in simplified characters, since there is an unavoidable loss of information. When more than one edition is listed, the first is the one cited except when specified.

Annotations justify datings or explain why a seldom-used work is important. Sometimes they elucidate a title the meaning of which may not be obvious to a modern reader, or tell why my translation of a title differs in some significant way from those in previous publications in Western languages. I also mention useful editions that I did not have occasion to cite.

Bibliography B includes all other sources, cited in the body of this book by author, editor, or compiling organization, and date. Translations of some of the names of organizations do not correspond to official English versions, since some of the latter are unavailable and others are not in standard English. My use of "ed." and "et al." is not entirely consistent, since in general it reflects usage in the original publications. I use "et al." for works with more than two authors. Published English translations of book or article titles are provided in quotation marks when available, except in a few cases when a straightforward English equivalent of the Chinese title is more informative. Annotations usually provide information about the contents of a source or remark on its strengths or limitations.

Wade-Giles romanization is used as elsewhere in this book. Within a single entry, initial letters are used as abbreviations to

449

minimize repetition; for instance, *Chin kuei yao lueh fang lun* is followed by CK *yü han* YLFL, which means *Chin kuei yü han yao lueh fang lun*. In bibliography B, Chinese and Japanese orthography reflect that of the source.

"1027–1029" means "the years 1027–1029 inclusive"; "1027/1029" means "some time within the period 1027–1029."

Abbreviations

Collections Cited in Bibliography A

BSS   *Basic Sinological Series (Kuo-hsueh chi-pen ts'ung-shu* 國 學 基 本 叢 書)

CP   *[Tseng pu] chen pen i shu chi ch'eng* 增 補 珍 本 醫 書 集 成

HY   Harvard-Yenching Institute Sinological Index Series

ITCM   *I t'ung cheng mai ch'üan shu* 醫 統 正 脈 全 書 (Beijing, 1907; repr., Taipei, 1975)

TIZ   *Tōyō igaku zempon sōsho* 東 洋 医 学 善 本 叢 書 (see Kosoto et al., ed. 1981)

Editorial Abbreviations

a.p.	author's preface dated
attrib.	attributed to
C	century (1C = first century)
comp.	compiled by
compl.	completed
ed.	edited, editor
e. p.	editor's preface dated
pr.	printed
prob.	probably
publ.	published (not necessarily printed)
repr.	reprinted
rev.	revised
simpl. chars.	simplified characters
tr.	translated by, translator, translation

Bibliography A
Sources in East Asian Languages before 1900

Ch'an chien 產 鑑 [Mirror of obstetrics]. Wang Hua-chen 王 化 貞 , a.p. 1618. CC chu shih 注 释 , Kaifeng, 1982.
Critical edition of rare work, censored and with mediocre annotations.

Chen chiu chia i ching 鍼 灸 甲 乙 经 . See *Huang ti chia i ching* 黃 帝 甲 乙 经 .

Cheng chih chun sheng 證 治 準 繩 [Water level and line marker (i.e., standards) of diagnosis and therapy]. Wang K'en-t'ang 王 肯 堂 , a.p. 1602–1608. Reprint of first eds., 6 vols., Shanghai, 1957–1959.
An important collection, largely oriented toward clinical practice, by a scholar active in defining medical orthodoxy.

Ch'eng fang ch'ieh yung 成 方 切 用 [Practical prescriptions]. Wu I-lo 吳 儀 洛 , pr. 1761. P'ing hua shu wu 瓶 花 書 屋 edition of 1847.

Cheng-ho sheng chi tsung lu 政 和 聖 濟 總 録 [Medical encyclopedia: A sagely benefaction of the Regnant Harmony era]. Shen Fu 申 甫 et al., eds. by imperial order, issued 1122. Reprint, 2 vols., Beijing, 1952, 1982.
Title reflects imperial patronage.

Ch'i ching pa mai k'ao 奇 経 八 脉 考 [On the extraordinary tracts]. Li Shih-chen 李 時 珍 , pr. 1578. Printed with *Pents'ao kang mu* 本 草 綱 目 .

Chia i ching 甲 乙 経 . See *Huang ti chia i ching* 黃 帝 甲 乙 経 .

Ch'ien chin fang 千 金 方 . See *Pei chi ch'ien chin yao fang* 備 急 千 金 要 方 .

Ch'ien k'un t'i i 乾 坤 體 義 [Cosmological epitome]. Matteo Ricci 利 瑪 竇 , compl. 1608. Photograph of Ssu k'u ch'üan shu 四 庫 全 書 MS in Jimbun kagaku kenkyūsho, Kyoto.

Chin kuei yao lueh fang lun 金 匱 要 畧 方 論 [Essentials and discussions of prescriptions in the golden casket].

451

Usually referred to as CK *yao lueh*. One of the three books into which *Shang han tsa ping lun* 傷 寒 雜 病 論 was divided in the official edition of 1064/1065. In ITCM under the title as in the latter edition, CK *yü han* 玉 丞 YLFL.
See *Shang han tsa ping lun* entry below.

Ching shih cheng lei Ta-kuan pen-ts'ao 経 史 證 類 大 觀 本 草 [Materia medica of the Great Prospect era, classified and verified from the classics and histories]. Ai Sheng 艾 晟 ed., pub. 1108. Reprint of 1302 edition, Tokyo, 1970.

Ching-yueh ch'üan shu 景 岳 全 書 [Collected treatises]. Chang Chieh-pin 張 介 賓 , 1624. Reprint of Yueh ssu lou 岳 峙 樓 edition, Taipei, 1972.

Chou i 周 易 [Book of changes]. Anon., ca. 800 B.C. HY.

Chu ping yuan hou lun 諸 病 源 候 論 [Origins and symptoms of medical disorders]. Ch'ao Yuan-fang 巢 元 方 , compl. 610. Reprint of 1891 edition, Beijing, 1955.
For critical edition in simpl. chars. see Nan-ching Chung-i hsueh-yuan 南 京 中 医 学 院 ed. 1980.

Chu-tzu yü lei 朱 子 語 類 [Classified discourses]. Chu Hsi 朱 喜 (1130–1200), posthumously compiled 1270. *CTYL ta ch'üan* 大 全 . Reprint of 1688 Yamashinaya 山 形 屋 edition, 8 vols., Taipei, 1973.

Ch'uan ya 串 雅 [The penetrator improved]. Chao Po-yun 趙 栢 雲 . Chao Hsueh-min 趙 學 敏 ed., e.p. 1759. Kowloon, 1957. The volumes of selections cited here are Fu-chien sheng i-yao yen-chiu-so 福 建 省 医 药 研 究 所 ed. 1977, Ch'ang-ch'un Chung-i hsueh-yuan 长 春 中 医 学 院 ed. 1980, and Yü Ch'uan 于 船 et al., eds. 1982. "Penetrator" was itinerant doctors' slang for drugs of downward-tending function, mostly purges. The title, given the book by its eminent editor, refers to his effort to make the work of his itinerant friend respectable by choosing remedies from the latter's repertory that would not be offensive to an elite reader-ship. The title also suggests the broad purview of the dictionary *Erh ya* 爾 雅 (probably early Han), which ultimately became one of the Confucian classics.

Chuang-tzu 莊 子 [The works of Chuang-tzu]. Attributed to Chuang Chou 莊 周 , second half of 4C B.C., but parts are much later; collected 1C B.C., reached final form ca. A.D. 300. HY. See Graham 1981: 27.

Ch'un ch'iu fan lu 春 秋 繁 露 ["Abundant dew" interpretation of the *Spring and Autumn Annals*]. Tung Chung-shu 董 仲

舒 , ca. 135 B.C. *CCFL i cheng* 義 證 , a.p. 1909, first edition of 1910; reprint, Kyoto, 1973.

Chung tsang ching 中 藏 經 [Canon kept in the palace repository]. Attrib. Hua T'o 華 佗 (d. A.D. 208?), but prob. N. Sung. ITCM.

Fu k'o yü ch'ih 婦 科 玉 尺 [Jade footrule of obstetrics and gynecology]. Shen Chin-ao 沈 金 鼇 , a.p. 1774. Typeset edition, one item censored, simpl. chars., Shanghai, 1983.
"Jade footrule" implies "precious standard."

Hsi yuan chi lu 洗 冤 集 錄 [Collected record of the washing away of wrongs]. Sung Tz'u 宋 慈 , a.p. 1247. Critical edition by Chia Ching-t'ao 賈 靜 濤 based on Yuan recension, Shanghai, 1981.
The oldest extant manual of forensic medicine. The title refers to punishing criminals through accurate determination of the cause of death. See McKnight trans. 1981.

Hsiao erh yao cheng chih chueh 小 兒 藥 證 直 訣 [Direct instructions for pediatric manifestation types and medicines]. Ch'ien I 錢 乙 and Yen Chi-chung 閻 季 忠 (also known as Hsiao-chung 孝 忠) eds., compl. 1119. In Wu-ying-tien chü-chen-pan ts'ung-shu 武 英 殿 聚 珍 版 叢 書 .
Important for early form of visceral manifestation type determination (*chüan* 1) and for pediatric case histories (*chüan* 2).

Hsin hsiu pen-ts'ao 新 修 本 草 [Revised materia medica]. Su Ching 蘇 敬 , compl. 650/659. Critical reconstruction by Okanishi Tameto 岡 西 為 人 , *Ch'ung chi* 重 輯 HHPT, rev. edition, Kawanishi, 1978.

Hsing se wai chen chien mo 形 色 外 诊 简 摩 [Simplified study of external diagnosis]. Chou Hsueh-hai 周 學 海 , 1894. In Chou shih i hsueh ts'ung-shu 周 氏 醫 學 叢 書 . Reprint, Beijing, 1960.

Hsun-tzu 荀 子 [Collected writings]. Hsun Ch'ing 荀 卿 , fl. 298–238 B.C. HY.

Huai-nan-tzu 淮 南 子 [The writings of the King of Huai-nan]. Comp. under the patronage of Liu An 劉 安 , 164/139 B.C. Collected commentary of Liu Wen-tien 劉 文 典 , *HN hung lieh chi chieh* 鴻 烈 集 解 , pr. 1923.

Huang ti chia i ching 黃 帝 甲 乙 经 ["A-B" canon of the Yellow Lord]. Huang-fu Mi 皇 甫 謐 , compl. 256/282. In ITCM under the title of the official N. Sung edition, *HT chen chiu* 鍼 灸 CIC.

For variora see Shan-tung Chung-i hsueh-yuan 山 东 中 医
学 院 ed. 1979. Collects and orders the three major "Yellow
Lord" texts extant in its time. Discusses circulation tracts and
acupuncture loci identified with the Six Warps. Uses yin-yang
and Five Phases theories systematically. Note that this book is
contemporary with the equally important *Mai ching*. Most
modern editions are entitled *Chen chiu chia i ching*. The "A-B"
in the title refers to the designation of the 10 original chapters
by a series of cyclical characters roughly equivalent to Latin letters. The chapters are so cited in *Wai t'ai pi yao*.

Huang ti nei ching 黄 帝 内 經 [Inner canon of the Yellow
Lord]. Anon., prob. 1C B.C. *HTNC su wen* 素 問 and *HTNC
ling shu* 靈 樞 are generally considered the surviving parts of
this work, but see Keegan forthcoming. *HTNC t'ai su* 太 素
is a late recension. See individual titles for references, and additional titles *s.v.* HTNC *Ling shu, Su wen*.

Huang ti nei ching ling shu 黄 帝 内 經 靈 樞 [Inner Canon
of the Yellow Lord: Divine pivot]. Wang Ping 王 冰 ed. 762.
Typeset reprint of early or mid-Ming edition, Beijing, 1956,
1982. For critical edition in simpl. chars. see Kuo Ai-ch'un 郭
靄 春 1982 (bibliography B).

Huang ti nei ching ling shu chu cheng fa wei 黄 帝 内 經 靈
樞 注 證 發 微 [The divine pivot: Elucidation of subtleties
with critical notes in the form of a commentary]. Ma Shih 馬
蒔, a.p. 1580. Oldest extant complete commentary. In *Ku chin
t'u shu chi ch'eng*, "I pu" 古 今 圖 書 集 成 醫 部
(*q.v.*).

Huang ti nei ching su wen 黄 帝 内 經 素 問 [Inner Canon of
the Yellow Lord: Basic questions]. Wang Ping ed., e.p. 762.
Critical text based on Ssu pu ts'ung k'an 四 部 叢 刊 edition, Beijing, 1956, 1982. For more extensively based critical
edition in simpl. chars. see Kuo Ai-ch'un 1981. A good recent
collection of classical annotations is Ch'eng Shih-te 程 士 德
ed. 1982.

My tr. of the title is based on the first commentator, Ch'üan
Yuan-ch'i 全 元 起 (6C), who glosses *su* as *pen* 本 . The
several prevalent translations are derived from forced explanations by later commentators ("plain questions") or are imagina-
tive interpretations rather than translations ("questions [and
answers] about living matter").

Huang ti nei ching su wen chi chu 黃帝內經素問集註 [Basic questions, with collected annotations]. Chang Chih-ts'ung 張志聰 , a.p. 1670, pr. 1672. Shanghai, 1959. Does not identify sources of particular annotations, and often philologically deficient, but an important commentary.

Huang ti nei ching t'ai su 黃帝內經太素 [Inner Canon of the Yellow Lord: Grand basis]. Yang Shang-shan 楊上善 , 666/683? Critical edition, Beijing, 1965. This edition omits many extant portions of the Ninnaji MS, which I cite from the TIZ photographs.

The usual dating of ca. 600 depends on late sources. Evidence for the date adopted here is summarized in Maruyama Toshiaki 1981: 63–65; see also Ch'ien Ch'ao-ch'en 钱超尘 1982. Maruyama's case is not conclusive, but he failed to consider Yang's entire official title. The latter rules out any date earlier than 650, and tallies with evidence that further narrows the span. The name of the book refers to a stage of cosmogony.

Huang ti pa-shih-i nan ching 黃帝八十一難經 [Canon of eighty-one problems (in the Inner canon) of the Yellow Lord]. Anon., prob. 2C A.D. In *Nan ching pen i* 難經本義 , *q.v.*

Huang ti su wen chih chieh 黃帝素問直解 [Basic questions: A direct commentary]. Kao Shih-shih 高世栻 , pr. 1695. Critical edition based on 1695 and 1887 versions, Beijing, 1980.

Synthesis of the views of Kao's teacher Chang Chih-ts'ung and his predecessors.

I chi k'ao 醫籍考 [Studies of medical books]. Taki Mototane 多紀元胤 (*or* Tamba no Mototane 丹波元胤), compl. 1819, pr. 1831. Reprint with added indexes, *Chung-kuo* 中国 *ICK*, Beijing, 1956.

A pastiche of bibliographical descriptions, critical notes, prefaces, etc., for a broad range of medical literature. A more detailed work of similar content for books through the end of the Sung is Okanishi 1958. Both are in Chinese.

I fang chi chieh 醫方集解 [Collected explanations of medical prescriptions]. Wang Ang 汪昂 , pr. 1682. Taipei, 1973.

Nearly 700 prescriptions are arranged under Wang's comprehensive system of 21 rubrics, from which most 20C classifications are descended.

I hsueh ch'i yuan 醫學啟源 [Basic medical studies for beginners]. Chang Yuan-su 張元素 , late 12C. Critical edition by Jen Ying-ch'iu 任应秋 based on 1472 ed., Beijing, 1978.

A basic textbook, prob. written down by Chang's leading disciple Li Ming-chih 李明之 .

I hsueh ch'uan teng 醫學傳燈 [Transmission of the lamp of medical studies]. Ch'en Ch'i 陳岐 , a.p. 1700. CP.
"Transmission of the lamp" implies "orthodox tradition."

I hsueh hsin wu 醫學心悟 [The awakening of the mind in medical studies]. Ch'eng Kuo-p'eng 程國彭 , a.p. 1732. Ch'eng shu tzu t'ang 程樹滋堂 edition of 1732, reprint, Beijing, 1955.
An influential, aphoristic work.

I hsueh ju men 醫學入門 [Introduction to medical studies]. Li Ch'an 李梴 , a.p. 1575. Ch'ing yun lou 青雲樓 edition, reprint, Taipei, 1973.

I hsueh shih-tsai i 醫學實在易 [Medicine is really simple]. Ch'en Nien-tsu 陳念祖 , compl. 1808. Annotated critical edition, simpl. chars., Fuzhou, 1982.
A greatly simplified general text for beginners.

I hsueh yuan-liu lun 醫學源流論 [Topical discussions of the history of medicine]. Hsu Ta-ch'un 徐大椿 , a.p. 1757. In *Hsu Ling-t'ai i shu ch'üan chi* 徐靈胎醫書全集 , 4 vols., Taipei, 1972.

I i hsiao ts'ao 醫醫小草 [Jottings for the doctoring of medicine]. Pao Hui 寶輝 , a.p. 1901. CP.
Very short essays on a broad variety of medical topics.

I kuan 醫貫 [The pervading unity of medicine]. Chao Hsien-k'o 趙獻可 , 1617? Critical edition, Beijing, 1959.

I lin kai ts'o 醫林改錯 [Corrections of errors in the forest of medicine, i.e., among physicians]. Wang Ch'ing-jen 王清任 , pr. 1830. Kowloon, 1964.
A radical reevaluation of traditional views of the viscera and circulation.

I men pang ho 醫門棒喝 [To awaken the doctors]. Chang Nan 章楠 , a.p. 1825. Reprint of Wang Meng-ying 王孟英 ed., 1909, 2 vols., Taipei, 1973.
Pang ho is a Buddhist term for a blow and a shout to awaken a drowsy disciple from error.

I pien 醫碥 [Stepping-stone to medicine]. Ho Meng-yao 何夢瑤 , pr. 1751. Reprint of 1751 T'ung wen t'ang 同文堂 edition, Shanghai, 1982.

I shu 醫述 [The medical heritage]. Ch'eng Wen-yu 程文囿 , compl. 1826, pr. 1833. Hofei, 1983.

The title is an allusion to Confucius' claim to be a transmitter and not a creator (*shu erh pu tso* 述 而 不 作). A general introduction to medicine in the form of an anthology compiled from more than 320 sources, with attention to both theory and therapy.

I tsung pi tu 醫 宗 必 讀 [Essential readings for the orthodox line of physicians]. Li Chung-tzu 李 仲 梓 , a.p. 1637. Taipei, 1971.

I yuan 醫 原 [The bases of medicine]. Shih Shou-t'ang 石 壽 棠 , pr. 1861. Critical edition, Nanjing, 1983.

Iseki kō 醫 籍 考 . See *I chi k'ao*.

Ko-chih yü lun 格 致 餘 論 [Supplementary discussions for the perfection of understanding through investigation of phenomena]. Chu Chen-heng 朱 震 亨 , 1347. CP.

Chu was one of the few leading physicians to be an initiate in a school of Confucianism. The title refers to a Neo-Confucian ideal.

Ku chin i an an 古 今 醫 案 按 [Medical case histories old and new, with analytical comments]. Yü Chen 俞 震 , a.p. 1778. Shanghai, 1959.

Leading anthology, from the first writings in this genre in the Sung until the beginning of the Ch'ing.

Ku chin t'u shu chi ch'eng: "I pu" 古 今 圖 書 集 成 " 醫 部 " [Encyclopedia collected from sources old and new: "Section on medicine"]. Chiang T'ing-hsi 蔣 廷 錫 et al., compl. 1725. *KCTSCCIP ch'üan shu* 全 書 , 16 vols., Pan-ch'iao, Taiwan, 1977.

The Beijing, 1959–1962 edition, under the title *KCTSCCIPC lu* 錄 , is reset in simpl. chars. and censored. Part of the great Ch'ien-lung encyclopedia, reprinted separately as the largest premodern medical encyclopedia. Tends to cite classical sources from later works, and relies heavily on the Ming orthodox tradition rather than giving a balanced view of medicine. It has little value for its texts, which were not rare and are not always cited faithfully, but a good deal for its systematic and chronological presentation of therapy.

Lao-tzu 老 子 [The writings of Lao-tzu]. Anon. Existed in some form by ca. 300 B.C.; reached more or less present form by 200 B.C. Cited by chapter nos. as in D. C. Lau 1982: 140, which includes Chinese texts.

Lei ching 類 經 [The classified canon]. Chang Chieh-pin 張 介 賓 , a.p. 1624. *Ssu k'u ch'üan shu chen pen wu chi* 四 庫 全 書 珍 本 五 集 , Vols. 182–91.
A topical arrangement of the *Su wen* and *Ling shu* with excellent annotations.

Ling shu 靈 樞 . See *Huang ti nei ching* 黃 帝 内 經 *ling shu*.

Lü shih ch'un ch'iu 呂 氏 春 秋 [Annals of Mr. Lü]. Compilation attributed to Lü Pu-wei; *Chi* 紀 portions completed 241 B.C., remainder by 235. *LSCC chiao shih* 校 釋 of Ch'en Ch'i-yu 陳 奇 猷 , 4 vols, Shanghai, 1984.
On the dates, see this edition, IV. 1885–1892.

Lun yü 論 語 [Analects]. Anon., recorded early 5C B.C. and subsequently edited. HY.

Mai ching 脈 經 [Canon of the pulse]. Wang Shu-ho 王 叔 和 , ca. A.D. 280. ITCM ed.
For critical ed. see Fu-chou shih jen-min i-yuan 1984 in bibliography B. On date see Kosoto et al. 1981. A synthesis of earlier canons. Kosoto et al. claim that the title refers to circulation channels rather than pulse, but the organization of the book and even the preface greatly emphasize pulse diagnosis. The issue is not either/or. Unlike the contemporary *Huang ti pa-shih-i nan ching*, this work does not alter the texts it quotes, but mainly depends on selection, to reconcile differences.

Mo-tzu 墨 子 [The writings of Mo-tzu (i.e., of the Mohist movement)]. By Mo Ti 墨 翟 and his disciples, ca. 350 B.C. The *Mo ching* 墨 經 sections are from ca. 300. HY.

Nan ching 難 經 . See *Huang ti pa-shih-i nan ching* 黃 帝 八 十 一 難 經 .

Nan ching cheng i 難經正義 [Canon of problems: Correct meanings]. Yeh Lin 葉 霖 , a.p. 1895. CP.

Nan ching chi chu 難 經 集 註 [Canon of problems: Collected annotations]. Wang Chiu-ssu 王 九 思, et al., compl. 1505. *Isson sōsho* 佚 存 叢 書 edition of 1789/1816, with added collation notes; reprint, Beijing, 1956.
Oldest extant collected annotations, incorporating T'ang and Sung commentaries.

Nan ching ching shih 難 經 經 釋 [Canon of problems explained through the *Inner Canon*]. Hsu Ta-ch'un 徐 大 椿 , a.p. 1727. In *Hsu Ling-t'ai i shu ch'üan chi*.

Nan ching pen i 難 經 本 義 [Canon of problems: Original meanings]. Hua Shou 滑 壽 , a.p. 1361, pr. 1366. Taipei, 1976.

Excellent text and what is generally considered the best commentary. ITCM is less complete than the edition cited.

Nei ching su wen Wu chu 內 經 素 問 吳 注 [*Basic Questions* with Wu's commentary]. Wu K'un 吳 崐 , a.p. 1594. Variorum ed. by Chang Shu-p'u 張 舒 普 , Jinan, 1984. Simpl. chars.

Pai hu t'ung 白 虎 通 [Comprehensive discussions in the White Tiger Hall]. Pan Ku 班 固 , A.D. 80? *PHT shu cheng* 疏 證.
Summary of discussions held in 80, but possibly a forgery compiled by 245.

Pao-p'u-tzu nei p'ien 抱 朴 子 內 篇 [Inner chapters of the Holding-to-Simplicity Master]. Ko Hung 葛 洪 , ca. A.D. 320.

P'ing chin kuan ts'ung-shu 平 津 館 叢 書 ·
Pei chi ch'ien chin yao fang 備 急 千 金 要 方 [Essential prescriptions worth a thousand, for urgent need]. Sun Ssu-mo (*or* Ssu-miao) 孫 思 邈 , compl. 650/659. Reprint of Edo igaku 江 戶 醫 學 edition of 1849, Taipei, 1965.
The book is cited in all early bibliographies as *Ch'ien chin fang*, but the longer title is given in the author's preface. For its meaning see Sivin 1968: 51, n. 32.

Pen-ts'ao ching chi chu 本 草 經 集 注 [The Divine Husbandman's canon of materia medica, with collected annotations]. T'ao Hung-ching 陶 弘 景 , ca. 500. Incomplete Six Dynasties or T'ang MS, reprint, Shanghai, 1955.
Based on *Shen-nung pen-ts'ao* 神 農 本 草 ·

Pen-ts'ao kang mu 本 草 綱 目 [Systematic materia medica]. Li Shih-chen 李 時 珍 , comp. 1552–1593, pr. 1596. Reprint, 4 vols., Beijing, 1930, 1959.
See also critical edition, simpl. chars., 4 vols., Beijing, 1975–1981. The standard handbook, but not reliable for citations of predecessors. Some Chinese sources claim the first edition was pr. 1590, but the preface of that year does not say that the book is about to be printed. *Kang mu* refers to major divisions and subdivisions of a systematic arrangement.

Pen-ts'ao kang mu shih i 本 草 綱 目 拾 遺 [Systematic materia medica: Supplement]. Chao Hsueh-min 趙 學 敏 , comp. 1760–1803 or later, pr. 1871. Corrected edition based on 1885 version, 2 vols., Shanghai, 1955.

Pen-ts'ao yen i 本 草 衍 義 [Dilatations on the materia medica]. K'ou Tsung-shih 寇 宗 奭 , compl. 1116, pr. 1119. Shanghai, 1937; reprint, Beijing, 1959.

Original title, *PT kuang* 廣 *i*, changed in the 1195 edition to avoid a taboo on the emperor's name.

Pin-hu mai hsueh 瀕 湖 脉 學 [Pulse studies from the lakeside hermitage]. Li Shih-chen, a. p. 1564. Repr. in *Pen-ts'ao kang mu*.

The author was often referred to by the name of his studio as given in this title.

San yin chi i ping yuan lun ts'ui 三 因 極 一 病 源 論 粹 [The three causes epitomized and unified: The quintessence of doctrine on the origins of medical disorders], usually referred to as *San yin fang* 三 因 方 [The three-type etiology formulary]. Ch'en Yen 陳 言 , 1174 or slightly later. Beijing, 1957, entitled *SYCI ping cheng fang lun* 病 證 方 論 ·

After *Chu ping yuan hou lun*, the most influential treatise on etiology, more oriented toward therapy than the latter.

Shang han hai ti yen 傷 寒 海 底 眼 [The submarine eye on the *Treatise on Cold Damage Disorders*]. Ho Yuan 何 淵 , preface 1416. Shanghai, 1984.

Comments on a variety of topics in the next item, with special attention to the modification of prescriptions. The editor of the modern version, a twenty-second-generation descendant of Ho, is unable to explicate the title.

Shang han lun 傷 寒 論 [Treatise on cold damage disorders]. For description see *SH tsa ping* 雜 病 *lun*. No definitive text of this work exists. Critical edition based on 4 recensions, including a Japanese MS of 1058/1064, in Ōtsuka 1966.

For passages rejected by Ōtsuka see the Shanghai 1923/1924 repr. of the Chao K'ai-mei version, based on the pr. edition of 1088.

Shang han lun t'iao pien 傷 寒 論 條 辨 [*Treatise on Cold Damage Disorders*: Systematic critical examination]. Fang Yu-chih 方 有 執 , a.p. 1589, pr. 1592. In *Ssu k'u ch'üan shu chen pen wu chi*, Vols. 193–94.

An important attempt to reconstitute *Shang han tsa ping lun* as it was before Wang Shu-ho and the Sung editors revised it. Served as the basis for *Shang lun p'ien* 尚 論 篇 , *q.v.*

Shang han tsa ping lun 傷 寒 雜 病 論 [Treatise on Cold Damage and miscellaneous disorders]. Attrib. Chang Chi 張 機 , 196/220. For citations see *Shang han lun* and *Chin kuei yao lueh fang lun*.

This work was lost by the late 3C. It was reconstituted with considerable revision near that end of that century by Wang

Shu-ho 王叔和 , and drastically edited in 968/975 and 1064/1065. In the last major revision the extant recensions were divided into three books, *Shang han lun, Chin kuei yü han ching* 金匱玉函経 , and *Chin kuei yao lueh fang lun*. The latter is derived from the portion on miscellaneous disorders. A pre-Sung fragment has been published in Miki 1959. For the history of the text see Ōtsuka 1966: 17–45 and Okanishi 1974: 19–32.

Shang lun p'ien 尚論篇 . See the next item.

Shang lun Chang Chung-ching Shang han lun ch'ung pien san-pai-chiu-shih-ch'i fa 尚論張仲景傷寒論重編三百九十七法 [A respectful discourse on the *Shang han lun* of Chang Chi, in which the (original) 397 therapeutic prescriptions are reconstituted]. Yü Ch'ang 喻昌 , pr. 1648. In *Ssu k'u ch'üan shu chen pen erh chi* 四庫全書珍本二集 , Vols. 192–93.

The best attempt so far to reconstitute the classic.

Shang shu 尚書 [Book of documents, lit., "venerable documents"]. Anon., collected possibly as early as 500 B.C.; present recension dates from ca. A.D. 320, with much later corruption. In *SS t'ung chien* 通檢 concordance, Beijing, 1982.

Shen-nung pen-ts'ao 神農本草 [The Divine Husbandman's materia medica]. Anon., late 1C, or 2C A.D. Reconstruction in *Hsin hsiu pen-ts'ao*.

The word *ching* 経 was added by an editor to mark the book's canonical status. Dating of original based on lack of mention in Han standard history's bibliography (comp. after A.D. 50), use of early E. Han place names, and first quotation by Hsi K'ang 嵇康 , 223–62. There is no proof, despite assertions to the contrary, that any part of this treatise was written earlier than the rest. The Okanishi restoration used an early MS that proved parts of the introduction formerly considered commentary are actually part of this work.

Sheng chi ching 聖濟経 [Canon of sagely benefaction]. Compiled by command of Emperor Hui-tsung 徽宗 , promulgated for school use 1118. CP.

This is a general theoretical work which draws on religious Taoist sources concerned with hygiene and longevity as well as on medical writings. The title refers to imperial patronage.

Sheng chi tsung lu 聖濟總錄. See *Cheng-ho sheng chi tsung lu*.

Shih chi 史 記 [Records of the Grand Historian]. Ssu-ma Ch'ien
司 馬 遷 , compl. 100/90 B.C. *Shiki kaichū kōshō* 史 記
會 註 考 證 , 10 vols., Tokyo, 1932–34.
Shih ming 釋 名 [Explanations of names]. Liu Hsi 劉 熙 ,
ca. A.D. 100. Citations in *T'ai-p'ing yü lan* 太 平 御 覽 .
Ssu chen chueh wei 四 診 抉 微 [Selection of subtleties in diagnostic technique]. Lin Chih-han 林 之 翰 , a.p. 1723. Beijing, 1957, 1981.
  Mostly a compilation, with many quotations from relatively late
  authors as well as the classics.
Su wen 素 問 . See *Huang ti nei ching* 黃 帝 内 経 *su wen.*
Su wen ching chu chieh chieh 素 問 経 注 節 解 [Basic ques-
tions: Canon and commentaries, reordered and explained]. Jao
Shao-yü 姚 紹 虞 , a.p. 1677. Beijing, 1983.
  Title alludes to *Chou i,* hexagram 60, "T'uan chuan" 周 易
  象 傳 , and refers to the author's rearrangment of the text
  and excision of redundant and corrupt portions.
SW. See *Su wen.*
Ta-kuan pen-ts'ao 大 觀 本 草 . See *Ching shih cheng lei Ta-
kuan pen-ts'ao.*
T'ai-p'ing sheng hui fang 太 平 聖 惠 方 [Imperial grace for-
mulary of the Great Peace and Prosperous State era]. Wang
Huai-yin 王 懷 隱 et al., comp. 978–992. Critical edition,
Beijing, 1958.
  See Okanishi 1974: 103–10. "T'ai-p'ing" is short for the reign
  title "T'ai-p'ing hsing kuo" 太 平 興 國 .
T'ai-p'ing yü lan 太 平 御 覽 [Encyclopedia of the Great Peace
and Prosperous State era for imperial scrutiny], comp. Li Fang
李 昉 et al. 977–983. Critical edition, 4 vols., Beijing, 1960.
  Major source for lost early works and parts of works.
T'ai su. See *Huang ti nei ching t'ai su.*
TS. See *T'ai su.*
Tso chuan 左 傳 [The Tso tradition of interpretation of the *Spring
and Autumn Annals*]. Attrib. Tso Ch'iu-ming 左 丘 明 ,
ca. 500 B.C., but prob. compiled ca. 350. HY.
Tsu pi shih-i mai chiu ching 足 臂 十 一 脉 灸 経 [Moxibus-
tion canon for the eleven foot and arm vessels]. Anon., before
168 B.C. In Ma-wang-tui 1979; cf. Ma-wang-tui 1975.
  Important studies are Ho Tsung-yü 何 宗 禹 1981, 1984,
  Yao Ch'un-fa 姚 纯 发 1982.
Tz'u shih nan chih 此 事 難 知 [This is no simple matter]. Li
Kao 李 杲 , ed. Wang Hao-ku 王 好 古 , e.p. 1308. ITCM.

Mainly concerned with *Shang han lun.*

Wai t'ai pi yao 外 台 秘 要 [Arcane essentials from the imperial library]. Wang T'ao 王 燾 , a.p. 752. Beijing, 1955, based indirectly on Ch'eng Yen-tao 程 衍 道 edition of 1640. A major T'ang work on therapy. The title has often been mistranslated, by myself among others. The first two words may refer to certain administrative posts with censorial duties, or to the Imperial Library Department. There is no reason to believe that the author served as a censor. In his preface (p. 22a) he says " . . . in more than twenty years in scholarly posts in the palace I was long acquainted with the prescription books and other holdings of the Institute for the Advancement of Literature." See Yü Chia-hsi 余 嘉 錫 1958: 660–63 and Okanishi 1974: 94.

Wen i lun 溫 疫 論 [Treatise on Warm Factor Epidemic Disorders]. Wu Yu-hsing 吳 有 性 , a.p. 1642. Reprint of 1897 edition, Beijing, 1955. See also the critical and annotated edition based on 1709 version, simpl. chars., Beijing, 1977. Wu originated the idea that Warm Factor Epidemic heteropathy enters through the mouth and nose, but kept the old belief that Cold Damage and other heteropathy enters through the pores.

Wen je lun 溫 热 論 [Treatise on Heat Factor Disorders]. Yeh Kuei 葉 桂 , prob. taken down by Ku Ching-wen 顧 景 文 , ca. 1740? Annotated edition in *I men pang ho* (Part 2, 1835, published separately as *Shang han lun pen chih* 傷 寒 論 本 旨), 6: 36a-51b (II, 749–78), under title *Yeh T'ien-shih wen ping lun* 葉 天 士 溫 病 論 . Unannotated edition in simpl. chars., slightly variant, in *Wu i hui chiang, 1:* 3–11. Another early title, often used today, is *Wai kan wen je p'ien* 外 感 溫 热 篇 .

Wen ping t'iao pien 溫 病 條 辨 [Systematic manifestation type determination in Heat Factor Disorders]. Wu T'ang 吳 瑭 , compl. 1798. Chengdu, 1957.

Wu hsing ta i 五 行 大 義 [General significances of the Five Phases]. Hsiao Chi 蕭 吉 , shortly after 581. In Nakamura 1973. Cited in T'ang standard histories as *WH chi* 五 行 紀 .

Wu i hui chiang 吳 醫 滙 講 [Collected discourses of Suzhou physicians]. Comp. T'ang Ta-lieh 唐 大 烈 , 1792–1801. Critical edition by Ting Kuang-ti 丁 光 迪 based on 1814 and other editions, Shanghai, 1983.

Published 1 *chüan* a year—a precursor of medical journals. Superior collection of medical informal essays, scholarly and hortatory, some published for the first time.

Wu shang hsuan yuan san t'ien yü t'ang ta fa 無 上 玄 元 三 天 玉 堂 大 法 [Great rites of the jade hall, a Mysterious Prime Triple Heaven revelation of the Most High]. Preface 1158. Said to have been divinely revealed to Lu Shih-chung 路 時 中 in 1120, but the book is largely composed of earlier documents. In *Cheng-t'ung Tao tsang* 政 統 道 藏 , Vols. 100–4 (Schipper no. 220).
See Liu Ts'un-yan 1971 in bibliography B.

Wu-shih-erh ping fang 五 十 二 病 方 [Prescriptions for 52 ailments]. Anon., prob. 2C B.C., definitely before 168 B.C. In Ma-wang-tui 1979.
See Harper 1982. The earliest extant collection of medical prescriptions.

Wu-wei Han-tai i chien 武 威 汉 代 医 简 [Han medical documents on wooden slips from Wuwei, Gansu]. Anonymous, mid-1C A.D.? Beijing, 1975.

Yin-yang shi-i mai chiu ching 陰 陽 十 一 脈 灸 经 [Moxibustion canon for the eleven yin and yang vessels]. In Ma-wang-tui 1979.
See Akahori 1981.

Ying-t'ung lei ts'ui 嬰 童 類 萃 [Classified essentials of pediatrics]. Wang Ta-lun 王 大 倫 , a.p. 1622. Beijing, 1983.

Bibliography B

Other Sources

Academy of Traditional Chinese Medicine. 1975. *An Outline of Chinese Acupuncture*. Beijing.
Written for foreigners.

Ågren, Hans. 1972. "Medical Science in China: A Compendium." *Science*, 178 (27 October 1972): 394–95.
Review of Hu-nan i-hsueh-yuan 湖南医学院 ed. 1971.

_____. 1975. "Patterns of Tradition and Modernization in Contemporary Chinese Medicine." Pp. 37–59 in Kleinman et al. 1975.
Papers from a conference on the comparative study of traditional and modern medicine in Chinese societies.

_____. Forthcoming. "Chinese Traditional Medicine: Temporal Order and Synchronous Events." Pp. 211–18 in Fraser et al. forthcoming.

Akahori, Akira 赤堀昭. 1978a. "Shin shutsudo shiryō ni yoru Chūgoku iyaku koten no minaoshi" 新出土資料に於る 中國医薬古典の見直し [Chinese medical classics reconsidered in the light of recently excavated materials]. *Kampō no rinsō* 漢方の臨床 25, nos. 11–12: 1–16.

_____. 1978b. "Bu'i Kandai ikan ni tsuite" 武威漢代醫簡について [On the Han medical texts on wooden strips from Wuwei, Gansu]. *Tōhō gakuhō* 東方學報 (Kyoto) 50: 75–107.

_____. 1979a. "On'yō jūichi myaku kyūkyo to Somon—Somon no seiritsu ni tsuite no ikkōsatsu" '陰陽十一脈灸経'と ─'素問─素问'の成立について乙の一考察 [Chapters of *Huang ti nei ching su wen* derived from *Yin-yang shih-i mai chiu ching*]. *Nihon ishigaku zasshi* 日本醫史學雜誌 25, no. 3: 277–90.

_____. 1979b. "Kleiner Beitrag: Medical Manuscripts Found in Han Tomb No. 3 at Ma-wang-tui." *Sudhoffs Archiv* 63: 297–301.

_____. 1981. "On'yō jūichi myaku kyūkyo no kenkyū" 陰 陽 十 一 脉 灸 経 の 研 究 [A study of the *Moxibustion Canon for the Eleven Yin and Yang Vessels*]. *Tōhō gakuhō* (Kyoto) 53: 299–339.

  See *Yin-yang shih-i mai chiu ching* in bibliography A.

Akhtar, Shahid. 1975. *Health Care in the People's Republic of China: A Bibliography with Abstracts* (IDRC-038e). Ottawa.

  Mainly but not exclusively English-language books and articles, primarily for people working in development studies. No listings for basic clinical medicine or biomedical research, but there is a section on history of medicine.

Anonymous. 1973. *A Bibliography of Chinese Sources on Medicine and Public Health in the People's Republic of China: 1960–1970* (Geographic Health Studies, John E. Fogarty International Center for Advanced Study in The Health Sciences. DHEW Publication [NIH]: 73–439). Bethesda, Maryland.

  Books and articles, the latter almost entirely those abstracted or translated by the Joint Publications Research Service. The largest bibliography of its kind, but still very incomplete.

_____, ed. 1977. *Chung hsi i chieh-ho chih ping ching-yen hui-pien* 中 西 醫 結 合 治 病 經 驗 滙 編 [An anthology of clinical experience in combined Chinese and Western therapy]. Hong Kong.

  Collection of 39 articles from Chinese medical journals selected by the publisher.

Basalla, George. 1962. "William Harvey and the Heart as a Pump." *Bulletin of the History of Medicine* 36: 467–70.

  Partly superseded by Webster 1965.

Bauer, Wolfgang, ed. 1979. *Studia Sino-Mongolica: Festschrift für Herbert Franke*. Münchener ostasiatische Studien, 25. Wiesbaden.

Beijing College of Traditional Chinese Medicine et al. 1980. *Essentials of Chinese Acupuncture*. Beijing.

  Translation of a Chinese book. Unlike Academy of Traditional Chinese Medicine ed. 1975, this includes a section on theory, including yin-yang and Five Phases.

Berger, Peter, and Thomas Luckmann. 1966. *The Social Construction of Reality: A Treatise in the Sociology of Knowledge*. Garden City, New York.

A basic work, written at a high level of abstraction.

Bridgman, Robert F. 1955. "La médecine dans la Chine antique, d'après les biographies de Pien-ts'io et de Chouen-yu Yi." *Mélanges chinois et bouddhiques*, 10: 1–213.

Bridgman's interpretations are penetrating from the medical point of view, but his linguistic understanding is not reliable.

_____. 1981. "Les fonctions physiologiques chez l'homme dans la Chine antique." *History and Philosophy of the Life Sciences* 3, no. 1: 3–30.

An attempt to summarize Chinese physiological knowledge up to 200 B.C.

Bullock, Mary Brown. 1980. *An American Transplant: The Rockefeller Foundation and Peking Union Medical College*. Berkeley.

Burnet, John. 1930. *Early Greek Philosophy*. 4th edition. London. First published 1892.

Caplan, Arthur L., et al., eds. 1981. *Concepts of Health and Disease: Interdisciplinary Perspectives*. Reading, Massachusetts.

Few of the 48 essays in this book are interdisciplinary. They capably present the views of specialists in a variety of fields.

Ch'ang-ch'un Chung-i hsueh-yuan 长 春 中 医 学 院 (Changchun College of Chinese Medicine), ed. 1980. *Ch'uan ya nei p'ien hsuan chu* 串 雅 内 篇 选 注 [Annotated selections from the "Inner Chapters" of *Ch'uan ya*]. Beijing.

Includes about three-fifths of the "Inner Chapters."

Chang Hsueh-yung 张 学 庸 et al., eds. 1979. *Chung hsi i chieh-ho chien-ming nei-k'o-hsueh* 中 西 医 结 合 简 明 内 科 学 [Simplified internal medicine for combined Chinese and Western therapy]. Vol. 1. Xi'an.

Introduction to traditional concepts, including manifestation types, combined with modern diagnosis.

Chang Sheng-hsing 张 晟 星 , ed. 1983. *Chen-chiu chih-liao shou-ts'e* 针 灸 治 疗 手 册 [Handbook of acupuncture and moxibustion therapy]. Shanghai.

Revision of Shang-hai-shih chen-chiu yen-chiu-so 上 海 市 针 灸 研 究 所 ed. 1970, with significant changes in theoretical viewpoint.

Chao P'u-shan 赵 璞 珊 . 1983. *Chung-kuo ku-tai i-hsueh* 中 国 古 代 医 学 [Ancient Chinese medicine]. Beijing.

Largely anecdotal but useful.

Che-chiang Chung-i hsueh-yuan 浙 江 中 医 学 院 . 1983. *Chung-i nei-k'o shou-ts'e* 中 医 内 科 手 册 [Handbook of Chinese internal medicine]. Hangzhou.

Ch'en Chu-yu 陈竹友 . 1979. *I yung ku Han-yü* 医用古汉语 [Medical classical Chinese]. Fuzhou.
Often neglects to gloss difficult phrases.

Ch'en Meng-chia 陳夢家 . 1938. "Wu-hsing chih ch'i-yuan" 五行之起源 [Origin of the Five Phases]. *Yen-ching hsueh-pao* 燕京學報 24: 35–53.

Ch'en Pang-hsien 陳邦賢 . 1937. *Chung-kuo i-hsueh shih* 中國醫學史 [History of Chinese medicine]. Shanghai.

Ch'en Tse-lin 陳澤霖. 1982. "She chen shih kai shu" 舌诊史概述 ["An introduction to the history of lingual examination"]. *Chung-hua i shih tsa-chih* 12, no. 1: 1–4.

Ch'eng Shih-te 程士德 , ed. 1982. *Su wen chu shih hui ts'ui* 素问注释汇粹 [The *Basic Questions* with selected commentaries]. 2 vols. Beijing.
A good comprehensive digest of textual variations and explanatory annotations. Simplified characters.

Ch'eng-tu Chung-i hsueh-yuan 成都中医学院 (Chengdu College of Chinese Medicine), ed. 1978. *Chung-yao-hsueh* 中药学 [Chinese pharmacology]. Shanghai.

Chi-lin i-k'o ta-hsueh 吉林医科大学 (Jilin Medical University), ed. 1977. *Ch'ih-chiao i-sheng chiao-ts'ai* 赤脚医生教材 [Training manual for barefoot doctors]. 2 vols. Beijing.

Chia Te-tao 賈得道 . 1979. *Chung-kuo i-hsueh shih lueh* 中国医学史略 [Outline history of Chinese medicine]. Taiyuan.
Substantial introductory history.

Chiang Ch'un-hua 姜春华 et al., eds. 1970. *Chung hsi i chieh ho chih "shen hsu"* 中西医结合治"肾虚" [Combined Chinese and Western therapy for renal system depletion]. Hong Kong.

Chiang-su hsin i-hsueh-yuan 江苏新医学院 (Jiangsu New Medical College), ed. 1977–1978. *Chung yao ta-tz'u-tien* 中药大辞典 [Unabridged dictionary of Chinese materia medica]. 3 vols. Shanghai.
Makes previous publications of its kind obsolete.

Chiang-su sheng wei-sheng-t'ing 江苏省卫生厅 (Bureau of Public Health, Jiangsu Province), ed. 1980. *Chung-i chi-ch'u* 中医基础 [Foundations of Chinese medicine]. Suzhou.
Revision of a 1977 publication of the same title.

Ch'ien Ch'ao-ch'en 錢超尘 . 1982. "Yang Shang-shan sheng yü Hou Wei tsu yü Sui *T'ai su* ch'eng yü Hou Chou shuo" 楊

上 善 生 于 后 魏 卒 于 隋 《 太 素 》 成 于 后 周 说 [On the propositions that Yang Shang-shan was born during the Later Wei period (534–549) and died during the Sui (581–617), and that the *Huang ti nei ching t'ai su* was completed during the Later Chou (557–80)]. Pp. 336–48 in Jen Ying-ch'iu 任 应 秋 and Liu Ch'ang-lin 刘 长 林 eds. 1982.

Ch'ien Mu 錢 穆. 1956. *Hsien Ch'in chu tzu hsi nien* 先 秦 諸 子 繫 年 [Studies in the chronology of Chou philosophers]. Revised edition, 2 vols. Hong Kong.
First published 1935.

Chiu, Martha Li. 1986. "Mind, Body, and Illness in a Chinese Medical Tradition." Ph.D. diss., Department of History and East Asian Languages, Harvard University.
On the diversity of concepts in *Huang ti nei ching t'ai su*.

Chou Chin-huang 周 金 黃 , ed. 1984. *Yao-li-hsueh* 药 理 学 [Pharmacology]. Revised edition. Hefei.
Includes modern as well as traditional drugs.

Ch'üan Han-sheng 全 漢 昇 . 1936. "Ch'ing mo Hsi-yang i-hsueh ch'uan-ju shih kuo-jen so ch'ih te t'ai-tu" 清 末 西 洋 醫 學 傳 入 時 國 人 所 持 的 態 度 [Attitudes taken by Chinese when Western medicine was transmitted at the end of the Ch'ing period]. *Shih huo pan-yueh-k'an* 食 貨 半 月 刊 3, no. 12: 43–53.

Chung, C. 1982. *Ah-shih Point. The Pressure Pain Point in Acupuncture. A Illustrated Diagnostic Guide to Clinical Acupuncture.* Taipei.
Discusses loci used in 51 cases chosen from the clinical experience of a physician originally trained in modern medicine.

Chung-hua jen-min kung-ho-kuo Wei-sheng-pu 中 华 人 民 共 和 国 卫 生 部 (Ministry of Public Health, P.R.C.). 1978–1979. *Chung-hua jen-min kung-ho-kuo yao-tien: 1977 pan* 中 华 人 民 共 和 国 药 典 : 1977 版 [Pharmacopoeia of the People's Republic of China: 1977]. 2 vols. Beijing.
Vol. 1 (1979): *Chinese Materia Medica*; Vol. 2 (1978): other.

Chung-i yen-chiu-yuan 中 医 研 究 院 (Academy of Traditional Chinese Medicine) et al., eds. 1964. *Ch'üan kuo Chung-yao ch'eng yao ch'u fang chi* 全 国 中 药 成 药 處 方 集 [Prescriptions for prepared Chinese medicines throughout China]. Beijing.
For a large number of common compound medicines, gives the recipes used in 25 main cities; shows considerable variation.

____. 1973. "Wu-wei Han-tai i-yao chien-tu tsai i-hsueh shih shang te chung-yao i-i" 武 威 汉 代 医 药 简 牍 在 医 学 史 上 的 重 要 意 义 [The important significance to medical history of the wooden slips concerning Han medicine found at Wuwei]. *Wen-wu* 文 物 12: 23–29, pl. 1–4.
Unreliable translation in *Chinese Sociology and Anthropology* 8 (1975): 55–81. For revised version, see *Wu-wei Han-tai i chien* in bibliography A.

____. et al., eds. 1973. *Chung-i ming-tz'u shu-yü hsuan shih* 中 医 名 词 术 语 选 释 [Glossary of selected Chinese medical terms]. Beijing.
Reprint in 1975 under the misleading title *CIMTSY tz'u-tien* [Dictionary of selected Chinese medical texts]. Hong Kong, 1975. Also reprinted in 1979 under the original title.

____. et al., eds. 1979. *Chien-ming Chung-i tz'u-tien* 简 明 中 医 辞 典 [Simplified dictionary of Chinese medicine]. Beijing. Differs considerably in content and coverage from the preceding item. Its greater size is due mainly to inclusion of materia medica and prescriptions.

____. et al., eds. 1982. *Chung-i ta-tz'u-tien: chi-pen li-lun fen-ts'e* 中 医 大 辞 典 ﹕ 基 础 理 论 分 册 [Unabridged dictionary of Chinese medicine: Basic theory]. Preliminary edition, Beijing.
Revision of the preceding item.

____. et al., eds. 1983. *Chung-i ta-tz'u-tien: fang-chi fen-ts'e* 中 医 大 辞 典 ﹕ 方 剂 分 册 [Unabridged dictionary of Chinese medicine: prescriptions]. Preliminary ed., Beijing.

____. and Pei-ching t'u-shu-kuan 北 京 图 书 馆 (Beijing Library), ed. 1961. *Chung-i t'u-shu lien-ho mu-lu* 中 医 图 书 联 合 目 录 [Union catalogue of books on traditional Chinese medicine]. N.p., 1961.
Lists 7,661 titles, mostly premodern, in 60 Chinese collections, with information on editions.

Chung-kuo jen-min chieh-fang-chün, Wu-han pu-tui hou-ch'in-pu wei-sheng-pu 中 国 人 民 解 放 军 武 汉 部 队 后 勤 部 卫 生 部 (Public Health Section, Rear Support Units, Wuhan Command, People's Liberation Army). 1972. *Chien-ming Chung-i-hsueh* 简 明 中 医 学 [Simplified Chinese Medicine]. Wuhan.

CL. See Lu and Needham 1980.

Cohen, Sir Henry. 1981. The evolution of the concept of disease. Pp. 209–19 in Caplan et al. eds. 1981.

Committee on Scholarly Communication with the People's Republic of China, ed. 1980. *Rural Health in the People's Republic of China: Report of a Visit by the Rural Health Systems Delegation. June 1978.* NIH Publication 81-2124. Bethesda, Maryland.

Croizier, Ralph C. 1968. *Traditional Medicine in Modern China: Science, Nationalism, and the Tensions of Cultural Change.* Harvard East Asian Series, 34. Cambridge, Massachusetts. Deals with China before 1949.

———. 1973. "Traditional Medicine in Modern China: Social, Political, and Cultural Aspects." Pp. 30-46 in Risse ed. 1973.

———. 1976. "The Ideology of Medical Revivalism in Modern China." Pp. 341-55 in Leslie ed. 1976.

DeGowin, Elmer L., and Richard L. DeGowin. 1981. *Bedside Diagnostic Examination.* Fourth edition. New York. First edition, 1965.

Douglas, Mary. 1970. *Natural Symbols: Explorations in Cosmology.* New York.

Dunglison, Robley. 1874. *Medical Lexicon: A Dictionary of Medical Science: Containing a Concise Explanation of the Various Subjects and Terms.* New edition, enlarged and thoroughly revised, ed. Richard J. Dunglison. Philadelphia. First published as *A New Dictionary of Medical Science and Literature* (2 vols., Philadelphia, 1833).

Dunstan, Helen. 1975. "The Late Ming Epidemics: A Preliminary Survey." *Ch'ing-shih wen-t'i* 3, no. 3: 1-59. Also concerned with *Wen i lun* 瘟 疫 論 (see bibliography A).

Eberhard, Wolfram, and Rolf Mueller. 1936. "Contributions to the Astronomy of the Han Period III: Astronomy of the Later Han Period." *Harvard Journal of Asiatic Studies* 1: 194-241. Reprinted in Eberhard 1970: 181-228.

———. 1970. *Sternkunde und Weltbild im alten China: Gesammelte Aufsätze.* Taipei.

Eliade, Mircea. 1956. *Forgerons et alchimistes.* Paris. English tr., *The Forge and the Crucible.* 1962. New York.

———. 1968. "The Forge and the Crucible: A Postscript." *History of Religions* 8, no. 1: 74-88.

———. 1978. *The Forge and the Crucible.* Tr. Stephen Corrin. 2nd ed. Chicago.

Epler, D[ean] C., Jr. 1980. "Blood-letting in Early Chinese Medicine and Its Relation to the Origin of Acupuncture." *Bulletin of the History of Medicine* 54: 337-67.

Evans, John R. 1984. "Medical Education in China." Paper presented at the Rockefeller Archive Center conference "Research and Education in 20th Century China," 23 May 1984.

Fan Hsing-chun 范 行 准 . 1944. "La médecine occidentale en Chine vers la fin des Ming (1644)." *Bulletin de l'Université l'Aurore* 5, no. 3: 671–84.

——. 1965. "Liang Han San-kuo Nan-pei-ch'ao Sui T'ang i fang chien lu" 两 漢 三 國 南 北 朝 隋 唐 醫 方 简 錄 [A simple list of medical prescriptions from the Han through the T'ang periods]. *Chung-hua wen shih lun-ts'ung* 中 華 文 史 論 叢 6: 295–347.
Actually a fairly general bibliography of medical works cited in early sources.

Fang Yao-chung 方 药 中 . 1979. *Pien cheng lun chih yen-chiu ch'i chiang* 辨 证 论 治 研 究 七 讲 [Seven lectures on therapeutic reasoning based on manifestation type determination]. Beijing.

Farquhar, Judith. 1986. "Knowledge and Practice in Chinese Medicine." Ph.D. diss., Department of Anthropology, University of Chicago.
Field observation of use of medical classics in contemporary teaching.

Fraser, J. T., ed. 1966. *The Voices of Time: A Cooperative Survey of Man's Views of Time as Expressed by the Sciences and by the Humanities.* New York.

——. Forthcoming. *The Voices of Time.* Vol. 5, *Time, Science and Society in East and West.* Amherst, Massachusetts.

Freidson, Elliott. 1970. *Profession of Medicine: A Study of the Sociology of Applied Knowledge.* New York.
The most intellectually substantial textbook of the sociology of medicine.

——. 1975. *Doctoring Together: A Study of Professional Social Control.* New York.

Fu-chien sheng i-yao yen-chiu-so 福 建 省 医 药 研 究 所 (Fujian Provincial Medical Research Institute), ed. 1977. *Ch'uan ya wai p'ien hsuan chu* 串 雅 外 篇 选 注 [Annotated selections from the Outer Chapters of *Ch'uan ya*]. Beijing.
About two-fifths of the "Outer Chapters."

Fu-chou shih jen-min i-yuan 福 州 市 人 民 医 院 . 1984. *Mai ching chiao shih* 脉 经 校 释 [Critical edition of the *Canon of the Pulse* with vernacular translation]. Beijing. Simplified characters.

Graham, A. C., trans. 1981. *Chuang-tzu: The Seven Inner Chapters and Other Writings from the Book by Chuang-tzu*. London.

Hansen, Chad. 1983. *Language and Logic in Ancient China*. (Michigan Studies on China, 8). Ann Arbor.
An important analysis of assumptions about substance in late Chou philosophical writngs, especially semantic texts, which the author views from the perspective of modern linguistics. An extension to scientific sources would be a major contribution.

Hao Yin-ch'ing 郝 印 卿 . 1982. "Lun shang han liu ching shih tsang-fu, ching-lo, ch'i-hua te yu-chi chieh-ho" 论 伤 寒 六 经 是 脏 腑，经 络，气 化 的 有 机 结 合 [On the Six Warps of the Treatise on Cold Damage Disorders as an organic combination of the visceral systems of function, the circulation tract system, and *ch'i* transformation processes]. *Chung-i tsa-chih* 中 医 杂 志 3: 4–9.

Harper, Donald J. 1976. "Mawangdui Tomb Three: Documents. Vol. 1, The Medical Texts." *Early China* 2: 68–69.
Summaries of six publications about excavated texts.

———. 1982. "The *Wu Shih Erh Ping Fang*: Translation and Prolegomena." Ph.D. diss., University of California, Berkeley.
A first attempt to translate the mutilated text of a recently excavated medical formulary, the earliest extant, with a valuable philological commentary.

Ho Chih-hsiung 何 志 雄 . 1983. "Shang han lun liu ching shih-chih t'an-t'ao" 伤 寒 论 六 经 实 质 探 讨 [An inquiry into the substance of the Six Warps in the *Shang han lun*]. *Hsin Chung-i* 新 中 医 2: 6–10.

Ho-pei hsin i ta-hsueh 河 北 新 医 大 学 (Hebei New Medical University), ed. 1974. *Chien-ming Chung-i-hsueh* 简 明 中 医 学 [Simplified Chinese Medicine]. Beijing.

Ho Tsung-yü 何 宗 禹 . 1981. "Ma-wang-tui i shu k'ao-cheng i-shih wen-t'i t'an-t'ao" 马 王 堆 医 书 考 证 译 释 问 题 探 讨 ["Study on the translation, interpretation, and textual research of medical works unearthed from Ma Wang Dui"]. *Chung-hua i shih tsa-chih* 中 华 医 史 杂 志 11, no. 2: 125–27. *See also* Yao Ch'un-fa 姚 纯 发 1982.

———. 1984. "Ma-wang-tui po shu Tsu pi shih-i mai chiu ching yu kuan te wen-t'i tsai t'an" 马 王 堆 帛 书 《 足 臂 十 一

脉 灸 经 》 有 关 的 问 题 再 探 [Restudy of some
problems relevant to the Mawangdui silk MS *Tsu pi shih-i mai
chiu ching*]. *Chung-hua i shih tsa-chih* 14, no. 3: 172–75.
Sums up arguments against interpreting this text as concerned
with the sinew system.

Hoeppli, R. 1959. *Parasites and Parasitic Infections in Early
Medicine and Science*. Singapore.
Comparative, but largely concerned with China. The author
had little overall understanding of Chinese medicine, but
provided copious translations from classical writings.

Hsiao Kung-ch'üan. 1979. *A History of Chinese Political Thought*.
Vol. 1, *From the Beginnings to the Sixth Century A.D.*
Tr. Frederick W. Mote. Princeton.
Translation of *Chung-kuo cheng-chih ssu-hsiang shih* 中 國
政 治 思 想 史. 2 vols., Chongqing, 1945; Shanghai, 1946.

Hsiao, William C. 1984. "Special Report: Transformation of
Health Care in China." *The New England Journal of Medicine*
310: 932–36.

Hsieh, E. T. 1921. "A Review of Ancient Chinese Anatomy."
Anatomical Records 20: 97–127.

Hsu, Francis L. K. 1952. *Religion, Science and Human Crises: A
Study of China in Transition and Its Implications for the West*.
International Library of Sociology and Social Reconstruction.
London.
Classic anthropological study of a cholera epidemic in a wartime
Yunnan town.

Hu-nan Chung-i hsueh-yuan 湖 南 中 医 学 院 (Hunan College of Chinese Medicine), ed. 1980–1981. *Ma-wang-tui i shu
yen-chiu chuan k'an* 马 王 堆 医 书 研 究 專 刊 [Spe-
cial number: studies of the Mawangdui medical writings]. 2
vols. Changsha.

Hu-nan Chung-i-yao yen-chiu-so ko-wei-hui 湖 南 中 医 药 研
究 所 革 委 会 (Revolutionary Committee, Hunan
Chinese Medicine Research Institute), ed. 1971. *Ch'ih-chiao i-
sheng shou-ts'e* 赤 脚 医 生 手 册 [Barefoot doctor's
manual]. Changsha.
Translation in Revolutionary Health Committee of Hunan
Province ed. 1977.

Hu-nan i-hsueh-yuan 湖 南 医 学 院 (Hunan Medical College),
ed. 1971. *Nung-ts'un i-sheng shou-ts'e* 农 村 医 生 手 册
[Village physician's handbook]. Fourth edition. Beijing.
Originally published 1959.

Hu-pei Chung-i hsueh-yuan 湖北中医学院 (Hubei College of Chinese Medicine), ed. 1978. *Chung-i-hsueh kai lun* 中医学概论 [Outline of Chinese medicine]. Shanghai.

Hu, Shiu-ying. 1981. *An Enumeration of Chinese Materia Medica.* Hong Kong.

Alphabetical list of about 2,000 substances by romanization (not always correct), giving scientific names, common names in English, and pharmaceutical designations.

Hu Tao-ching 胡道静. 1963. "Shen K'uo (*or* Kua) te nung-hsueh chu-tso Meng ch'i (*or* hsi) wang huai lu" 沈括的農學著作·夢溪忘懷錄 [On Shen K'uo's agricultural book *Record of Longings Forgotten at Dream Brook*]. *Wen shih* 文史 3: 221-25.

On one of the earliest sources for cultivated medicinal plants.

Hu Teh-wei. 1974. *An Economic Analysis of Cooperative Medical Services in the People's Republic of China.* Bethesda, Maryland.

Hymes, Robert P. 1987. "Not Quite Gentlemen? Doctors in Sung and Yuan." *Chinese Science* 8: 9-76.

Jamison, Dean T., et al. 1984. *The Health Sector in China.* Population, Health, and Nutrition Department, World Bank. Reports, 4664-CHA. Washington, D.C.

Based on findings of a World Bank rural health and medical education mission that visited China in September and October 1982, with further information supplied by the Chinese government. Exceptionally well informed.

Jen Ying-ch'iu 任应秋. 1960. *Yin-yang wu-hsing* 阴阳五行 [Yin-yang and the Five Phases in medicine]. Shanghai.

Introduction by China's leading historian of medical theory, who died in 1984.

_____. 1978. *Nei ching shih chiang* 内经十讲 [Ten lectures on the *Inner Canon of the Yellow Lord*]. Beijing.

Excellent brief but systematic introduction to the *Inner Canon* and to scholarship about it, with appendices on several technical topics.

_____, ed. 1980. *Chung-i ko chia hsueh-shuo* 中医各家学说 [Doctrines of the schools of classical Chinese medicine]. Shanghai.

Medical school textbook; analysis and anthology. Arranged topically. Pei-ching Chung-i hsueh-yuan et al. eds. 1961 and Pei-ching Chung-i hsueh-yuan 1964 are earlier versions. They are in chronological order and thus are less useful for tracing the evolution of concepts.

_____. and Liu Ch'ang-lin 刘 长 林 , eds. 1982. *Nei ching yen-chiu lun-ts'ung* 内 经 研 究 论 丛 [Collected studies on the *Inner Canon of the Yellow Lord*]. Wuchang.
  Fourteen essays.

Jenerick, Howard P., ed. 1974. *Proceedings* (NIH Acupuncture Research Conference. 28 February and 1 March 1973. Bethesda, Maryland. DHEW Publication [NIH] 74–165). Bethesda, Maryland.
  Documents the poorly informed clinical experimentation and assessment current in the U.S. at the time.

Kan-su sheng hsin i-yao-hsueh yen-chiu-so 甘 肃 省 新 医 药 学 研 究 所 (Gansu Provincial New Medical Research Institute), ed. 1982. *Chung yao hsueh* 中 药 学 [Chinese materia medica]. Beijing.

Kao To 高 铎 . 1984. "Ching-lo shih chih ch'ien lun" 经 络 实 值 浅 论 [The substantiality of the circulation tracts: A superficial discussion]. *Chung i yao hsueh-pao* 中 医 药 学 报 2: 10–14, 64.
  "On the basis of the analysis above, we can maintain that, although a distribution throughout the flesh is the formal manifestation of the *ching-lo*, with respect to substance the latter is a reflection of the level of organismic functioning of the visceral systems, *ch'i*, and *hsueh*" (page 64).

Kaptchuk, Ted J. 1983. *The Web that Has No Weaver: Understanding Chinese Medicine*. New York.
  An insightful introduction for laymen. The author has had some training in a proprietary school of traditional medicine on the periphery of China. Includes a fairly extensive bibliography of Chinese sources, most of which the author has obviously not read.

Keegan, David. Forthcoming. "The Forms of a Tradition: The Structure and History of the *Huang-ti nei-ching*." Ph.D. diss., University of California, Berkeley, due 1986.
  Separates the different texts brought together in the *Huang ti nei ching* and their combinations in various versions. Differs from Yamada 1979b and other Japanese publications in its concern for texts rather than schools.

Kenton, Charlotte. 1976. *Medicine and Health in China: January 1973 through December 1975*. NLM Literature Search 76–7. Bethesda, Maryland.

_____. 1982. *Medicine and Health in China: January 1979 through May 1982*. NLM Literature Search 82–5. Bethesda, Maryland.

These two bibliographies are neither selective nor thorough; they include mainly publications in English, with a few in French and German.

Kleinman, Arthur, et al., eds. 1975. *Medicine in Chinese Cultures: Comparative Studies of Health Care in Chinese and Other Societies.* Washington, D.C.

Papers from a "Conference on the Comparative Study of Traditional and Modern Medicine in Chinese Societies," Seattle, Washington, February 1974. A few important contributions, but most papers are poorly informed about medical aspects of Chinese culture and the history of health care in China and the West.

———. 1980a. "Traditional Doctors." Pp. 63–67 in Committee on Scholarly Communication with the People's Republic of China, ed. 1980.

———. 1980b. *Patients and Healers in the Context of Culture: An Exploration of the Borderland between Anthropology, Medicine, and Psychiatry.* Comparative Studies of Health Systems and Medical Care, 3. Berkeley.

Excellent field observation and analysis.

Kosoto, Hiroshi 小 曽 戸 洋 , et al. 1981. "Myakkyō sōsetsu" 脈 経 総 説 ["Studies on 'Mai Jing'"]. 8: 333–424 in Kosoto et al. eds. 1981.

———, et al., eds. 1981. *Tōyō igaku zempon sōsho* 東 洋 医 学 善 本 叢 書 [Collected rare books on Oriental Medicine]. 8 vols. Osaka.

High-quality reproductions, some halftone, of very rare recensions of Chinese medical classics from Japanese collections, with important reference tools in the form of indexes and analytical essays in vol. 8.

Ku Chen-sheng 谷 振 声 et al., eds. 1981. *Chung-i chi-ch'u hsueh* 中 医 基 础 学 [Foundation studies in Chinese medicine]. Hangzhou.

Revised for private study from *Hsi-i hsueh-hsi Chung-i shih yung chiao-ts'ai* 西 医 学 习 中 医 试 用 教 材 [Provisional teaching materials for Western physicians studying Chinese medicine]. Hangzhou, 1972.

Kuang-chou Chung-i hsueh-yuan 广 州 中 医 学 院 (Guangzhou College of Chinese Medicine), ed. 1979. *Fang-chi-hsueh* 方 剂 学 [Pharmacy]. Shanghai.

Kuang-chou pu-tui 广 州 部 队 后 勤 部 卫 生 部 (Public Health Section, Rear Support Units, Guangzhou Command) et al., eds. 1972. *Hsin pien Chung-i-hsueh kai yao* 新 編 中 医 学 概 要 [Revised outline of Chinese medicine]. Beijing.

The book translated above; cited as *Revised Outline*.

Kunst, Richard A. 1977. "More on *Xiu* 宿 and *Wuxing* 五 行 , with an Addendum on the Use of Archaic Reconstructions." *Early China* 3: 67–69.

See Major 1976, 1977.

Kuo Ai-ch'un 郭 靄 春 . 1981. *Huang ti nei ching su wen chiao chu yü i* 黄 帝 内 经 素 问 校 注 语 译 [Critical edition of the *Basic Questions* with vernacular translation]. Tianjin.

Simplified characters.

——. 1982. *Ling shu ching chiao shih* 灵 枢 经 校 释 [Critical edition of the *Divine Pivot*]. 2 vols. Beijing.

Simplified characters. Includes a translation into modern Chinese.

Kuo-chia ch'u-pan-chü 國 家 出 版 局 (National Publication Administrative Bureau, Acquisitions Library), ed. 1980. *Ku chi mu-lu: 1949 nien 10 yueh chih 1976 nien 12 yueh* 古 籍 目 錄 : 1949 年 10 月 至 1976 年 12 月 [Catalogue of ancient books reprinted October 1949 to December 1976]. Beijing.

Lists all reprints of premodern books, with notes on sizes of editions and annotations.

Kuroda, Genji 黑 田 源 次 . 1977. *Ki no kenkyū* 氣 の 研 究 [Researches on *ch'i*]. Tokyo.

Parts 1–4 originally published 1953–55.

Lampton, David M. 1974. "Health Policy during the Great Leap Forward." *China Quarterly* 60: 668–98.

——. 1977. *The Politics of Medicine in China: The Policy Process, 1949–1977*. Boulder, Colorado.

Mainly concerned with changes in the loci of decision-making.

Lau, D. C., trans. 1982. *Chinese Classics: Tao Te Ching*. Hong Kong.

Translation of *Lao-tzu*, originally published Harmondsworth, England, 1963, followed by translation of text edited from newly discovered MSS.

Lee, T'ao. 1943. "Medical Ethics in Ancient China." *Bulletin of the History of Medicine* 13: 268–77.

Leslie, Charles, ed. 1976. *Asian Medical Systems: A Comparative Study*. Berkeley. Papers of Burg Wartenstein Symposium

No. 53, Wenner-Gren Foundation for Anthropological Research, July 1971.
Few of the essays are comparative, but several are well-informed.

Li, C. P. 1974. *Chinese Herbal Medicine*. Bethesda, Maryland.
Informative introduction, written mainly for medical researchers.

Li Ching-wei et al. 1977. *Creating a New Chinese Medicine and Pharmacology*. Beijing.
Four essays, one general and three on experiments in combined Chinese and Western therapy. See Shang T'ien-yu 1977.

Li Guohao et al. 1982. *Explorations in the History of Science and Technology in China: Compiled in Honour of the Eightieth Birthday of Dr. Joseph Needham, FRS, FBA*. A special number of the "Collections of Essays on Chinese Literature and History" (i.e., *Chung-hua wen shih lun-ts'ung* 中 华 文 史 论 丛). Shanghai.
Includes three essays on medicine.

Li Hsiang-chung 李 相 中 . 1964. *Chung-yao-hsueh kai lun* 中 药 学 概 論 [Outline of Chinese materia medica]. Beijing.

Li Shuo-kuang 李 爍 光 , ed. 1976. *Min-chien shih-yen ling fang* 民 間 實 驗 靈 方 [Tested efficacious popular prescriptions]. 2 vols. Taipei.

Liao-ning Chung-i hsueh-yuan 辽 宁 中 医 学 院 (Liaoning College of Chinese Medicine), ed. 1972. *Chung-i-hsueh chiang-i* 中 医 学 讲 义 [Lectures on Chinese medicine]. Vol. 1. Liaoyang.
No further volumes published.

Ling I-k'uei 凌 一 揆 et al., eds. 1984. *Chung yao hsueh* 中 药 学 [Chinese materia medica]. Shanghai.
Briefer discussion of doctrine than in Ch'eng-tu Chung-i hsueh-yuan ed. 1978.

Liu Ch'ang-lin 刘 长 林 . 1982. *Nei-ching te che-hsueh ho Chung-i-hsueh te fang-fa* 内 经 的 哲 学 和 中 医 学 的 方 法 [The philosophy of the *Inner Canon* and the methodology of Chinese medicine]. Beijing.
Contains some original insights, but is often vitiated by specious reasoning. Preoccupied with such matters as proving that the Five Phases is a precursor of general systems theory.

Liu Chen-min 刘 振 民 et al. 1980. *I ku-wen chi-ch'u* 医 古 文 基 础 [Foundations of medical classical Chinese]. Beijing.
Medical school textbook.

Liu Heng-ju 刘 衡 如 . 1982. "Lun *Nei ching* san yin san yang ch'i hsueh to-shao te ch'ang-shu" 论 内 经 三 阴 三 阳 气 血 多 少 的 常 数 . . . [On the constant differences in the amounts of *ch'i* and *hsueh* in the three yin and three yang tracts in the *Inner Canon*], ed. Liu Shan-yung 劉 曜 曦 . Pp. 277–82 in Jen Ying-ch'iu and Liu Ch'ang-lin eds. 1982.

Liu Ts'un-yan. 1971. "The Taoists' Knowledge of Tuberculosis in the Twelfth Century." *T'oung Pao* (Leiden) 57: 285–301.
Argues that priests were observing microorganisms through compound microscopes, although the source states clearly that the demons responsible for the infectious disease (not identical with tuberculosis) are to be seen by visionary meditation.

Liu Yao-hsi 劉 曜 曦 . 1929. "Lun chiu i ching-lo chih chen chia" 論 舊 醫 經 絡 之 真 價 ["On the true value of *ching-lo* in the old medicine"]. *Min-kuo i-hsueh tsa-chih* 7: 235–43.
Skeptical evaluation by an M.D.

Lo Fu-i 罗 福 颐 . 1973. "Tui Wu-wei Han i-yao chien te i-tien jen-shih" 对 武 威 汉 医 药 简 的 一 点 认 识 ["Some notes on the Eastern Han dynasty wooden slips inscribed with medical prescriptions unearthed at Wuwei, Gansu province"]. *Wen-wu* 12: 30–31.
Unsatisfactory translation in *Chinese Sociology and Anthropology* 8 (1975): 82–88.

Lock, Margaret. 1980a. *East Asian Medicine in Urban Japan: Varieties of Medical Experience.* Comparative Studies of Health Systems and Medical Care, 4. Berkeley.
Based on extended field observation in a Chinese-style clinic.

_____. 1980b. "The Organization and Practice of East Asian Medicine in Japan: Continuity and Change." *Social Science and Medicine* 14B, no. 4: 245–54.

Loewe, Michael. 1974. *Crisis and Conflict in Han China: 104 B.C. to A.D. 9.* London.

Lu Gwei-djen and Joseph Needham. 1980. *Celestial Lancets: A History and Rationale of Acupuncture and Moxa.* Cambridge, England.

Lucas, AnElissa. 1982. *Chinese Medical Modernization: Comparative Policy Continuities, 1930s-1980s.* New York.

Ma Chi-hsing 马 继 兴 (Chung I-yen 钟 益 研 , pseud.) and Li Hsueh-ch'in 李 学 勤 (Ling Hsiang 凌 襄 , pseud.). 1975. "Wo kuo hsien i fa-hsien te tsui ku i-fang—po shu Wu-shih-erh ping fang" 我 国 现 已 发 现 的 最 古 医 方 － 帛 书 《 五 十 二 病 方 》 [The oldest prescriptions discovered so far in China: the silk MS "Prescriptions for Fifty-two Ailments"]. *Wen-wu* 9: 49–60.

Reprinted in Ma-wang-tui 1979: 179–208 under the authors' true names.

Ma K'an-wen 馬 堪 温. 1963. "Tsu-kuo Ch'ing tai chieh-ch'u te i-hsueh-chia Wang Ch'ing-jen" 祖 国 清 代 杰 出 的 医 学 家 王 清 任 [Wang Ch'ing-jen, outstanding physician of the Ch'ing period]. *K'o-chi-shih chi-k'an* 科 学 史 集 刊 6: 66–74.

Ma Po-ying 马 伯 英. [1982]. *Chung wai i-hsueh shih chiang-i* 中 外 医 学 史 讲 义 [Lectures on the history of medicine, Chinese and foreign]. Mimeographed, 3 vols. Shanghai. Vol. 1, *History of Chinese medicine.* Vol. 2, *History of medicine outside China.* Vol. 3, *Development of Chinese medicine after the importation of European medicine.*

Textbook used in Shanghai First Medical College.

Ma-wang-tui Han mu po shu cheng-li hsiao tsu 马 王 堆 汉 墓 帛 书 整 理 小 组 (Mawangdui Han Tombs Silk MSS Working Group). 1975. "Ma-wang-tui Han mu ch'u t'u i shu shih wen" 马 王 堆 汉 墓 出 土 医 书 释 文 ["Transcription of the silk manuscript of medical treatises found in the Tomb no. 3 at Mawangtui in Changsha"]. *Wen-wu* 6: 1–5; 9: 35–48.

See the revised version in the next item. Both must be consulted, since neither is definitive.

———. 1979. *Ma-wang-tui Han mu po shu: Wu-shih-erh ping fang* 马 王 堆 汉 墓 帛 书 ： 五 十 二 病 方 [Silk MSS from the Han tomb at Mawangdui: Prescriptions for fifty-two ailments]. Beijing.

Includes transcriptions of five MSS and three essays.

Maekawa Shōzō 前 川 捷 三. 1978. "Kōkotsubun, kimbun ni mieru ki" 甲 骨 文 金 文 に 見 元 る 氣 [Ch'i on oracle documents and early bronze inscriptions]. Pp. 13–29 in Onozawa Seiichi et al. 1978.

Major, John S. 1976. "A Note on the Translation of Two Technical Terms in Chinese Science: *Wu-hsing* 五 行 and *Hsiu* 宿." *Early China* 2: 1–3.

———. 1977. "Reply to Richard Kunst's Comments on *Hsiu* and *Wu hsing.*" *Early China* 3: 69–70.

See Kunst 1977.

Mann, Felix, et al. 1973. "Treatment of Intractable Pain by Acupuncture." *Lancet* (14 July 1973): 57–60.
Criticized for lack of attention to other therapies used on clinical subjects and for other failings in a letter by Arthur Taur (15 September 1973): 618.

Maruyama Masao 丸 山 昌 朗 . 1977. *Shinkyū igaku to koten no kenkyū: Maruyama Masao tōyō igaku ronshū* 鍼 灸 医 学 と 古 典 の 研 究 ：丸 山 昌 朗 東 洋 医 学 論 集 [Studies in medical acupuncture and moxibustion and their classics: Collected essays of Maruyama Masao on Oriental medicine]. Osaka.

Maruyama Toshiaki 丸 山 敏 秋 . 1979. "Somon igaku no shisō—Chūgoku dentō igaku no kihonteki kangaekata" '素 問 医 学 ' の 思 想 － 中 國 伝 統 医 学 の 基 本 的 考 元 力、た [The ideas of *Su wen* medicine: basic modes of thought of traditional Chinese medicine]. *Rinri shisō kenkyū* 倫 理 思 想 研 究 4: 1–18.

_____. 1980. "Chūgoku kodai ni okeru gogyōron no kōsatsu—shinkyū kei igaku ni tsuite" 中 国 古 代 医 学 に す け る 五 行 論 の 考 察 － 鍼 灸 系 医 学 に つ い て [A study of Five Phases theory in ancient Chinese medicine, with special reference to the acupuncture and moxibustion tradition]. *Rinri shisō kenkyū* 5: 1–18.

_____. 1981. "Yō Jōzen to Ō Hyō: Yō Ō ryō chū no hikakuteki kōsatsu" 楊 上 善 と 王 冰 ： 楊 王 両 注 の 比 較 的 考 察 [Yang Shang-shan and Wang Ping: A comparative study of their commentaries]. 8: 60–91 in Kosoto et al. eds. 1981.

McKeown, Thomas. 1971. "A Historical Appraisal of the Medical Task." Pp. 29–55 in McLachlan and McKeown eds. 1971.
Statistical assessment of the contribution of medicine to the growth of the English population from about 1700 on.

_____. 1979. *The Modern Rise of Population.* New York.

McKnight, Brian E. 1981. *The Washing Away of Wrongs: Forensic Medicine in Thirteenth-century China.* Science, Medicine, and Technology in East Asia, 1. Ann Arbor.
Translation of *Hsi yuan chi lu* 洗 冤 集 錄 (see bibliography A).

McLachlan, Gordon, and Thomas McKeown, eds. 1971. *Medical History and Medical Care: A Symposium of Perspectives Ar-*

ranged by the Nuffield Provincial Hospitals Trust and the Josiah Macy Jr. Foundation. London.

Physicians, civil servants, humanists and social scientists. Practical insights on the social history and prospects of medicine. Valuable discussions.

Mechanic, David. 1968. *Medical Sociology: A Selective View.* New York.

One of the better textbooks.

Miki Sakae 三木栄 . 1959. "Stein Tonkō bunsho . . . to genden Sōhan Shōkanron bemmyaku hō narabi ni Kinki gyokkan kyō bemmyaku to no hikaku. Fu . . . Heimyaku ryakurei スタ イン敦煌文書 British Museum Stein Rolls No. 202 と現伝'宋板傷寒論'辨脉法並に'金匱玉函経',辨脉との比較. 附. Stein Rolls No. 5614 and 6245 '平脉略例'" [A comparison of the pulse diagnosis methods in the Dunhuang documents of British Museum Stein Rolls No. 202 and in the extant Sung recensions of the *Shang han lun* and the *Chin kuei yü han ching*. Appendix: Stein Rolls No. 5614 and 6245, *P'ing mai lueh li*]. *Kampō no rinsō* 6, no. 5: 249–72.

Includes transcriptions of the MSS.

Miyasita Saburō. 1976. "A Historical Study of Chinese Drugs for the Treatment of Jaundice." *American Journal of Chinese Medicine* 4, no. 3: 239–43.

This important series of essays is mainly concerned with historical changes in drugs of choice for various remedies. This and 1980 are sometimes confusing because of careless editing.

_____. 1977. "A Historical Analysis of Chinese Formularies and Prescriptions: Three Examples." *Nihon ishigaku zasshi* 23, no 2: 283–300.

_____. 1979. "Malaria (*Yao*) in Chinese Medicine during the Chin and Yuan Periods." *Acta Asiatica* 36: 90–112.

On 瘧 , usually romanized as *nueh.*

_____. 1980. "An Historical Analysis of Chinese Drugs in the Treatment of Hormonal Diseases, Goitre, and Diabetes Mellitus." *American Journal of Chinese Medicine* 8, no. 1: 17–25.

Moran, Patrick E. 1983. "Key Philosophical and Cosmological Terms in Chinese Philosophy: Their History from the Beginning to Chu Hsi (1130–1200)." Ph.D. diss., Department of Oriental Studies, University of Pennsylvania.

Morohashi Tetsuji 諸 橋 轍 次   1957–1960. *Dai Kan-wa jiten* 大 漢 和 辭 與 [Unabridged Chinese-Japanese dictionary]. 13 vols. Tokyo.

Nakayama, Shigeru, and Nathan Sivin, eds. 1973. *Chinese Science: Explorations of an Ancient Tradition.* Cambridge, Massachusetts.

Nan-ching Chung-i hsueh-yuan 南 京 中 医 学 院 (Nanjing College of Chinese Medicine), ed. 1958. *Chung-i-hsueh kai lun* 中 醫 學 概 論 [Outline of Chinese medicine]. Beijing.

———, ed. 1964. *Chung-i fang-chi-hsueh chiang-i* 中 医 方 剂 学 讲 义 [Lectures on Chinese pharmacy]. Shanghai. Reprint, Hong Kong, 1971.

———, ed. 1980. *Chu ping yuan hou lun chiao shih* 诸 病 源 候 论 校 释 [Origins and symptoms of medical disorders: Critical annotated edition]. Beijing.
Simplified characters. Includes a translation into modern Chinese.

———, ed. 1983. *Chung-i-hsueh* 中 医 学 [Chinese medicine]. Nanjing.
Revised version of a book published by Chiang-su hsin i-hsueh-yuan (Nanjing, 1972), with increased emphasis on theory.

Nan-k'ai i-yuan 南 开 医 院 (Nankai Hospital), ed. 1972. *Chung Hsi i chieh-ho chih-liao chi-fu-cheng* 中 西 医 结 合 治 疗 急 腹 症 [Treatment of acute abdomen by combined Chinese and Western therapy]. Beijing.
The best-known book on combined therapy.

Needham, Joseph. *See also* Lu Gwei-djen.

———. et al. 1954- . *Science and Civilisation in China.* 7 vols. projected. Cambridge, England.

———. 1965. *Time and Eastern Man: The Henry Myers Lecture 1964.* London: Royal Anthropological Institute of Great Britain and Ireland. Reprinted in pp. 92–135 of Fraser ed. 1966 and in pp. 218–98 of Needham 1969.

———. 1969. *The Grand Titration: Science and Society in East and West.* London.
Collected essays.

———. 1970. *Clerks and Craftsmen in China and the West: Lectures and Addresses on the History of Science and Technology.* Cambridge, England.
Includes four important essays on medicine in collaboration with Lu Gwei-djen and Ho Ping-yü.

____, and Lu Gwei-djen. 1975. "Problems of Translation and Modernisation of Ancient Chinese Technical Terms: Manfred Porkert's Interpretations of Terms in Ancient and Mediaeval Chinese Natural and Medical Philosophy." *Annals of Science* 32: 491–502.

Comments on Needham and Lu's critique by Porkert, pp. 501–2. Stresses Porkert's tendency to translate into English words, such as "energy," which carry inappropriate modern scientific meanings. Needham and Lu overlook the qualifications attached to many of Porkert's translations and his emphasis that only his Latin translations are normative. They also sometimes introduce inappropriate modern senses into their own translations.

O'Connor, John, and Dan Bensky. 1981. *Acupuncture: A Comprehensive Text*. Chicago.

Translation of Shang-hai Chung-i hsueh-yuan 1974.

Okanishi Tameto 岡 西 為 人 . 1958. *Sung i-ch'ien i chi k'ao* 宋 以 前 醫 籍 考 [Studies of medical books through the Sung period]. Beijing.

A pastiche of information on most of the known pre-fourteenth-century medical books. Fundamental reference work.

____. 1974. *Chūgoku isho honzō kō* 中 國 醫 書 本 草 考 [Studies of Chinese books on medicine and materia medica]. Osaka.

Posthumously published essays by Japan's foremost scholar of Chinese medical bibliography.

Onozawa Seiichi 小 野 沢 精 一 et al. 1978. *Ki no shisō: Chūgoku ni okeru shizenkan to ningenkan no tenkai* 気 の 思 想: 中 国 に お け る 自 然 観 と 人 間 観 の 展 開 [The intellectual history of ch'i: The evolution of naturalistic and humanistic views in China]. Tokyo.

Seminar volume; thorough but uneven in quality, indexed.

Ōtsuka Keisetsu 大 塚 敬 節 . 1966. *Rinsō ōyō Shōkanron gaisetsu* 傷 寒 論 概 说 [Introduction to the *Shang han lun* for clinical use]. Osaka.

Includes carefully edited Chinese text, Japanese translation, and commentary oriented toward therapeutic applications, by the foremost Japanese authority.

____. 1976. *Kanpo: Geschichte, Theorie und Praxis der chinesisch-japanischen traditionellen Medizin*. Tokyo.

Translation by Ōtsuka Yasuo 大 塚 恭 男 of *Kampō igaku* 漢 方 醫 學 (Tokyo, 1976).

P. *See* Porkert 1974.

P'ang P'u 庞 朴 . 1977. "Ma-wang-tui po shu chieh-k'ai-le Ssu
Meng wu-hsing shuo chih mi: Po shu Lao-tzu chia pen chüan
hou ku i shu chih i te ch'u-pu yen-chiu" 马 王 堆 帛 书
解 开 了 思 孟 五 行 说 之 谜 ： 帛 书 ＂老 子 ＞
甲 本 卷 后 古 佚 书 之 一 的 初 步 研 究 [A silk
MS from Mawangdui solves the enigma of Tzu-ssu's 子 思,
and Mencius' *wu hsing*].
Introductory study of one of the lost books appended to the
Mawangdui *Lao-tzu* text A. *Wen-wu* 10: 63–69.
Demonstrates that in these books *wu-hsing* is an ethical notion
distinct from the well-known naturalistic concept.

Pei-ching Chung-i hsueh-yuan 北 京 中 医 学 院 (Beijing College of Chinese Medicine) et al., eds. 1961. *Chung-i ko chia
hsueh-shuo chi i an hsuan chiang-i* 中 医 各 家 学 说
及 医 案 选 讲 义 [Lectures on doctrines of the schools of
classical Chinese medicine and selected medical case histories].
Beijing.
See Jen Ying-ch'iu ed. 1980.

_____. 1964. *Chung-i ko chia hsueh-shuo* 中 医 各 家 学 说
[Doctrines of the schools of classical Chinese medicine].
Shanghai.

_____, ed. 1974. *Chung-i-hsueh chi-ch'u* 中 医 学 基 础 [Foun-
dations of Chinese medicine]. Shanghai.

_____. et al., eds. 1975. *Shih-yung Chung-i-hsueh* 实 用 中 医 学
[Practical Chinese medicine]. 2 vols. Beijing.

_____, ed. 1978. *Chung-i-hsueh chi-ch'u* 中 医 学 基 础 [Foun-
dations of Chinese medicine]. Shanghai and Beijing, with minor
differences.
Revision of 1974 version, also incorporating information from a
1977 book of the same title and a 1977 compilation of teaching
materials for specialists in modern medicine.

Peterson, Willard J. 1973. "Western Natural Philosophy Published
in late Ming China." *Proceedings of the American Philosophical
Society* 117, no. 4: 295–322.

Porkert, Manfred. 1974. *The Theoretical Foundations of Chinese
Medicine: Systems of Correspondence.* M.I.T. East Asian
Science Series, 3. Cambridge, Massachusetts.
The best analysis of Chinese medical terminology to date; deals
with certain physiological concepts in the *Inner Canon* tradition.

_____. 1976. *Lehrbuch der chinesischen Diagnostik.* Heidelberg.
Good for the clinical orientation of classical theory.

_____. 1977. "Chinese Medicine—A Science in Its Own Right." *Eastern Horizon* (February): 12–18.

_____. 1978. *Klinische chinesische Pharmakologie.* Heidelberg.

_____. 1979. "Die verschiedenen Fassungen der 'Allgemeinen Darstellung der chinesischen Medizin' (*Chung-i-hsueh kai-lun*) als Beispiel für den Wandel des Wissenschaftlichen Verständnisses der traditionellen Medizin in der Volksrepublik China." Pp. 417–26 in Bauer 1979.

_____. 1982a. "The Difficult Task of Blending Chinese and Western Science: The Case of Modern Interpretations of Traditional Chinese Medicine." Pp. 553–72 in Li Guohao et al. 1982.

_____. 1982b. *Die chinesische Medizin.* Düsseldorf.
A general introduction.

_____. 1983. *The Essentials of Chinese Diagnostics.* Zürich.

Quinn, Joseph R., ed. 1974. *China Medicine as We Saw It.* Bethesda, Maryland.
An anthology of reports by physicians and scientists who had visited China.

Revised Outline. See Kuang-chou pu-tui et al. eds. 1972.

Revolutionary Health Committee of Hunan Province, ed. 1977. *A Barefoot Doctor's Manual.* Revised and enlarged edition. Seattle.
Originally published Bethesda, Maryland, 1974. Translation of Hu-nan Chung-i-yao yen-chiu-so ko-wei-hui ed. 1971. The title of the editorial organization is not correctly translated.

Risse, Guenter B., ed. 1973. *Modern China and Traditional Chinese Medicine: A Symposium Held at the University of Wisconsin, Madison.* Springfield, Illinois.
Papers of widely varying quality.

Rosenberg, Charles E. 1977. "The Therapeutic Revolution: Medicine, Meaning and Social Change in Nineteenth-century America." *Perspectives in Biology and Medicine* 20: 485–506.

Rudolph, Richard C. 1977. "Early China and the West: Fertilization and Fetalization." Pp. 1–27 in Rudolph and Cammann 1977.

_____, and Schuyler van Rensselaer Cammann. 1977. *China and the West: Culture and Commerce.* Los Angeles.

Savill, Thomas Dixon. 1930. *A System of Clinical Medicine: Dealing with the Diagnosis, Prognosis, and Treatment of Disease: For Students and Practitioners.* 8th edition. New York.
First edition, 2 vols., London, 1903–1905.

Shan-tung Chung-i hsueh-yuan 山东中医学院 (Shandong College of Chinese Medicine), ed. 1976. *Chung-i nei-k'o-hsueh* 中医内科学 [Chinese internal medicine]. Jinan.
Largely based on T'ien-chin shih ed. 1974.

_____, ed. 1979. *Chen chiu chia i ching chiao shih* 针灸甲乙经校释 [Critical edition of the *A-B Canon*]. 2 vols. Beijing.
Variorum notes, glosses, translation into modern Chinese. Simplified characters.

Shang Chih-chün 尚志钧 . 1981. "Wu-shih-erh ping fang yü Shen-nung pen-ts'ao" 《五十二病方》与《神農本草》 [*Prescriptions for fifty-two ailments* and *The Divine Husbandman's Materia Medica*]. 2: 78–81 in Hu-nan Chung-i hsueh-yuan ed. 1980–81.

Shang T'ien-yu. 1977. "New Developments in Fracture Treatment." Pp. 21–42 in Li Ching-wei et al. 1977.

Shang-hai Chung-i hsueh-yuan 上海中医学院 (Shanghai College of Chinese Medicine), ed. 1960. *Chen-chiu-hsueh chiang-i* 针灸学讲义 [Lectures on acupuncture and moxibustion]. Shanghai.

_____, ed. 1965. *Chen-chiu shu-hsueh-hsueh* 针灸腧穴学 [The study of acupuncture and moxibustion loci]. Shanghai. Reprint, Hong Kong, 1970.

_____. et al., eds. 1970. *Ch'ih-chiao i-sheng shou-ts'e* 赤脚医生手册 [Barefoot doctors' handbook]. Shanghai.

_____. 1974. *Chen-chiu-hsueh* 针灸学 [Acupuncture and moxibustion]. Beijing.
For translation see O'Connor and Bensky 1981.

_____. et al., eds. 1978. *I ku-wen* 医古文 [Medical classical Chinese]. Shanghai.

_____, ed. 1979–80. *Nei-k'o-hsueh* 内科学 [Internal medicine]. 2 vols. Shanghai.
Textbook.

_____. 1980. Ku-wen chiao tsu 古文教组 (Classical Chinese teaching group), ed. *Ku-tai i-hsueh wen-hsuan* 古代医学文选 [Anthology of ancient Chinese medicine]. Shanghai.
Eighty selections; wide scope.

Shang-hai shih 上海市 (Commune Hospital, Jiangzhen Commune, Chuansha County, Shanghai), ed. 1977. *Ch'ih-chiao i-sheng chiao-ts'ai* 赤脚医生教材 [Training manual for barefoot doctors]. 2 vols. Beijing.
Second edition of a manual originally published in 1973.

Shang-hai shih chen-chiu yen-chiu-so 上 海 市 針 灸 研 究 所 (Shanghai Municipal Research Institute for Acupuncture and Moxibustion), ed. 1970. *Chen-chiu chih-liao shou-ts'e* 針 灸 治 疗 手 册 [Handbook of acupuncture and moxibustion therapy]. Shanghai.
See also Chang Sheng-hsing ed. 1983.

Shang-hai shih Chung-i hsueh-hui 上 海 市 中 医 学 会 (Shanghai Society for the Study of Chinese Medicine), ed. 1960. *Tsu-kuo i-hsueh ching-lo hsueh-shuo te li-lun chi ch'i yun-yung* 祖 国 医 学 经 络 学 说 的 理 论 及 其 运 用 [The theory and application of circulation tract doctrine in the medicine of the fatherland]. Shanghai.
Apparently an expansion of parts of Shang-hai Chung-i hsueh-yuan ed. 1960, without discussion of the anatomical status of the circulation system. Written for traditional and modern physicians.

Shang-hai shih wei-sheng-chü 上 海 市 衛 生 局 (Shanghai Municipal Public Health Bureau). 1958. *Chung-i Chung yao lin-ch'uang shih-yen hui-pien* 中 医 中 药 临 床 实 驗 汇 编 [Collected clinical experiments in Chinese medicine and drug therapy]. 2 vols. Shanghai.
Includes acupuncture experiments.

Shang-hai ti-i i-hsueh-yuan 上 海 第 一 医 学 院 (Shanghai First Medical College). 1971. *Tsu-kuo i-hsueh chi-pen chih-shih: Hsin i-liao fa ho Chung ts'ao-yao* 祖 国 医 学 基 本 知 识：新 医 疗 法 和 中 草 药 [Basic knowledge about the medicine of the fatherland: New therapies, and Chinese materia medica]. Shanghai.

Shih Hsueh-chung 师 学 忠，et al. 1983. *Chinese-English Terminology of Traditional Chinese Medicine.* Changsha.
The most comprehensive and least reliable of the generally unreliable Chinese-English dictionaries recently published in China.

Shryock, Richard Harrison. 1936. *The Development of Modern Medicine: An Interpretation of the Social and Scientific Factors Involved.* Philadelphia. Reprint, Madison, Wisconsin, 1979.
Classic social history.

Sidel, Victor W., and Ruth Sidel. 1973. *Serve the People: Observations on Medicine in the People's Republic of China.* New York.
Informative account based on two visits to China by a physician and a psychiatric social worker.

_____. 1982. *The Health of China.* Boston.

To some extent extends the preceding book on the basis of two further visits, but not as currently informed.

Sivin, Nathan. 1966. "Chinese Conceptions of Time." *The Earlham Review* 1: 82–92.

———. 1968. *Chinese Alchemy: Preliminary Studies*. Harvard Monographs in the History of Science, 1. Cambridge, Massachusetts.

Includes a critical study of the biography of the physician and alchemist Sun Ssu-mo 孫 思 邈 (*or* Ssu-miao, alive 673) and the dating of his works.

———. 1976. "Chinese Alchemy and the Manipulation of Time." *Isis* 67: 513–527. Reprinted in Sivin ed. 1977: 108–22.

———. 1977. "Social Relations of Curing in Traditional China: Preliminary Considerations." *Nihon ishigaku zasshi* 23: 505–32.

———, ed. 1977. *Science and Technology in East Asia* (History of Science: Selections from *Isis*). New York.

Includes medicine.

———. 1980. "The Theoretical Background of Elixir Alchemy." 5.4: 210–305 in Needham et al. 1954- .

Thomas, Robert. 1817. *The Modern Practice of Physic, Exhibiting the Characters, Causes, Symptoms, Prognostics, Morbid Appearances, and Improved Method of Treating the Diseases of All Climates*. Fourth American edition, New-York.

First published London, 1801.

Thomas, Clayton L., ed. 1973. *Tabor's Cyclopedic Medical Dictionary*. Twelfth edition. Philadelphia.

First published 1940.

T'ien-chin i-hsueh-yuan 天 津 医 学 院 (Tianjin Medical College) et al., eds. 1971. *Chung-i chien-i chiao-ts'ai* 中 医 简 易 教 材 [Simplified teaching materials on Chinese medicine]. Tianjin.

T'ien-chin shih Chung-i i-yuan 天 津 市 中 医 医 院 (Tianjin Municipal Hospital for Chinese Medicine). 1974. *Chung-i nei-k'o* 中 医 内 科 [Chinese internal medicine]. Tianjin.

TIZ. See Kosoto, et al., eds. 1981.

Topley, Marjorie. 1970. "Chinese Traditional Ideas and the Treatment of Disease: Two Examples from Hong Kong." *Man* 5, no. 3: 421–37.

T'ung Chün-chieh 僮 俊 杰 . 1980. "Ching-lo chih ch'i-yuan chi ch'i yü shu-hsueh kuan-hsi te t'an-t'ao" 经 络 之 起 源 及 其 与 腧 穴 关 系 的 探 讨 [Origins of the cir-

culation tract system and its relations to the acupuncture loci].
In Hu-nan Chung-i hsueh-yuan ed. 1980–81, 1: 33–37.

Unschuld, Paul Ulrich. 1973. *Pen-ts'ao* 本草 : *2000 Jahre traditionelle pharmazeutische Literatur Chinas.* München.
For English translation of the text of this illustrated book see 1977.

_____. 1975. *Medizin und Ethik: Sozialkonflikte im China der Kaiserzeit.* Münchener ostasiatische Studien, 11. Wiesbaden.
Suggestive but inadequate as sinology and sociology.

_____. 1977. "The Development of Medical-Pharmaceutical Thought in China." *Comparative Medicine East and West* 5, no. 2: 109–15; 2: 211–31.
See Unschuld 1973.

_____. 1978. "Das Ch'uan-ya und Die Praxis chinesischer Landärzte im 18. Jahrhundert." *Sudhoffs Archiv* 62, no. 4: 378–407.
On *Ch'uan ya* 串雅 see bibliography A.

_____. 1979. *Medical Ethics in Imperial China: A Study in Historical Anthropology.* Comparative Studies of Health Systems and Medical Care, 2. Berkeley.
Translation of 1975, somewhat revised. Not anthropological in approach.

_____. 1980. *Medizin in China. Eine Ideengeschichte.* München.
Little concerned with medical ideas.

_____. 1981. "Die amtlichen arzneibücher Chinas im 20: Jahrhundert." *Pharmazeutische Zeitung* 126: 684–95.
Description of the P.R.C. pharmacopoeia; see Chung-hua jen-min kung-ho-kuo Wei-sheng-pu 1978–79.

Wang Min-kang 汪敏刚 et al. 1970. "Chih-ch'i-kuan hsiao-ch'uan huan-che shen-shang-hsien-p'i-chih kung-neng yü tsu-kuo i-hsueh chung te shen hsu kuan-hsi te t'an-t'ao"
支气管哮喘患者肾上腺皮倾功能与祖国医学中肾虚关系的探讨 [Investigation of adrenocortical activity in patients with bronchial asthma and the relation of bronchial asthma to the traditional medical concept of renal system depletion]. Pp. 40–56 in Chiang Ch'un-hua et al. eds. 1970.

Watanabe Kōzō 渡邊幸三 . 1956. "Genson suru Chūgoku kinsei made no gozō rokufu zu no gaisetsu"
現存する中國近世まC の五藏六府圖の概説 [Extant classical Chinese diagrams of the visceral systems]. *Nihon ishigaku zasshi* 7: 88–182.

Webster, Charles. 1965. "William Harvey's Conception of the Heart as a Pump." *Bulletin of the History of Medicine* 39: 508–17.

Harvey "consistently emphasised that the theory was in accordance with Aristotelian vitalist physiology, and that the heart which propelled the blood was operated by a force which could not be expressed in physical terms and gave rise to non-mechanical effects . . . he in no way considered the circulatory system as a self-motivating machine" (page 517).

Wilhelm, Richard. 1928. *Frühling und Herbst des Lü Bu We: Aus dem Chinesischen verdeutscht und erläutert*. Jena.

Translation of *Lü shih ch'un-ch'iu* 呂·氏春秋 (bibliography A).

Wong, K. Chimin, and Wu Lien-teh. 1936. *History of Chinese Medicine: Being a Chronicle of Medical Happenings in China from Ancient Times to the Present Period*. Second edition, Shanghai.

First published Tientsin, 1932. Three quarters of this book is a valuable narrative of the influence of European medicine, with major attention to the twentieth century. The section on traditional medical history is hopeless.

Wu K'ao-p'an 吳考槃 . 1983. "Huang ti nei ching, Su wen, Ling shu k'ao" 《黃帝內經》《素問》《靈樞》考 ["A textual research on *Internal Classics of Yellow Emperor, Su Wen* and *Ling Shu*"], *Chung-hua i shih tsa-chih* 13, no. 2: 85–87.

Argues that there is no proof for identification of the extant *Su wen* and *Ling shu* with the original *Inner Canon of the Yellow Lord*.

_____. 1984. "Shang han lun pien cheng shih chih chien-hsi"《傷寒論》辨證施治簡析 [Concise analysis of manifestation type determination and therapeutic reasoning in *Shang han lun*]. *Chung-i-yao hsueh-pao* 中医药学报 , 2: 1–5.

Demonstrates that theoretical perspectives from the *Huang ti nei ching* pervade *Shang han lun*.

Wu Kuo-ting 吳國定 . 1967. *Nei ching chieh-p'ou sheng-li-hsueh* 内經解剖生理學 [Anatomy and physiology in the *Inner Canon*]. Taipei.

Arranges information about body structure and function under modern rubrics.

Xie Zhufan and Huang Xiaokai, eds. 1984. *Dictionary of Traditional Chinese Medicine* 中醫藥詞典 . Hong Kong. Revised

version of *Han-Ying ch'ang yung Chung-i-yao tz'u-hui* 汉英 常用中医药词彙 Beijing, [1981?].
Not a dictionary but a glossary with stroke-order index. The best available Chinese-English lexicon. Too concise to be reliable for use by novices.

Yamada Keiji 山田慶兒. 1978. *Shushi no shizengaku* 朱子の自然学 [Chu Hsi's studies of nature]. Tokyo.
Incorporates studies published by Yamada from 1964 on in *Tōhō gakuhō* (Kyoto).

———. 1979a. "Kōtei naikyō no seiritsu" '黄帝内経' の成立 [Formation of the *Huang ti nei ching*]. *Shisō*   , 662: 94–108.

———. 1979b. "The Formation of the *Huang-ti Nei-ching*." *Acta Asiatica* 36: 67–89.

———. 1980. "Kyukū hachifū setsu to Shoshiha no tachiba" 九宮八風説と少師派の立場 [The Nine Palaces-Eight Winds theory and the standpoint of the Shao shih school]. *Tōhō gakuhō* (Kyoto) 52: 199–242.
An attempt to identify textual constituents of the *Huang ti nei ching* with a particular school.

Yao Ch'un-fa 姚純发. 1982. "Ma-wang-tui po shu Tsu pi shih-i mai chiu ching ch'u t'an" 马王堆帛书《足臂十一脉灸经》初探 [Preliminary investigation of the Mawangdui MS Moxibustion Manual for the Eleven Foot and Arm Vessels]. *Chung-hua i shih tsa-chih* 12, no. 3: 171–74.
Argues that this text is concerned with the sinew system rather than the circulation system. See also Ho Tsung-yü 1981, 1984.

Yen K'un-ying 顔焜熒. 1980a. *Yuan se ch'ang yung Chung yao t'u chien* 原色常用中藥圖鑑 ["The illustrated Chinese materia medica: Crude drugs"]. Taipei.
Color photographs of samples of crude, dried drugs, with usual information, including notes on medical usage, in English, and other data in Chinese.

———. 1980b. *Yuan se Chung yao yin p'ien t'u chien* 原色中藥飲片圖鑑 ["The illustrated Chinese materia medica: Prepared drugs"]. Taipei.
The simples included are in general those that require processing for certain uses; photographs are mainly of raw substances.

Yen T'ien-shou 顔添壽, ed. 1968. *Min chien ku ch'uan shih-yen pi fang* 民間古傳實驗秘方 [Tested secret prescriptions long circulated among the people]. Taichung, Taiwan.

Yin Hui-ho 印 会 河 and Chang Po-no 张 伯 讷 , eds. 1984. *Chung-i chi-ch'u li-lun* 中 医 基 础 理 论 [Basic theories of Chinese medicine].
Thorough revision and expansion of portion on theory (chs. 1–4, 7) of Pei-ching Chung-i hsueh-yuan ed. 1978.

Yü Chia-hsi 余 嘉 錫 . 1958. *Ssu ku t'i yao pien cheng* 四 庫 提 要 辨 證 [Critical notes on the *Ssu k'u ch'üan shu tsung mu t'i yao*]. Revised edition, Beijing, 1958; Hong Kong reprint, 1974. First edition 1937.

Yü Ch'uan 于 船 et al., eds. 1982. *Ch'uan ya shou i fang* 串 雅 兽 医 方 [Veterinary prescriptions from *Ch'uan ya*]. Beijing.

Yuan Han-ch'ing 袁 翰 青 . 1956. *Chung-kuo hua-hsueh-shih lun-wen chi* 中 国 化 学 史 论 文 集 [Collected papers on the history of Chinese chemistry]. Beijing.
Includes alchemy, industrial chemistry, and iatrochemistry.

496

Chao P'u-shan, 197n
chaos (*luan*), 100n
Che-chiang Chung-i hsueh-
yuan, 115n
che pei (Zhejiang fritillary;
Fritillaria thunbergii), 397
ch'en (sunken pulse), 316
chen ch'i (inborn vitality), 98;
(true *ch'i*), 237, 238n
chen ch'ien (yang latensification), 240
chen ch'ien an shen (yang latensification and sedation), 192,
240n
Chen chiu chia i ching, see
Huang ti chia i ching
ch'en ch'ü (sunken reading),
314
Ch'en Chu-yu, 27n
chen han (genuine perspiration), 104n
ch'en han chi leng (submerged
cold and accumulated chill
factors), 279
chen je chia han (true hot-false
cold), 336
Ch'en Meng-chia, 75
Chen Pang-hsien, 141n
Ch'en Tse-lin, 176n
chen yin (Realized Yin, renal
Water), 394
cheng (manifestation type),
329; (symptom), 106, 107n;
(to steam), 294n, 389, 409n
cheng ch'i (orthopathic *ch'i*), 49,
102, 237, 238n
cheng chih (normal therapy),
417
Cheng chih chun sheng (Water
level and line marker of
diagnosis and therapy), 277n

cheng ching (regular or cardinal
tracts), 249
Ch'eng fang ch'ieh yung (Practical Prescriptions), 192n
Cheng-ho sheng chi tsung lu
(Medical encyclopedia: A
sagely benefaction of the
Regnant Harmony era),
107n
cheng hsu hsieh luan (orthopathy depleted and
heteropathy causing confusion), 424
Ch'eng Kuo-p'eng, 101
Ch'eng Shih-te, 26n, 98n,
163n, 286n
chi (disease), 106
ch'i (sectors), 379–391;
(vitalities), 235n; (essences),
14; (hurried), 174; (tense),
174; (vitalities, energies),
xxvii, 43–53, 149–162, 237–
240
active, sector, 379, 381
admission of (na *ch'i*), 228
admission of, to the renal
system (*na ch'i kuei shen*),
374
augmenting the (*i ch'i*), 412
backflow (*ch'i ni*), 239
bringing down the (*chiang
ch'i*), 240, 421
circulating (*ching ch'i*), 251
constructive (*ying*), 152, 239
constructive and defensive
(*ying-wei*), 152–160, 380–
391
constructive, sector (*ying*),
389–391
defensive, sector (*wei*), 152,
224, 382–384
depletion of (*ch'i hsu*), 239

532

ADDENDA ET CORRIGENDA

Traditional Medicine in Contemporary China

Page/Par. or Sec./Line	Error	Correction
x/6.2.	Visual Inspection	Inspection
xi/7.	Manifestation	Eight Rubrics Manifestation
xii/8.3.6.	preponderance	preponderance; Stomach system yin depletion
xiv/10.5.1.	Adjusting medication	Adjusting treatment
xviii/2/7	David	Cai Jingfeng, David
51/5/2	*hsueh*	*hsueh* 穴
160/n. 53/1	Shih Hsueh-chung	Shuai Hsueh-chung
202/ll. 14-17	Chinese Medicine	Traditional Chinese Medicine
202/ll. 19-23	Hospital	Medical College
202/l. 24	Publishers	Publishing House
212/2/6	reinforcement	mutual reinforcement
219/4/1	muscles	muscles, fascia
226/2/5	fluid metabolism	water metabolism
230/1/6	urinary bladder	urinary bladder,
240/1/2	or vomiting	or hiccups with vomiting; in hepatic system *ch'i* backflow one observes dizziness, fainting, or vomiting
240/4/6	coagulates	coagulates (*or* stagnates)
241/3/6	sensations	sensations without rise in body temperature
249/end	sytem	system
254/2/2	ventral	anterior
254/3/1	palmar (medial)	flexor
254/3/5	dorsal (lateral)	extensor
254/4/1	proximal	medial
254/4/6	outside	lateral side
265/1/8	plexes	plexuses
275/3/12	migraine	more rarely migraine
281/5/3-4	vaginal disorders	vaginal discharges
300/6.2.	Visual Inspection	Inspection
329/7.	Manifestation	Eight Rubrics Manifestation
365/1/1	hepatitis	hepatitis with jaundice
419/10.5.1.	Adjusting medication	Adjusting treatment
420/4/3	drugs of chilling	drugs of warming character; that due to hot heteropathy be treated with drugs of chilling
481/2/4	*K'o-chi-shih*	*K'o-hsueh-shih*
489/5/1	Shih Hsueh-chung	Shuai Hsueh-chung